Telepediatrics: Telemedicine and Child Health

Edited by Richard Wootton and Jennifer Batch

Telepediatrics: Telemedicine and Child Health

Edited by

Richard Wootton

Centre for Online Health, University of Queensland, Brisbane, Australia

Jennifer Batch

Department of Endocrinology, Royal Children's Hospital, Brisbane, Australia

Foreword by

Don Roberton

McGregor Reid Professor of Paediatrics, University of Adelaide, Adelaide, Australia
President Paediatrics and Child Health, Royal Australasian College of Physicians

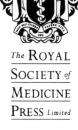

The ROYAL
SOCIETY *of*
MEDICINE
PRESS *Limited*

British Library Cataloguing in Publication Data
A catalogue record for this book is available from the British Library.

ISBN 1-85315-645-0

Distribution in Europe and Rest of World:
Marston Book Services Ltd
PO Box 269
Abingdon
Oxon OX14 4YN, UK
Tel: +44 (0)1235 465 500
Fax: +44 (0)1235 465 555

Distribution in the USA and Canada:
Royal Society of Medicine Press Ltd
c/o Jamco Distribution Inc
1401 Lakeway Drive
Lewisville, TX 75057, USA
Tel: +1 800 538 1287
Fax: +1 972 353 1303
E-mail: jamco@majors.com

Distribution in Australia and New Zealand:
Elsevier Australia
30–52 Smidmore Street
Marrickville, NSW 2204
Australia
Tel: + 61 2 9517 8999
Fax: + 61 2 9517 2249

Typeset by Phoenix Photosetting, Chatham, Kent
Printed in Great Britain by Bell & Bain Ltd, Glasgow

▶ Contents

Section 2: Primary and Community Services 211

▶ List of Contributors

Marcus D Atlas Lions Ear and Hearing Institute, University of Western Australia, Sir Charles Gairdner Hospital, St John's Hospital, Perth, WA, Australia

Tina Babineau Maritime Medical Genetics Service, IWK Health Centre, Halifax, Nova Scotia, Canada

Judith Barbour Child and Youth Health, Adelaide, SA, Australia

Jennifer Batch Department of Endocrinology, Royal Children's Hospital, Brisbane, Australia

Mark Bensink Centre for Online Health, University of Queensland, Royal Children's Hospital, Brisbane, Australia

Deborah Burton University of Kentucky Chandler Medical Center, Kentucky, Lexington, US

Liam Caffery Department of Medical Imaging, Royal Brisbane and Women's Hospital, Brisbane, Australia

Debra Caswell Kids Help Line, Brisbane, Australia

Fung Yee Chan Department of Maternal Fetal Medicine, University of Queensland, Mater Mothers' Hospital, South Brisbane, Australia

Ian Constable Lions Eye Institute, University of Western Australia, Perth, WA, Australia

David Dossetor Department of Psychological Medicine, The Children's Hospital, Westmead, NSW, Australia

Robert H Eikelboom Lions Ear and Hearing Institute, University of Western Australia, Perth, WA, Australia

Robert Ferguson Child Health Line, Riverton Early Parenting Centre, Brisbane, Australia

John P Finley Children's Heart Centre, Izaak Walton Killam Health Centre; and Dalhousie University, Halifax, Nova Scotia, Canada

Niall Higgins Education Centre, Royal Children's Hospital, Brisbane, Australia

Beth Hudson Carnarvon Regional Hospital, Carnarvon, WA, Australia

Helen Irving Paediatric Oncology Service, Royal Children's Hospital, Brisbane, Australia

Alan Isles Royal Children's Hospital and Health Service District, Brisbane, Queensland, Australia

Robert Justo Prince Charles Hospital, Brisbane, Queensland, Australia

Roy Kimble University of Queensland Department of Paediatrics and Child Health, Stuart Pegg Paediatric Burns Centre, Royal Children's Hospital, Brisbane, Australia

Sajeesh Kumar Lions Eye Institute, University of Western Australia, Perth, WA, Australia

Edward Lemaire Institute for Rehabilitation Research and Development, The Rehabilitation Centre, Ottawa, Ontario, Canada

Mark D Ludman Maritime Medical Genetics Service, IWK Health Centre; and Division of Medical Genetics, Department of Pediatrics, Dalhousie University, Halifax, Nova Scotia, Canada

James P Marcin Department of Pediatrics, University of California Davis Children's Hospital, University of California Davis, USA

Robert McCrossin Medical Services, Royal Children's Hospital, Brisbane, Australia

Grant G Miller Department of Surgery, University of Saskatchewan, Saskatoon, Canada

Philip O Ozuah Department of Pediatrics, Children's Hospital at Montefiore, Albert Einstein College of Medicine, Bronx, New York, USA

Wendy Reid Kids Help Line, Brisbane, Australia

Marina Reznik Department of Pediatrics, Children's Hospital at Montefiore, Albert Einstein College of Medicine, Bronx, New York, USA

Michael J Romano Department of Pediatrics, West Virginia University School of Medicine, Morgantown, West Virginia, USA

Anthony C Smith Centre for Online Health, University of Queensland, Royal Children's Hospital, Brisbane, Australia

Barbara Soong Centre for Maternal Fetal Medicine, Mater Mothers' Hospital, South Brisbane, Australia

Michael South Department of General Medicine, Department of Paediatrics, University of Melbourne, Royal Children's Hospital, Victoria, Australia

Ryan Spaulding Centre for Telemedicine and Telehealth, University of Kansas Medical Center, Kansas, USA

Deborah Stanley Department of Pediatrics, University of Kentucky Chandler Medical Center, Kentucky, Lexington, USA

Jean Starling Department of Psychological Medicine, The Children's Hospital, Westmead, NSW, Australia

Pat Swinfen Swinfen Charitable Trust, Canterbury, UK

Roger Swinfen Swinfen Charitable Trust, Canterbury, UK

Mei-Ling Tay Kearney Lions Eye Institute, University of Western Australia, Perth, WA, Australia

Pamela Whitten Department of Telecommunications, Michigan State University, Michigan, USA

Michael L Williams Child and Adolescent Health Service, Mackay Base Hospital, Mackay, Queensland, Australia

Richard Wootton Centre for Online Health, University of Queensland, Royal Children's Hospital, Brisbane, Australia

Kanagasingam Yogesan Lions Eye Institute, University of Western Australia, Perth, WA, Australia

Karen Youngberry Centre for Online Health, University of Queensland, Royal Children's Hospital, Brisbane, Australia

▶ Foreword

Most healthcare professionals would find it inconceivable to think of life without the telephone as part of their day-to-day work. Our ubiquitous pagers and mobile phones have also become intimate attachments in recent decades. We rarely give them a second thought as we grab them each morning, although the urgency with which they demand our attention earns the occasional unprintable words! We also need to remember, however, that communication between health professionals and those they care for remains difficult in many parts of the world. Health services may be completely inaccessible for many, and others may face days of trekking through difficult terrain to reach even the most rudimentary of health facilities.

What then is telehealth? Essentially, it involves the potential for communication at a distance between health professionals and those being cared for. It may be a very simple and brief communication, lasting only a few seconds, or alternatively it may involve long and complex interactions through a range of telecommunications media. An extreme, reported avidly by the media, is the ability for physical interventions, and even surgery, using complex equipment directed from a remote site.

In *Telepediatrics: Telemedicine and Child Health*, the emphasis is on providing information and reviews from experienced paediatric health professionals who use telemedicine in their own professional workplace. Their experience has been hard won, with error and success often in equal measure. The approaches have been diverse, with variation according to health needs, geography and available infrastructure. Important lessons have been learned, and children and their families have contributed strongly. There have been frustrations and remarkable successes.

Telepediatrics: Telemedicine and Child Health brings together a wide range of telehealth applications, both clinical and educational. Despite its broad scope, the structure of the book lends itself to easy use. Section 1, on specialist services, provides an overview and practical examples from many different domains of specialty child healthcare. Section 2 provides information that relates to use of telepaediatrics in non-hospital, ambulatory and community based services. Here, there is appropriate emphasis on interactions with children and families for counselling, guidance and other needs. Section 3, entitled Education, addresses the ways in which information can be made available. This may be through professional education and training, parent support group interactions or websites that provide high quality information for professionals and for children and their families.

The editors of this book, based in Brisbane, Australia, are recognized as world leaders in telemedicine and child health. The vast geography of Australia, with settlements and population centres at great distances from each other, has meant an early and deep interest in telepaediatrics for the editors. They have drawn widely from their experience and connections for contributors of chapters. This has led to a highly interesting and wide ranging text. All who work in the many and varied disciplines of child health will find something of importance and relevance in these pages.

Don Roberton
McGregor Reid Professor of Paediatrics, University of Adelaide and
President Paediatrics and Child Health, Royal Australasian College of Physicians, 2004

▶ Preface

This is the fifth book in the Royal Society of Medicine's telemedicine series. Its predecessors are:

- *The Legal and Ethical Aspects of Telemedicine*, BA Stanberry, 1998
- *Introduction to Telemedicine*, R Wootton and J Craig (eds), 1999
- *Teledermatology*, R Wootton and AMM Oakley (eds), 2002
- *Telepsychiatry and e-Mental Health*, R Wootton, P Yellowlees and P McLaren (eds), 2003

The present volume describes how telemedicine applies to paediatrics and child health generally. The book represents an eclectic collection of essays from contributors who work in a variety of medical, technical and administrative specialties. The majority are practising clinicians with substantial practical experience of telemedicine and health informatics.

The aim of the book is to present the collective experience of practitioners with a wide range of telepaediatric and related applications. Most of the contributors come from North America and Australasia. There is considerable and positive experience of telepaediatrics in Australia, and in Queensland in particular, and it is a pleasure to acknowledge the support of the Royal Children's Hospital Foundation in the production of the book. We think that anyone involved in telemedicine will find the material interesting, because much of it is relevant to other fields, rather than simply paediatrics and child health.

The aim of the book is principally to allow those who are involved in paediatrics and child health to begin to assess how telemedicine might be applied to their working practice. Clinicians should find it particularly useful, of course, but many chapters are also relevant to health service managers, planners and information technology staff. Parts of the book may also be useful to patients and their families.

The book is divided into three sections:

- Section 1 deals with specialist services, eg those delivered from tertiary centres by telemedicine.
- Section 2 describes primary and community paediatric services, as delivered by telemedicine.
- Section 3 concerns education at a distance: education of the patient, the family and also the healthcare professional.

Technical matters have been relegated to an appendix, so as not to disrupt the body of the text.

We hope you enjoy reading it.

Richard Wootton and Jennifer Batch
Brisbane, Australia
August 2004

▶ Glossary

Term	In full	Notes
ADSL	Asymmetric Digital Subscriber Line	A form of high-speed Internet connection, in which the digital signals are transmitted through the public telephone network. These digital signals are sent at a higher frequency than voice signals, so there is no interference between them. The bandwidth of an ADSL connection ranges from 256 kbit/s to 1.5 Mbit/s. The asymmetric nature of ADSL means that the quoted bandwidth is normally for the download speed (ie to the user). The upload speed is typically limited to 64 kbit/s.
Bandwidth		The capacity of a transmission pathway, eg a telecommunications line. The bandwidth of a digital line is measured in bits per second (usually kbit/s or Mbit/s).
Bit		Basic unit of computer storage. A bit can store only two values (eg 0 or 1).
Bitmap		An image format.
Byte		A larger unit of computer storage. Generally, a byte is composed of eight bits, and can therefore store up to 256 different values.
Cable		Cable Internet employs the coupled fibre-optic and coaxial cable that is used by pay-TV services for data transfer. The speed of cable Internet is affected by traffic using the service but data transmission is in the range of 5–10 Mbit/s.
CIR	Committed Information Rate	The guaranteed speed of transmission in a frame-relay network.
CODEC	COder-DECoder	Technology for compressing and decompressing data (usually images). Codecs can be implemented in software or hardware, or a combination of both.

DCT	Discrete Cosine Transform	The discrete cosine transform is closely related to the fast Fourier transform. It is used in coding images, eg in the widely used standard JPEG compression technique.
DICOM	Digital Imaging and Communication in Medicine	A standard for medical image storage and transmission.
DWT	Discrete Wavelet Transform	The discrete wavelet transform is another method of coding images, similar to the DCT and Fourier transform.
Internet		The Internet is a global communications network consisting of thousands of computer networks all working to a common communications protocol (TCP/IP).
Intranet		A private computer network belonging to an organization using similar communications protocols to the Internet, ie an intranet appears to the members of the organization like a private version of the Internet.
IP	Internet Protocol	Part of the communication protocol (TCP/IP) used on the Internet.
ISDN	Integrated Services Digital Network	A digital telecommunications network. The bandwidth of a basic rate ISDN connection is 128 kbit/s, because it is made up of two 64 kbit/s data channels. The different channels of ISDN can be used concurrently for voice or data, or both.
ITU	International Tele-communication Union	The international organization responsible for setting telecommunications standards.
JPEG	Joint Photographic Experts Group	The JPEG committee defined the widely-used data compression techniques for still images.
kb	kbit	Approximately 1000 bits.
kB	kByte	Approximately 1000 bytes.
LAN	Local Area Network	A network connecting computers within a single building.
LP	Line Pairs	In optical specifications, a pair of straight stripes of equal width with a defined degree

		of contrast used as a means of determining resolution.
MAN	Metropolitan Area Network	A network connecting computers within a city, ie interconnecting LANs in separate buildings.
Mb	Megabit	Approximately one million bits.
MB	MegaByte	Approximately one million bytes.
Modem	MOdulator/DEModulator	A modem allows computers to communicate by converting digital data into analogue signals and transmitting them across the public telephone network. Modems have an advertised capacity of 56 kbit/s but are limited by the quality of telephone lines and will often transfer data at around 45–50 kbit/s. There are also overheads in converting the digital data to analogue signals, retransmitting data packets (affected by interference on the telephone lines) and the time taken to establish a connection, ie to dial the phone number of the receiving application.
PACS	Picture Archiving and Communication System	A filmless X-ray system, in which images are stored and displayed digitally. Image capture may be from plain film (by scanning it) or there may be direct digital capture from the appropriate imaging modality.
PGP	Pretty Good Privacy	A data-encryption standard.
PSTN	Public Switched Telephone Network	The ordinary telephone network. Although the links between telephone exchanges are now digital, the connections to private houses are still analogue.
PVC	Permanent Virtual Circuit	A predefined network path connecting two computers.
RLE	Run Length Encoding	A primitive compression method for reducing the size of image files.
SSL	Secure Socket Layer	A protocol for transmitting private documents through the Internet.
Switched 56		A digital telecommunications standard, mainly used in North America, originally

		where ISDN was not available. Now becoming less common.
T-1		A North American and Japanese standard for telecommunication. A T-1 line has a bandwidth of 1.54 Mbit/s. The communications line comprises 24 data channels, each of 64 kbit/s bandwidth.
TIE	Telemedicine Information Exchange	An independent source of information on telemedicine and telehealth, including a bibliography of telemedicine literature (see http://tie.telemed.org).
TIFF	Tag Image File Format	An image format.
WAN	Wide-Area Network	A wide-area network, by definition, connects computers separated by long distances, eg in different cities or in different countries. These networks can be private or public networks. Private networks offer a secure means of interconnecting two sites. The data speeds vary from 64 kbit/s to 1000 Mbit/s.

Section 1: Specialist Services

1. **Introduction**
   Jennifer Batch and Richard Wootton

2. **Telepaediatrics – A Review**
   Richard Wootton and Alan Isles

3. **Telepaediatrics in Queensland**
   Anthony C Smith

4. **Telecardiology in Canada and Australia**
   John Finley and Robert Justo

5. **The Applications of Telehealth in Medical Genetics**
   Tina Babineau and Mark D Ludman

6. **Telemedicine in Advanced Fetal Diagnosis and Therapy**
   Fung Yee Chan and Barbara Soong

7. **Child and Adolescent Telepsychiatry**
   Jean Starling and David Dossetor

8. **Diabetes and Telemedicine**
   Jennifer Batch and Anthony C Smith

9. **Telemedicine Applications in the Management of Asthma**
   Michael J Romano

10. **Post-acute Burns Care for Children**
    Roy Kimble and Anthony C Smith

11. **Telemedicine in Paediatric Surgery**
    Grant G Miller

12. **Telemedicine in Physical and/or Sexual Abuse**
    Philip O Ozuah, James P Marcin, Deborah Burton and Deborah Stanley

▶ 1

Introduction

Jennifer Batch and Richard Wootton

Telemedicine

Telemedicine is the delivery of healthcare and the exchange of healthcare information across distances. Telepaediatrics is thus telemedicine that is relevant to the health and wellbeing of children, young people and families. As with telemedicine, telepaediatrics encompasses the whole spectrum of medical activities performed when distance is an issue; these include diagnosis, treatment and prevention of disease, continuing education of healthcare providers and consumers, and research and evaluation. In the literature, a range of terminology is used to describe distance medicine, including telemedicine, telehealth, e-health and online health. These terms have been used variably by the contributors to the different sections of this book and reflect local usage.

Telemedicine has a long history that certainly predates the electronic age. The arrival of the PC and cheap digital communication in the 1980s, however, made telemedicine practicable. A still-growing body of work has resulted.[1] Although telemedicine has been in used in various forms for over 20 years, remarkably little work has been done in telepaediatrics specifically. The scope of current telepaediatric activity globally is reviewed in Chapter 2.

Why telepaediatrics?

Paediatric and adolescent medical practice is generally considered to include care provided from birth to 18 years. As such, paediatric and adolescent medicine constitutes a relatively small part of the total provision of healthcare services across a person's lifespan. One consequence of the size of paediatrics as a medical subspecialty is that paediatric resources are less available and generally are aggregated in major regional centres, state and provincial capital cities, and tertiary paediatric facilities. Another consequence is the relative dearth of paediatric subspecialists compared with the number of subspecialists in adult medicine. Both of these factors mean that access to a range of paediatric and adolescent healthcare services is often limited. These limitations may become more significant when issues of geography and distance are taken into account, as it is most uncommon to have specialized paediatric medical, nursing or allied health resources available outside tertiary centres.

Telepaediatrics in its many forms thus has the potential to provide equity of access to a range of paediatric healthcare resources for children and families from metropolitan and rural and remote areas.[2] It also provides the opportunity for continuing education and professional support for healthcare providers involved in paediatric healthcare and for the delivery of information on health related matters to children and their families.

Telepaediatrics and multidisciplinary healthcare

The practice of paediatrics always involves at least a three-way interchange between the practitioner, the child and the child's parent or guardian. In addition, many areas of paediatric practice involve multidisciplinary team management, particularly where a chronic disease exists. All of these factors could potentially complicate the practice of telepaediatrics. As is evident from many of the chapters in this book, however, telepaediatrics in its many forms accommodates, and indeed facilitates, multidisciplinary team involvement from tertiary and remote clinical team members.

Medicolegal issues

Although telepaediatrics may provide a solution to the problem of delivering specialist paediatric services to remote areas, a number of legal and ethical issues must be considered. These issues include security and confidentiality, professional accountability and responsibility, technical and clinical standards, intellectual property rights, licensure, reimbursement and other problems arising from the cross-border potential of telepaediatrics.[3] The medicolegal status of distance consultations needs to be considered, including requirements for appropriate record keeping and documentation, security of electronic files and transmission of patient data. The professional registration and indemnity of the healthcare providers must also be considered, particularly if the consultation occurs across state or national boundaries. In this context, medicolegal responsibility for implementation of treatment recommendations must be considered carefully.

Evaluation of the standards of healthcare delivered by telepaediatrics is an area of obvious importance and current research. The main body of literature on telepaediatrics to date has concentrated on the feasibility and acceptability of telepaediatrics rather than the quality per se of the healthcare delivered. Although telepaediatrics is accepted by families and practitioners alike, few studies rigorously assess the healthcare delivered by telepaediatrics compared with face-to-face delivery of a clinical service. The issue of quality of telepaediatric healthcare standards thus remains poorly studied, and no recognized standards of care for telepaediatrics have yet been established.

Finally, in most instances, reimbursement for practitioners involved in telepaediatrics remains an unresolved issue. The practice of telepaediatrics in many areas thus is confined to practitioners who do not require payment or remuneration for each consultation.

Barriers to development of telepaediatric services

The barriers to the development of telepaediatrics are similar to those of telemedicine in general. Many of these relate to clinician issues and have been summarized by Treister.[4] The issues include clinician reaction to change, failure to begin with an adequate physician base of support, lack of a user-friendly interface, concerns about the quality of the clinical interaction, physician technophobia, inadequate training of physicians in the use of the technology and lack of leadership by respected physicians. Other barriers may include concerns about medicolegal and reimbursement matters.

Aims of this book

This book aims to outline examples of the practice of telepaediatrics as it relates to delivery of medical, nursing and allied health services – including education – to children, families and health professionals who are remote from the source of the expertise. Every effort has been made to include the areas in which significant published work in telepaediatrics exists. (If we have overlooked any areas in which significant published work exists, then it is an error on our part.)

The first section of the book concentrates on the delivery of specialist services ranging from cardiology to child sexual abuse. The second section of the book provides information on community-based care, support and education for children and their families. The final section of the book contains examples of how telepaediatrics can provide education and information for children, families and staff at a distance.

The focus of this book is clinical. Those interested in the technical aspects of telemedicine as applied in paediatric work can find further information in Appendix 1.1.

Conclusion

Telepaediatrics is rapidly becoming an important part of the provision of paediatric healthcare services to children and families separated by distance from the healthcare source. In addition, telepaediatrics plays an important role in the provision of information and education for consumers and professionals alike.

References

1   Moser PL, Hauffe H, Lorenz IH, *et al.* Publication output in telemedicine during the period January 1964 to July 2003. *Journal of Telemedicine and Telecare* 2004; **10**: 72–7.
2   Spooner SA, Gotlieb EM. Committee on Clinical Information Technology; Committee on Medical Liability. Telemedicine: paediatric applications. *Pediatrics* 2004; **113**: e639–e643.
3   Stanberry B. Medicolegal aspects of telemedicine. In *Introduction to Telemedicine.* Wootton R, Craig J, eds. London: Royal Society of Medicine Press, 1999: 159–175.
4   Treister NW. Physician acceptance of new medical information systems: the field of dreams. *Physician Executive* 1998; **24**: 20–24.

Appendix to Chapter 1: Technology

Richard Wootton

Introduction

A common mistake in planning a new telemedicine application is to become focused on the technology. As a result, insufficient emphasis is placed on the human and organizational factors, and the almost inevitable consequence is a failed application. The history of telemedicine is littered with expensive technological failures.

Ten or twenty years ago, little readily available technology was suitable for telemedicine. The situation now is quite different: telecommunications are faster, cheaper and much more widely available. Telemedicine equipment of various kinds can be purchased off the shelf. It is important therefore to realize that the technology is the easy part of setting up a new application! A successful telemedicine system requires much more effort to be spent on the human factors and organizational aspects.[1] In this respect, the technology is almost irrelevant.

Components of a telemedicine system

In the context of the technology, any telemedicine system needs three essential components (four components, if the people are included). The three technical components are:

▶ **Devices for information input.** For example, the ordinary telephone is a rather under-rated telemedicine system by which advice can be obtained from a specialist. The information input device in this case is the microphone in the telephone handset. Generally speaking, the type of information to be transmitted in a telemedicine application may be audio, documents or text, still images or moving images (video). Each type of information may require a specialized input device.

▶ **Means of information transport.** Once the information has been captured, it needs to be transmitted to the other end of the telemedicine link. For example, a telephone call needs a telephone circuit to be established between the two parties. The amounts of information to be transmitted will determine the best type of telecommunications to use.

▶ **Devices for information display.** After the information has been transmitted to the remote party, it needs to be displayed. For example, in the case of a telephone call, the 'display' device is the loudspeaker in the telephone handset. Much of the information in telemedicine applications is visual and is often displayed on various kinds of television screen or computer monitor.

Telecommunications

Some form of telecommunication is required for telemedicine, and a wide variety of telecommunications media are now available. The variety is so wide, in fact, that the choice is often bewildering.

Local area telemedicine

For local area telemedicine – within a building, or between buildings on a campus – the transmission of information using the Internet Protocol (IP) is becoming increasingly common. That is, the telecommunications medium is a computer network of some kind. As an organization will usually have a computer network installed as part of its IT infrastructure, using it for telemedicine may seem attractive, as its use may be free of charge (or at least the charge will be borne by other parts of the organization).

Furthermore, the possibility exists of using IP transmission in the wide area as well. Thus the Internet can be used for telemedicine between countries, for example. Alternatively, an organization may operate a private network – an intranet – that can be used for IP transmission between cities or countries.

Internet Protocol transmission can work well in telemedicine; however, two main problems need to be dealt with. First, IP transmission on a computer network is data transmission on a shared medium – it is fundamentally different from sending data on a telephone line where there is a private circuit between sender and recipient for the duration of the call. It is possible therefore for other users of the network to create problems inadvertently, eg by transferring large files and causing transmission bottlenecks. This can have serious effects on the quality of real-time video pictures, in particular, which are sensitive to the amount of bandwidth available and also to any network delays. Although methods are being developed by which a quality of service can be guaranteed in advance, such techniques are not yet agreed internationally and tend to be proprietary to particular manufacturers of network equipment.

The second potential problem concerns data security. Again, by virtue of a computer network being a shared medium, the possibilities for electronic eavesdropping are much higher. Well-established techniques exist for encrypting computer traffic, but all of them come at a cost.

Wide area telemedicine

For wide area telemedicine – for example between two hospitals – the common choices are:

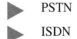 PSTN

ISDN

▶ broadband (eg ADSL)

▶ other (eg satellite).

PSTN

This is the ordinary telephone network. It has the huge advantages of being available almost everywhere and of being relatively cheap. It can be used to transmit voice (audio) obviously, as that was what it was originally designed for. It can also be used to transmit simple static images with a fax machine.

The telephone network is an under-rated transmission medium for telemedicine. Transmission of still images has been used successfully in isolated locations such as the Antarctic.[2] Electrocardiographic charts can also be sent with a fax machine.[3]

Finally, the PSTN can be used for low-speed digital transmission by attaching a modem to the network. The purpose of the modem is to convert digital bits and bytes from a computer into audio tones suitable for transmission through the telephone network. The only real disadvantage is that the data transmission speed is relatively slow. Data transmission speeds of only 28–56 kbit/s can be achieved in practice. Although this is rapid enough for the transfer of small files, such as email messages, it is insufficient for large image files or real-time video pictures

ISDN

The ordinary telephone network was designed originally to transmit analogue signals. The ISDN on the other hand, was designed from the outset as a digital network. Like the PSTN, when a call is placed, a private circuit is established from the caller to the recipient. In this respect, the likelihood of electronic 'eavesdropping' is much less than when medical information is transmitted on the Internet.

ISDN capacity is made available to users by bundling together one or more data channels. Each data channel can transmit 64 kbit/s of information. For low-speed data transfer, a single data channel may suffice; while for high-speed data transfer, such as the transmission of high-quality video pictures, perhaps 32 or more data channels may be needed (ie 2.048 Mbit/s).

Telephone companies sell ISDN capacity in a similar way to telephone services. There is normally an installation fee for the line and a monthly rental charge. On top of that, there are call charges for the time that the circuit is used; the call charges being higher for long-distance and international calls. Finally, ISDN is commonly sold in units of two data channels (known as a Basic Rate Interface) or 32 data channels (known as a Primary Rate Interface). Sometimes intermediate capacities are also available. One common requirement in videoconferencing is for data transmission at 384 kbit/s, which is achieved by the simultaneous use of three BRI lines. The use of multiple lines is known as ISDN multiplexing.

Broadband (eg ADSL)

Medium-speed digital connections are beginning to be offered by telephone companies to subscribers who live within a few kilometres of the nearest telephone exchange. Use of special equipment at the exchange allows a digital service to be delivered to the subscriber's premises through the existing (analogue) wiring. This may represent an effective compromise between the cost of laying a special digital cable and the desire for high-speed transmission. Different forms of DSL technology (digital subscriber line) exist; a common form is ADSL. Here, the A stands for Asymmetric, as the speed of data transmission to the exchange generally is lower than the speed at which data is sent in the other direction. Data rates for ADSL of 128 kbit/s to the exchange and 256 kbit/s from the exchange are common.

As well as allowing faster transmission of digital data, a broadband service such as ADSL represents a permanent connection. There is no need to dial a recipient each time it is used: it is always on. Broadband services therefore are sold in a different way to the PSTN. There is generally an installation fee and a monthly rental. After that, usage is either free or free up to a certain data transfer threshold, after which further charges are made. For example, a download 'cap' of 500 MBytes per month may be specified: if the user exceeds this limit, then the service provider will charge for each additional MByte of information transferred.

Other (eg satellite)

Although the telecommunications media mentioned above are widely available, there will always be areas where providing wired access is uneconomic or impractical. In these circumstances, satellite telecommunications can be used. The type of satellite service, and therefore its cost, is determined by whether the user wants one-way or two-way communication. In the former case, signals are sent to a satellite ground station, which causes them to be broadcast to satellite receiver units over a large portion of the earth's surface. This is a useful method for delivering lectures to several countries at once, for example. At one time, the EuroTransMed organization was delivering weekly medical seminars to about 250 hospitals in 27 countries in western Europe by satellite broadcast.[4]

If two-way communication is needed, a different form of satellite service is required. Such services are usually based on satellite telephony. For example, the Inmarsat organization offers a 64 kbit/s data link through small, portable telephone units (Fig. A1.1).

Unfortunately, because of the cost of providing satellite infrastructure and the relatively low volume of usage, satellite telecommunications tend to be expensive. Other forms of radio transmission, such as very high frequency (VHF), may be worth considering if circumstances permit.

Videoconferencing standards

Most videoconferencing for medical purposes takes place using equipment that conforms to various internationally agreed standards. This removes the need to purchase equipment from a particular manufacturer. The principal standards are:

 H.320: the original international standard for videoconferencing on circuit-switched networks, such as the ISDN. H.320 establishes the common formats

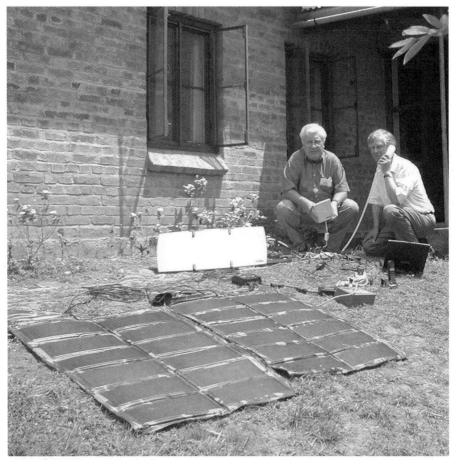

Fig. A1.1 Portable satellite phone in use at a hospital in Nepal (running on solar power). Picture courtesy of the Swinfen Charitable Trust.

necessary to make audio and video inputs and outputs compatible, for example.

▶ H.323: developed from the H.320 standard to define videoconferencing over packet-switched networks, such as IP-based computer networks

▶ H.324 defines videoconferencing over low-bandwidth networks, such as the ordinary telephone network.

Until recently, the dominant form of videoconferencing for telemedicine was undoubtedly H.320 using ISDN lines. A national survey conducted by the Association of Telehealth Service Providers (ATSP) in the US showed that about one-third of the 88 networks surveyed used ISDN.[5] IP videoconferencing is becoming more popular because the running costs are lower. Most modern equipment is capable of videoconferencing using either ISDN or IP connections.

Videoconferencing systems

Historically, most videoconferencing for telemedicine was done using purpose-built equipment, usually sold commercially in the form of a videoconferencing system. Such systems comprised either fixed equipment (a 'room-based' system, Fig. A1.2) or equipment mounted on castors so that they were movable ('rollabout' units, Fig. A1.3).

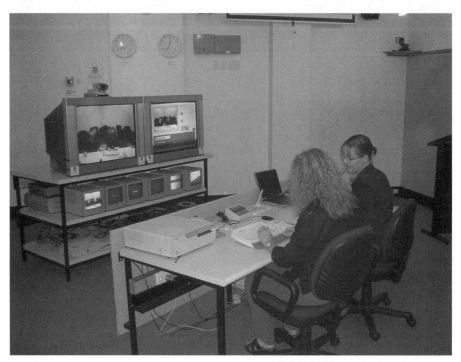

Fig. A1.2 Fixed videoconferencing equipment (a 'room-based' system).

Room-based and rollabout systems were designed for group videoconferencing, in which groups of say 6–12 people might be present in any one location. The equipment was relatively expensive. Recent miniaturization, and the economies of volume production, have meant that the equipment has become smaller and cheaper. The latest units are referred to as 'set-top', because the components are contained in a unit designed to be placed on top of the television set used to display the pictures (Fig. A1.4).

The inexorable rise of the personal computer (PC) has also seen it used as a platform for videoconferencing. Early PC-based videoconferencing required special cards

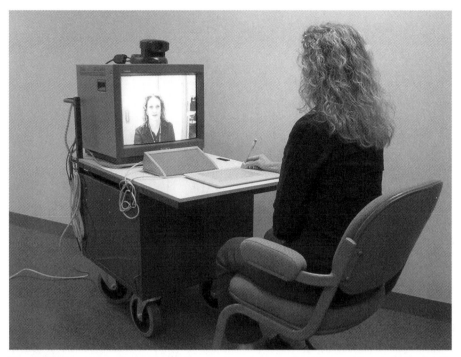

Fig. A1.3 Videoconferencing equipment mounted on castors so that it is movable (a 'roll-about' unit).

containing a hardware codec, but the increase in PC processor power now means that the codec function can be performed by software in the PC.

Personal computer-based videoconferencing can certainly be made to work, although it works best mainly for personal (ie single-person) videoconferencing. It should be borne in mind, however, that successful videoconferencing needs a great deal of attention to detail: a suitable environment is necessary, with appropriate lighting, acoustics and so on. Purchasing a PC instead of a set-top videoconferencing unit will not automatically lead to successful videoconferences. It may, in the long run, turn out to be false economy.

Video telephones

Videoconferencing using the ordinary telephone network is technically possible, although the picture quality achievable is severely constrained by the limited bandwidth of the connection. Videophones were introduced commercially in the 1960s but were not a success. Technical developments allowed further miniaturization, and they are again available (Fig. A1. 5). Telemedical work is certainly possible using videophones,[6–10] albeit of a limited nature, and they have the advantage for home nursing of not needing special telecommunications lines to be installed in a patient's house. Videophones have not proved as popular as one might have expected, however, either in telemedicine or in society generally. This may be partly because of unrealistic expectations of their technical performance.

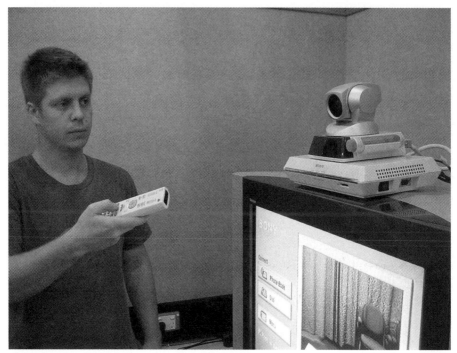

Fig. A1.4 Set-top videoconferencing equipment can be placed on top of the TV set used to display the pictures.

Video quality

Transmitting television pictures requires a high data rate. Studio-quality television pictures require a data rate of about 100 Mbit/s. Over the next few years, this sort of transmission rate will become more common on computer networks in organizations, so that transmission of raw television pictures (ie uncompressed) will become feasible. It will be years, however, before such transmission speeds will become generally available in places such as patients' homes.

Because of restricted bandwidth, most videoconferencing uses compressed video. At the sending end, a device called a codec compresses the pictures. At the receiving end, a similar device de-compresses them. (Hence, 'codec': <u>co</u>mpression– <u>dec</u>ompression). The more the video pictures are compressed, the lower the data rate needed to transmit them. The disadvantage is that the more they are compressed, the more their quality is reduced. As compression ratios get higher, the pictures may become jerky and 'blocky'.

Historically, much early telemedicine work took place using a single ISDN line, giving a bandwidth of 128 kbit/s. In other places, such as the US, early telemedicine work tended to use digital lines with a bandwidth of 1.54 Mbit/s, which produced much better video quality. It is interesting to observe that, for reasons of cost, there has

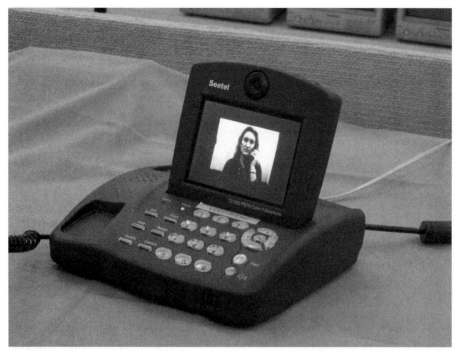

Fig. A1.5 Videophone designed for use on the ordinary telephone network.

been a shift in the US over the last few years to the use of lower bandwidth. An intermediate rate – 384 kbit/s – seems to represent a reasonable compromise between cost and quality.

Certain telemedicine applications, such as the transmission of fetal ultrasound video pictures, have been trialled under laboratory conditions at different bandwidths. Diagnostic accuracy may be seriously impaired if a bandwidth lower than 384 kbit/s is used.[11,12]

Compression of still pictures

Just as video pictures require compression to reduce the bandwidth needed for transmission, still images may also need to be compressed. For example, if images are being sent by email, their transmission through the international gateways cannot be guaranteed if the message size rises much above 1 MByte. The most common way of compressing still images is to use the JPEG algorithm (see Chapter 14). Although such compression results in some loss of image detail, if done carefully there will be no significant loss of diagnostic information.[13]

Peripherals

Videoconferencing for medical purposes usually needs various special devices depending on the exact purpose of the conference. For example, an educational conference may need a document camera to transmit pictures of paper documents. Document cameras can also be used to transmit pictures of X-rays, although the resolution is not high enough for primary diagnosis (Fig. A1.6). A video player may be needed to replay pre-recorded video tapes. A clinical conference may need some means of transmitting heart sounds (an electronic stethoscope) or perhaps video pictures from the ear (a video otoscope) (Fig. A1.7).

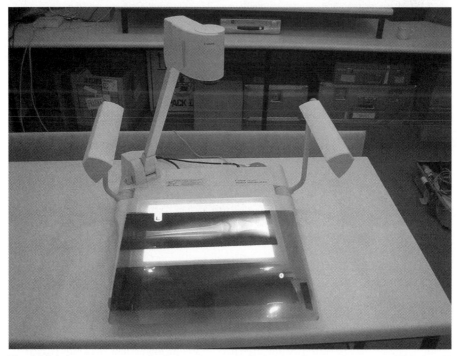

Fig. A1.6 A document camera is designed to transmit pictures of paper documents. With the aid of a back-light, it can also send pictures of X-ray films.

It is easy to lose sight of the cost of such peripherals. Unless they are used intensively, they will be difficult to justify economically.[14]

Advice

The choice of technology for telemedicine often creates problems for potential customers. Where can a prospective purchaser obtain disinterested advice? Useful sources of information include:

▶ national telemedicine societies

▶ the Telemedicine Information Exchange

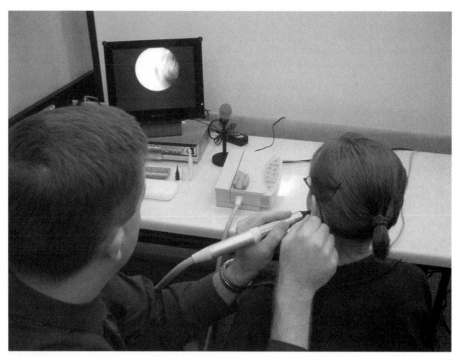

Fig. A1.7 Video otoscope for transmitting pictures suitable for ear, nose and throat telemedicine.

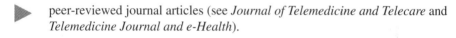 peer-reviewed journal articles (see *Journal of Telemedicine and Telecare* and *Telemedicine Journal and e-Health*).

The predominant body for national telemedicine societies is the International Society for Telemedicine (http:http://www.isft.org/).

Conclusion

When considering telemedicine technology, do not believe what the salesmen say! Remember that the history of telemedicine is littered with the expensive carcasses of unused technology. It is almost always better to plan a modest pilot trial and expand things if it is successful than to plan a grand scheme that will almost certainly end in disaster. It is also well worth consulting the literature to draw on the experience of others. A good place to start is the Telemedicine Information Exchange (http://tie.telemed.org).

References

1   Wootton R. Telemedicine: a cautious welcome. *British Medical Journal* 1996; **313**: 1375–1377.

2   Hyer RN. Telemedical experiences at an Antarctic station. *Journal of Telemedicine and Telecare* 1999; **5** (suppl. 1): 87–89.

3   Srikanthan VS, Pell AC, Prasad N, *et al.* Use of fax facility improves decision making regarding thrombolysis in acute myocardial infarction. *Heart* 1997; **78**: 198–200.

4   Young HL. Medical education by satellite: the EuroTransMed experience. *Journal of Audiovisual Media in Medicine* 1995; **18**: 75–78.

5   Grigsby B. *2004 TRC Report on US Telemedicine Activity*. Kingston, NJ: Civic Research Institute, 2004.

6   Mickus MA, Luz CC. Televisits: sustaining long distance family relationships among institutionalized elders through technology. *Aging and Mental Health* 2002 ;**6**: 387–396.

7   Nakamura K, Takano T, Akao C. The effectiveness of videophones in home healthcare for the elderly. *Medical Care* 1999; **37**: 117–125.

8   Guilfoyle C, Perry L, Lord B, *et al.* Developing a protocol for the use of telenursing in community health in Australia. *Journal of Telemedicine and Telecare* 2002; **8** (suppl. 2): 33–36.

9   Arnaert A, Delesie L. Telenursing for the elderly. The case for care via video-telephony. *Journal of Telemedicine and Telecare* 2001; **7**: 311–316.

10   Doolittle GC, Yaezel A, Otto F, Clemens C. Hospice care using home-based telemedicine systems. *Journal of Telemedicine and Telecare* 1998; **4** (suppl. 1): 58–59.

11   Wootton R, Dornan J, Fisk NM, *et al.* The effect of transmission bandwidth on diagnostic accuracy in remote fetal ultrasound scanning. *Journal of Telemedicine and Telecare* 1997; **3**: 209–214.

12   Chan FY, Whitehall J, Hayes L, *et al.* Minimum requirements for remote realtime fetal tele-ultrasound consultation. *Journal of Telemedicine and Telecare* 1999; **5**: 171–176.

13   Szot A, Jacobson FL, Munn S, *et al.* Diagnostic accuracy of chest X-rays acquired using a digital camera for low-cost teleradiology. *International Journal of Medical Informatics* 2004; **73**: 65–73.

14   Bergmo TS. An economic analysis of teleconsultation in otorhinolaryngology. *Journal of Telemedicine and Telecare* 1997; **3**: 194–199.

▶2

Telepaediatrics – A Review

Richard Wootton and Alan Isles

Introduction

What is telepaediatrics? Telemedicine can be defined as any medical activity that involves a distance element (see Chapter 1). A generic definition of this sort avoids the semantic confusion that surrounds terms like telehealth, online health, e-health, etc. There is no generally accepted definition of telepaediatrics, but by extrapolation it would be reasonable to classify it as any paediatric activity that involves a distance element, eg clinical, educational or research and administrative work, in which the parties concerned may not be present in the same space or time.

In clinical work, telepaediatrics therefore encompasses the delivery of specialist services to regional sites, using techniques such as videoconferencing, email or the humble telephone.

Literature review

What is known about telepaediatrics? Articles relating to telepaediatric work were identified in the Medline database, excluding those without abstracts, with a simple search: "Telemedicine AND (Pediatrics OR Child Health) AND HasAbstract". Although 3734 articles related to telemedicine generally, only 82 (2%) related to paediatrics or child health specifically. Telepaediatrics therefore seems to be a relatively under-researched area of telemedicine.

The 82 paediatric telemedicine articles were classified according to their main topic (Table 2.1). The largest single category of paper concerned reviews of various types – mostly those that advocated the benefits of using telemedicine in paediatric work. The next most common article concerned the use of the telephone, mainly for telephone helplines of various kinds.

Common telepaediatric applications

The two most common telepaediatric applications identified in the literature review were telephone helplines and telecardiology. Telephone helplines in paediatrics may provide advice for parents, for the children themselves or for health staff. Almost all of the 13 reports about telephone use concerned telephone triage. Telephone helplines for

Table 2.1. Telepaediatric articles categorized according to main topic

Topic	Articles
Review	15 (18%)
Telephone	13 (16%)
Cardiology	11 (13%)
Not relevant*	11 (13%)
General clinical consultations (videoconferencing)	7 (9%)
Education	4 (5%)
Child protection, including sexual abuse	3 (4%)
School	3 (4%)
Email	2 (2%)
Pathology	2 (2%)
Psychiatry	2 (2%)
Radiology	2 (2%)
Surgery	2 (2%)
Asthma	1 (1%)
Home	1 (1%)
Neurology	1 (1%)
Oncology	1 (1%)
User satisfaction	1 (1%)
Total	**82 (100%)**

*'Not relevant' includes papers describing theoretical work, such as planning.

general medical queries are growing in popularity, and in some countries, such as the UK, they are being implemented on a national basis. As yet, little evidence supports their cost-effectiveness, although they clearly provide members of the public with a new method of making contact with healthcare professionals, particularly outside normal working hours. This may be a major reason for their popularity. In paediatrics, telephone helplines are also becoming more common. There are concerns, however, about the quality of advice given.[1,2] There are also questions about the long-term economics of operating paediatric helplines. An American survey of 30 hospitals with a paediatric telephone triage and advice programme showed that all were operating at a substantial financial loss.[3] Despite these caveats, telephone helplines appear to be here to stay and, in the right circumstances, seem to be highly successful (see Chapters 24 and 25).

Almost all of the 11 reports on telecardiology concerned the real-time transmission of echocardiographic images. There is now extensive experience in doing this, and if a telemedicine link of high enough quality is used, the diagnostic accuracy is acceptable. In circumstances in which a baby with a heart problem may need to be transferred a considerable distance to a tertiary centre for evaluation and treatment, carrying out a consultation with an expert by telemedicine has many advantages. These aspects are explored in Chapter 4. Studies that show the cost-effectiveness of this form of telecardiology are beginning to appear.[4]

The next most common topic in the literature is general clinical teleconsultation, usually involving videoconferencing. This is addressed in Chapters 3, 11 and 20. In Queensland, there is a growing body of experience with teleconsultation.

Is telepaediatrics different from telemedicine in general?

Telepaediatrics is an application of telemedicine. It is not different in the sense that medical activities take place at a distance; however, it *is* different in the sense that for clinical work, the parent as well as the patient has to travel if telepaediatrics is not used. This may make the economics of the latter more favourable than for other telemedicine applications. There is not much work on the economics of telemedicine generally, and even less about telepaediatrics specifically. Two recent studies, however, examined the economics of paediatric telemedicine from the point of view of the families concerned.[5,6] Both studies found – perhaps as might be expected – that it is much cheaper and more convenient for families to attend a videoconference in a local facility than travel long distances for a face-to-face consultation in a specialist hospital.

Telepaediatrics is also different in the sense that for educational work, the subsequent benefits of the education may be realized for a longer period (and may therefore be more important economically) than in the case of adults. Note that there is the potential for both child and parent education.

Where is telepaediatrics being done?

Analysis of the country of origin of the articles identified in the literature search shows that most of the work being reported – more than half – is from the US (Table 2.2). This of course may not necessarily indicate where the majority of telepaediatrics is being practised.

No systematic worldwide survey of telemedicine practice has been done, so it is not possible to say definitively where telepaediatrics is being performed. The best data about practice in a given country comes from the US: a recent survey of telemedicine networks there found that 38% of respondents reported paediatrics as an application.[7] Paediatrics was the third most common clinical application after mental health and cardiology. There is also significant telepaediatric work in Queensland.[5,8–12]

Advantages and disadvantages of telepaediatrics

In the right circumstances, telepaediatrics can clearly work very well – saving patient and staff travel, improving access and perhaps even reducing costs.[5] There are as yet, however, very few studies that show strict cost-effectiveness. There is thus a danger that inappropriate use of resources will deter future investment in the technique. The history of telemedicine is littered with expensive failures, and one would hope that telepaediatrics could be developed in a cautious and sensible way. The key questions about telepaediatrics of interest to planners are:

▶ Can it provide diagnostic and management advice comparable to conventional practice?

Table 2.2. Telepaediatric articles categorized according to country of origin (excluding those classified as non-relevant*)

Country	Articles
US	43 (61%)
Australia	6 (9%)
Canada	5 (7%)
India	3 (4%)
France	2 (3%)
Japan	2 (3%)
Spain	2 (3%)
UK	2 (3%)
Bosnia and Herzegovina	1 (1%)
Germany	1 (1%)
Greece	1 (1%)
Israel	1 (1%)
Russia	1 (1%)
Switzerland	1 (1%)
Total	**71 (100%)**

*'not relevant' includes papers describing theoretical work, such as planning

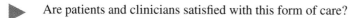
Are patients and clinicians satisfied with this form of care?

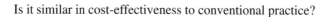
Is it similar in cost-effectiveness to conventional practice?

These questions are similar to those relating to the possible use of telemedicine generally.

The answers to the first two of these questions are almost certainly, yes – as much of the material in this book attests. Most studies of user satisfaction with telemedicine, for example, show that patients and clinicians are happy with it; the few studies of telepaediatrics are also positive.[13–17] There is, however, rather limited evidence about cost-effectiveness. Again, this is an observation that is also true for telemedicine generally.

The future

What forms will telepaediatrics take in the future? Various applications look promising, including teleconsulting in general (eg telecardiology, telepsychiatry and surgery consultations), care of schoolchildren (in the US) and teledentistry. The area of chronic disease monitoring (asthma and diabetes in particular), using relatively low-cost technology, may turn out to be especially successful in due course.

Perhaps because most telepaediatric work reported to date has emanated from the US, the American Academy of Pediatrics recently reviewed the use and limitations of telemedicine in paediatrics.[18] Their conclusion is that, although the evidence base is weak at present, telemedicine may be important for accessing paediatric subspecialty services, for improving communication with parents of sick and chronically ill children, and for extending the boundaries of the 'medical home'.

It is important that telepaediatric work continues in a careful but rigorous way. Those involved in telepaediatric projects have, in our view, a responsibility to include formal evaluation and cost-effectiveness measures in each project, so that the evidence base for telepaediatrics can be expanded. An evidence base that ultimately shows telepaediatrics to be clinically effective and cost-effective is, in the end, the only way of developing sustainable service models.

Further information

Wootton R, Craig J (eds). *Introduction to Telemedicine*. London: Royal Society of Medicine Press, 1999.

Journal of Telemedicine and Telecare. http://www.rsmpress.co.uk/jtt.htm (last checked 15 August 2004).

Telemedicine Information Exchange. http://tie.telemed.org (last checked 15 August 2004).

References

1   Oberklaid F. Paediatric telephone advice: a major gap in quality service delivery. *Journal of Paediatrics and Child Health* 2002; **38**:6–7.

2   Andrews JK, Armstrong KL, Fraser JA. Professional telephone advice to parents with sick children: time for quality control! *Journal of Paediatrics and Child Health* 2002; **38**: 23–26.

3   Melzer SM, Poole SR. Computerized pediatric telephone triage and advice programs at children's hospitals: operating and financial characteristics. *Archives of Pediatrics and Adolescent Medicine* 1999; **153**: 858–863.

4   Sicotte C, Lehoux P, Van Doesburg N, *et al*. A cost-effectiveness analysis of interactive paediatric telecardiology. *Journal of Telemedicine and Telecare* 2004; **10**: 78–83.

5   Smith AC, Youngberry K, Christie F, *et al*. The family costs of attending hospital outpatient appointments via videoconference and in person. *Journal of Telemedicine and Telecare* 2003; **9** (suppl. 2): 58–61.

6   Bynum AB, Irwin CA, Cranford CO, Denny GS. The impact of telemedicine on patients' cost savings: some preliminary findings. *Telemedicine Journal and e-Health* 2003; **9**: 361–367.

7   Grigsby B. *2004 TRC Report on US Telemedicine Activity*. Kingston, NJ: Civic Research Institute, 2004.

8   Smith AC, Williams M, Van der Westhuyzen J, *et al*. A comparison of telepaediatric activity at two regional hospitals in Queensland. *Journal of Telemedicine and Telecare* 2002; **8** (suppl. 3): 58–62.

9   Smith AC, Kimble R, Mill J, *et al*. Diagnostic accuracy of and patient satisfaction with telemedicine for the follow-up of paediatric burns patients. *Journal of Telemedicine and Telecare* 2004; **10**: 193–198.

10 Smith AC, Youngberry K, Mill J, *et al*. A review of three years experience using email and videoconferencing for the delivery of post-acute burns care to children in Queensland. *Burns* 2004; **30**: 248–252.

11 Smith AC, Batch J, Lang E, Wootton R. The use of online health techniques to assist with the delivery of specialist paediatric diabetes services in Queensland. *Journal of Telemedicine and Telecare* 2003; **9** (suppl. 2): 54–57.

12 Smith AC, Isles A, McCrossin R, *et al*. The point-of-referral barrier—a factor in the success of telehealth. *Journal of Telemedicine and Telecare* 2001; **7** (suppl. 2): 75–78.

13 Marcin JP, Ellis J, Mawis R, *et al*. Using telemedicine to provide pediatric subspecialty care to children with special health care needs in an underserved rural community. *Pediatrics* 2004; **113**: 1–6.

14 Kopel H, Nunn K, Dossetor D. Evaluating satisfaction with a child and adolescent psychological telemedicine outreach service. *Journal of Telemedicine and Telecare* 2001; **7** (suppl. 2): 35–40.

15 Elford DR, White H, St John K, *et al*. A prospective satisfaction study and cost analysis of a pilot child telepsychiatry service in Newfoundland. *Journal of Telemedicine and Telecare* 2001; **7**: 73–81.

16   Dick PT, Filler R, Pavan A. Participant satisfaction and comfort with multidisciplinary pediatric telemedicine consultations. *Journal of Pediatric Surgery* 1999; **34**: 137–141;discussion 141–142.

17   Blackmon LA, Kaak HO, Ranseen J. Consumer satisfaction with telemedicine child psychiatry consultation in rural Kentucky. *Psychiatric Services* 1997; **48**: 1464–1466.

18   Spooner SA, Gotlieb EM. Committee on Clinical Information Technology; Committee on Medical Liability. Telemedicine: pediatric applications. *Pediatrics* 2004; **113**: e639–e643.

▶3

Telepaediatrics in Queensland

Anthony C Smith

Introduction

Queensland is the second largest state in Australia, spanning about 1600 km from east to west and 2400 km from north to south (Fig. 3.1). Queensland has a population of about 4 million people: about 2.5 million people live in the southeast corner and one million in larger towns along the east coast. The remainder of the population is dispersed widely in small rural townships throughout the state. Many of the smaller towns have developed among rural properties or farms, mine sites or aboriginal communities. The long distances in Queensland add to the challenges of providing health services beyond the metropolitan area and to people living in rural and remote communities. A logical reason for developing telemedicine in Queensland is that most of the tertiary services, including the two paediatric hospitals, are situated in the far southeast of the state, in Brisbane.

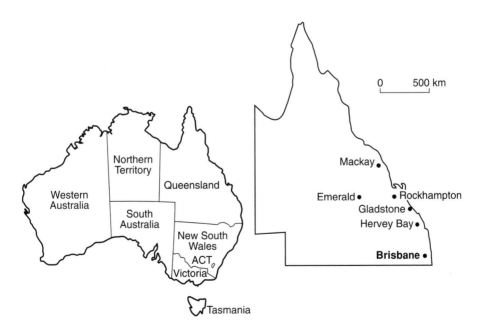

Fig. 3.1. Most tertiary paediatric services in Queensland are concentrated in Brisbane.

Throughout Australia, telemedicine projects or pilot services have proven the feasibility of online techniques such as videoconferencing for the delivery of health services. However, very few have become integrated into mainstream practice. The factors that have contributed to the limited uptake of telemedicine include lack of funding, limited incentives, inconvenience and lack of coordination and support.

Videoconferencing

In Queensland, the health department has established a large network of about 250 videoconferencing systems. Most equipment has been placed in hospitals, community health centres and civic centres throughout the state. The most recent report on the usage of the network was published in May 2000.[1] This indicated that about 1200 hours of videoconferencing were conducted per month, mainly for education (71%) with relatively little use for clinical services (8%). In the US, a report published by the Association for Telehealth Service Providers (ATSP) on telehealth usage estimated that about 48% of total usage was related to clinical applications. The relatively low proportion of clinical usage in Queensland suggests that the existing videoconference network has not reached its full potential.

Outreach services

For most families who live in rural and remote areas of Queensland, a referral to a specialist has usually meant significant disruption for the family. Quite often, the family need to travel long distances by car, bus or train (up to 20 hours), spend time away from home and take time off work. Some costs, such as those associated with travel and accommodation, are met by the health department through a patient travel subsidy scheme (PTSS).[2] In 2003, the health department spent $25 million on patient travel in Queensland.[3]

The health department also provides outreach services to regional areas by sending specialist teams from the tertiary hospitals to the regional hospitals on an intermittent basis (eg every three or six months) to see patients that have been referred. This is suitable for less urgent cases that do not require immediate treatment. The cost of sending the specialist and other staff for an outreach clinic can be justified when there is a substantial group of patients (eg in diabetes, paediatric surgery or cardiology). In comparison with sending patients to Brisbane, this method is less costly for the health department and much more convenient for the family. Apart from the costs, other important benefits of sending specialist teams to remote areas include education, training and professional support of isolated health professionals.

Telepaediatrics in Queensland

When children situated outside the metropolitan area need a specialist appointment, the costs generally are greater than for adults, as the child will also be accompanied by a parent or guardian. In effect, the travel costs are usually double those of a single adult patient who can travel independently. Travel to the specialist centre is inconvenient for these families, often disrupting family life and schooling, and resulting in time off work. Even if intangible, there are also emotional and social costs.

Telepaediatrics was shown to work in a feasibility study conducted in 1998.[4] This showed that videoconferencing could be used to provide specialist consultations to patients in a range of subspecialties. Subsequently, the adoption of telepaediatrics as a routine method of service delivery failed to occur. Apart from educational programmes, clinical activity largely ceased (Fig. 3.2). One reason for the lack of integration of telepaediatrics into mainstream practice was that organizing a videoconference typically required more effort and planning on the part of the referring clinician than the conventional method of patient transfer to Brisbane.

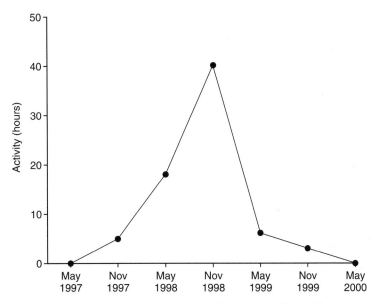

Fig. 3.2. Telepaediatric activity (hours per month) from May 1997 to May 2000.

New model

In 2000, a novel telepaediatric service was established as part of a research trial, offering a centralized service to selected sites in Queensland. The aim of the service was to make it as easy as possible for regional staff to make telepaediatric referrals. A single toll-free telephone number was offered to each site, giving them a direct link to a telepaediatric coordinator based in Brisbane. Regional staff were encouraged to refer all queries to the service. Once a referral was made, the coordinator took full responsibility for handling each referral and guaranteed a response by an appropriate specialist, usually within 24 hours. Responses included returned telephone calls, email or appointments via videoconference. About 85% of all referrals made to the telepaediatric service resulted in an appointment via videoconference.

Technical requirements

Most telepaediatric services were provided from the telemedicine studios in the Centre for Online Health (COH), which is situated conveniently in the Royal Children's Hospital (RCH) in Brisbane. The studio was the main base for the telepaediatric coordinators who provided all technical support (Fig. 3.3). In order for telepaediatric activity to take place in the chosen regional sites, improved videoconferencing facilities were needed. In each of these areas, minor room modifications were made, including additional room lighting, floor carpeting and the painting of walls in a neutral colour. Standard videoconference systems were installed (1600P or PCS-11P, Sony), as well as peripheral equipment such as a backlit video document camera, PC scan-converter and an extra S-video input to allow connection of a local ultrasound machine (Fig. 3.4). Videoconference consultations were conducted using the ISDN at a preferred minimum bandwidth of 384 kbit/s. Independent ISDN lines were installed at each site.

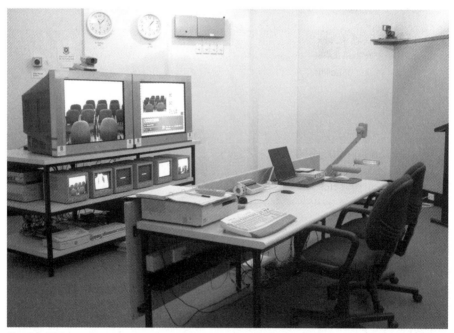

Fig. 3.3. Videoconferencing facilities at the Centre for Online Health in Brisbane (the hub site for the telepaediatric network).

Clinical activity

Since the start of the telepaediatric service, telepaediatric activity has grown steadily. The average number of consultations increased from 20 per month in 2000 to about 55 in 2004 (Fig. 3.5). More than 1500 patient consultations were conducted during the

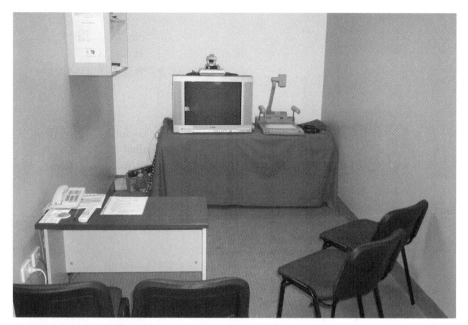

Fig. 3.4. Telepaediatric facilities in Mackay, one of the referring sites.

first three years of operation, making it the largest telepaediatric service reported in the literature. The telepaediatric service has facilitated the delivery of a broad range of services involving 30 different paediatric subspecialties. The most common applications have been for the delivery of post-acute burns care and specialist consultations in diabetes, oncology and cardiology (Fig. 3.6). Other fields have included psychiatry, gastroenterology, nephrology, neurology, orthopaedics and general medical care.

Post-acute burns care

Queensland's only specialist burns centre, the Stuart Pegg Paediatric Burns Centre (SPPBC), is based at the RCH and receives about 400 admissions annually from Queensland and northern New South Wales. Each year, about 1300 outpatient appointments are conducted in the SPPBC outpatient department. When patients are discharged from the SPPBC, a medical referral is sent to the referring general practitioner (GP) and regional occupational therapist. The family is usually sent home with the dressings and drugs needed for a two-week period and then returns for an outpatient appointment in the centre. During each follow-up appointment, the family will be seen by nurses, allied health staff and the treating doctor. After this appointment, the frequency of additional outpatient appointments will depend on the severity of the injury and treatment needs. This may constitute treatment lasting for many years.

The provision of post-acute care for children with burns has emerged as a significant development of the telepaediatric service.[5,6] We have established a routine programme

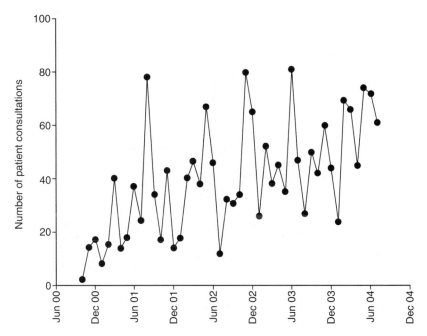

Fig. 3.5. Telepaediatric activity (number of patient consultations) from October 2000 to April 2004.

of virtual outpatient clinics that allows patients in rural and remote areas of Queensland to travel to their local hospital and be seen by the specialist burns team via videoconference. These clinics are held every month by each of the four consultants in the centre. During a videoconference appointment, routine follow-up can be conducted by discussing any concerns with the patient and family, and observing close-up images of the burn injury. Images are generally suitable for the assessment of scarring, contractures and breakdowns (Fig. 3.7). If high-quality images are required, these are sent via email for review by the burns centre (Fig. 3.8) (see Chapter 10).

Diabetes and endocrinology

Before the telepaediatric service was available, specialists in Brisbane would travel to regional hospitals and conduct outreach clinics every 3–4 months. Videoconferencing has complemented the delivery of specialist diabetes and endocrine services to children living outside the metropolitan area. Instead of travelling to the regions several times per year, the specialist makes an annual site visit and conducts videoconference clinics every 2–3 months in between. During videoconference clinics, routine reviews of patients can be conducted collaboratively with the regional paediatrician. The family is also able to discuss any concerns they may have with the specialist. All information can be shared via videoconference, including a progressive medical history, blood sugar readings, haemoglobin A_{1c} (HbA$_{1c}$), height and weight. Injection sites in areas such as the abdomen can also be examined via videoconference (see Chapter 8).

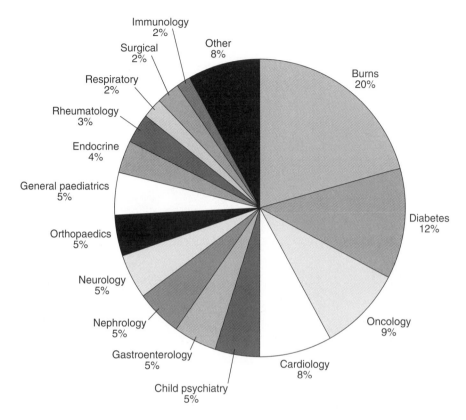

Fig. 3.6. Telepaediatric activity: the top 15 paediatric subspecialties in 1000 consultations.

Oncology

Specialist paediatric oncology services are also located in Brisbane, which means that patients who need treatment will be transferred from their regional hospital. Normally, routine follow-up (excluding treatment) requires travel to Brisbane to meet members of the oncology team. Staff from the oncology unit have reduced some of the travelling to Brisbane by providing outreach services to selected regional hospitals in Queensland. Outreach visits normally occur every three or six months. As part of the telepaediatric service, videoconferencing has been used alongside regional outreach visits, reducing the frequency of regional trips for staff, while maintaining their contact with their regional colleagues. During videoconference appointments, each patient can be reviewed and advice given to the regional paediatrician about interim management between treatments (Fig. 3.9).

Videoconferencing has also been a valuable method of coordinating discharge planning to regional sites before patients return home from the specialist hospital. These sessions are interactive and allow staff in the regional site to better prepare for pending admissions. The social benefits of videoconferencing have also been shown

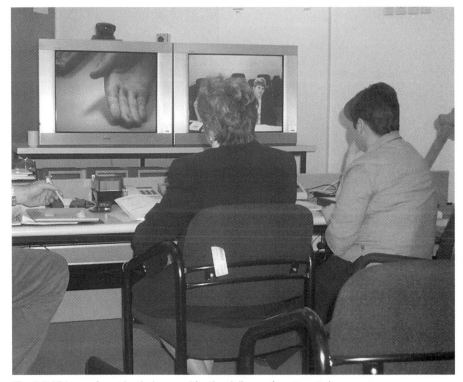

Fig. 3.7. Videoconferencing being used for the delivery of post-acute burns care.

by linking patients with family and friends, especially during long periods of hospitalization and time away from home (Fig 3.10).

Cardiology

The use of videoconferencing has also proved valuable for the diagnosis and clinical management of children with suspected cardiac defects.[7] We have conducted more than 100 cardiac studies via videoconference by transmitting the real-time ultrasound images direct to a paediatric cardiologist (Fig. 3.11). These sessions are interactive, allowing the specialist in Brisbane to provide guidance to the sonographer during the study and discuss the preliminary diagnosis and appropriate clinical management with the referring paediatrician and family (see Chapter 4).

Referral trends

One way of measuring the effect of the service is to examine whether or not fewer patients are being sent to the tertiary hospital as a result of telepaediatrics. Data were obtained for each intervention site and compared with all other hospitals that did not

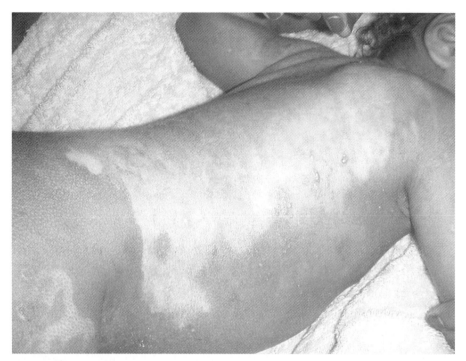

Fig. 3.8. Digital images sent via email are valuable for detailed assessment of burn injuries.

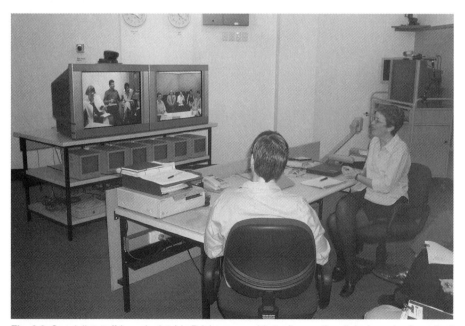

Fig. 3.9. Specialist staff (oncologists) in Brisbane are able to discuss the clinical needs of a patient with staff in a regional hospital before discharge.

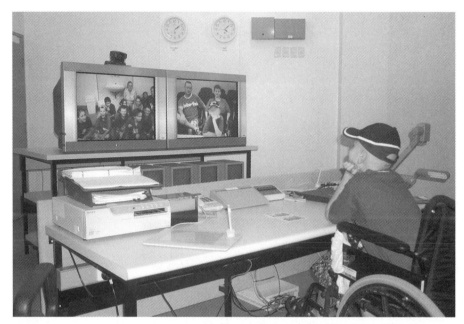

Fig. 3.10. Videoconferencing has social benefits for patients in Brisbane, who can stay in touch with school friends during long periods of hospitalization.

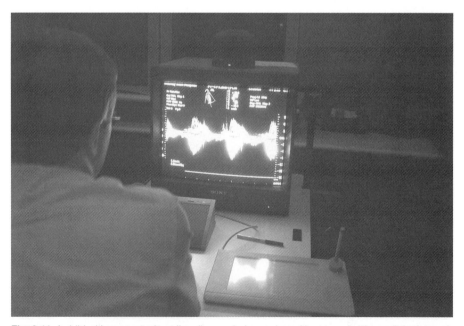

Fig. 3.11. A child with suspected cardiac disease being reviewed by a paediatric cardiologist: real-time echocardiography in progress.

have direct access to the service. In one site with considerable telepaediatric activity, marked reductions were seen in the number of children travelling to Brisbane for an outpatient appointment (Fig. 3.12). During the same period, a substantial increase was noted in the number of children accessing telepaediatric services from their local hospital (Fig. 3.13). It is likely that patients in this region were not being automatically sent to Brisbane to see the specialist and instead were able to see the specialist via videoconference at their local hospital with the regional paediatrician.[8]

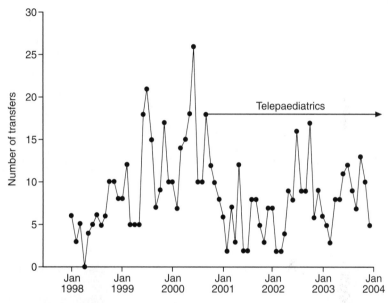

Fig. 3.12. Number of children being transferred from Mackay per month for admission at the RCH.

User satisfaction

Evaluations have been conducted to measure the satisfaction of staff involved in telepaediatrics and the satisfaction of patients and their families after a telepaediatric appointment. The results are typical of most satisfaction surveys in telemedicine.[9] A very high level of satisfaction was reported by both clinicians and families. Most families agreed that their telepaediatric consultation saved them money, time and stress.

Economics

The costs and potential savings associated with telepaediatrics have been examined from the perspective of the health service provider and also the family. All costs below are given in Australian dollars (A\$ is US\$0.76).

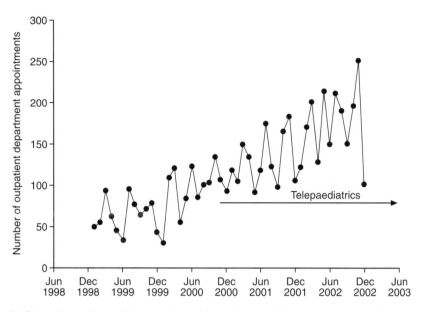

Fig. 3.13. Local outpatient activity – number of outpatient appointments per month in Mackay.

Health service

For the health department, there are considerable savings when patients are seen via videoconference instead of being transferred to the specialist hospital. A preliminary cost analysis showed that during a three-year period, the costs of providing telepaediatric services (975 patient consultations) was about $740 000 compared with estimated costs of almost $1.1 million had all patients been transferred to Brisbane for their appointment (Table 3.1). The most significant costs for the telepaediatric service related to infrastructure costs. The most significant costs associated with the conventional method related to patient travel.

Family

We have completed a study involving 400 families to compare the costs of attending an outpatient appointment in person at the RCH with the costs of attending an outpatient appointment via videoconference at a regional hospital close to home. The results are summarized in Table 3.2. Outpatient appointments conducted via videoconference were much less costly and more convenient for families than the conventional method of attending outpatient appointments at the specialist hospital.[10]

Funding

The absence of long-term funding for telehealth is often identified as a contributing factor in telehealth services that fail to continue beyond the pilot phase.[11-13] In some

Table 3.1. Actual costs for telepaediatrics and the potential costs of providing conventional outpatient services in Brisbane

Costs	Telepaediatrics ($)	RCH OPD ($)
Fixed costs		
Equipment	179 408	
Coordinator salaries	282 000	
Telecommunications	44 190	
Subtotal	505 598	0
Variable costs		
Telecommunications	45 960	0
Staff salaries	164 690	107 240
Patient travel and accommodation	0	952 991
Miscellaneous	24 000	
Subtotal	234 650	1 060 231
Total	**740 248**	**1 060 231**

Table 3.2. Average costs reported by families who attended an outpatient appointment, either face-to-face (FTF) at the tertiary hospital or by videoconference (VC) at their local hospital

Variable	FTF	VC
Travel time (minutes)	148	50
Distance travelled (km)	222	44
Direct costs ($)	37	2
Time off work (minutes)	133	31
Time off work (minutes) – second family member	50	24

cases, the cessation was perfectly reasonable, as the pilot work was designed to test the feasibility of new ideas or services before major decisions were made with regard to their adoption. One of the main reasons that organizations do not commit to ongoing funding is thought to be the lack of evidence to demonstrate cost-effectiveness.[14–20]. As described above, it is likely that the telepaediatric service has led to significant savings for the state health department through reduced patient travel. Ideally, a proportion of the savings generated through the use of telehealth should be used to defray the operating costs of the telehealth service. This would help to make the service sustainable.

Reimbursement

Reimbursement for services provided via telehealth is a matter of concern, especially in cases in which funding relies on rebates provided by the government (eg Medicare). Again, it has been suggested that one of the main reasons for the lack of committed funds for health provider reimbursement is the dearth of evidence related to the efficacy and cost-effectiveness of telemedicine.[21,22] The remuneration system for health professionals in Australia is different for the two forms of healthcare – private and public. In the private system, clinicians are paid on a fee-for-service basis. In the public system, clinicians are paid a set salary and are responsible for the delivery of services to patients through public hospitals and healthcare centres. Under very specific conditions in private care, it is possible for clinicians to claim Medicare reimbursement for case conferences that are conducted in person or via telephone or video link.[23] Conditions include the purpose of the consultation, the duration of session, the number of attendees and the involvement of a general practitioner. Apart from case conferencing, telepsychiatry is the only specialist field that has item numbers approved under the Medicare scheme.[24] No other clinical telehealth services in Australia are covered under the present Medicare funding arrangement.

Conclusions

The model used for the coordination of telepaediatric services in Queensland has worked very well, allowing the telepaediatric service to emerge as a routine method of delivering specialist paediatric services in parts of Queensland. A noticeable shift has been seen in the manner in which patients are referred to the service. With experience, specialists in Brisbane are becoming proactive in identifying patients suitable for the service and more confident in managing them at a distance.

Telepaediatric consultations are useful for obtaining specialist opinions without the need for extensive travel. Although the service is not designed to prevent all transfers to Brisbane, it has reduced the number of such transfers. A reduction in travel to Brisbane means significant savings for the state health service and the family.

References

1   Hornsby D. Videoconference Usage Report: May 2000. Brisbane: Queensland Telemedicine Network (Queensland Health), 2000.

2   Queensland Health. *Patient Travel Subsidy Scheme.* http://www.health.qld.gov.au/services/community/ptss/ (last checked 4 June 2004).

3   Queensland Health. *Queensland Health Annual Report 2002–2003.* Brisbane: Queensland Government; 2003.

4   Brommeyer M. *Telepaediatric Service – Final Report.* Brisbane: Royal Children's Hospital and Health Service District; 1998.

5   Smith AC, Youngberry K, Mill J, *et al.* A review of three years experience using email and videoconferencing for the delivery of post-acute burns care to children in Queensland. *Burns* 2004; **30**: 248–252.

6   Smith AC, Kairl JA, Kimble R. Post-acute care for a paediatric burns patient in regional Queensland. *Journal of Telemedicine and Telecare* 2002; **8**: 302–304.

7   Smith AC, Williams M, Justo R. The multidisciplinary management of a paediatric cardiac emergency. *Journal of Telemedicine and Telecare* 2002; **8**: 112–114.

8   Smith AC, Williams M, Van der Westhuyzen J, *et al.* A comparison of telepaediatric activity at two regional hospitals in Queensland. *Journal of Telemedicine and Telecare* 2002; **8** (suppl. 3): 58–62.

9   Mair F, Whitten P. Systematic review of studies of patient satisfaction with telemedicine. *British Medical Journal* 2000; **320**: 1517–1520.

10   Smith AC, Youngberry K, Christie F, *et al.* The family costs of attending hospital outpatient appointments via videoconference and in person. *Journal of Telemedicine and Telecare* 2003; **9** (suppl. 2): 58–61.

11   Farmer JE, Muhlenbruck L. Telehealth for children with special health care needs: promoting comprehensive systems of care. *Clinical Pediatrics* 2001; **40**: 93–98.

12   Preston J. Texas Telemedicine Project: a viability study. *Telemedicine Journal* 1995; **1**: 125–132.

13   Charles BL. Telemedicine can lower costs and improve access. *Healthcare Financial Management* 2000;

54: 66–69.

14   Crowe BL. Cost-effectiveness analysis of telemedicine. *Journal of Telemedicine and Telecare* 1998; **4** (suppl. 1): 14–17.

15   Falsone JJ, Moidu K, Sheehan CA, *et al*. Is telemedicine justifiable? *Connecticut Medicine* 1998; **62**: 423–427.

16   Hakansson S, Gavelin C. What do we really know about the cost-effectiveness of telemedicine? *Journal of Telemedicine and Telecare* 2000; **6** (suppl. 1): 133–136.

17   Mair FS, Haycox A, May C, Williams T. A review of telemedicine cost-effectiveness studies. *Journal of Telemedicine and Telecare* 2000; **6** (suppl. 1): 38–40.

18   Scott RE, Coates K, McCarthy GF. The value of an evaluation framework for telehealth initiatives. *Studies in Health Technology and Informatics* 1999; **64**: 39–45.

19   Jennett PA, Hunter BJ, Husack JP. Telelearning in health: a Canadian perspective. *Telemedicine Journal* 1998; **4**: 237–247.

20   Puskin DS, Sanders JH. Telemedicine infrastructure development. *Journal of Medical Systems* 1995; **19**: 125–129.

21   Hersh W, Wallace J, Patterson P, *et al*. Telemedicine for the Medicare population. *Evidence Report/Technology Assessment* 2001; **24**: 1–6.

22   Hersh W, Wallace J, Patterson P, *et al*. Telemedicine for the Medicare population: pediatric, obstetric, and clinician-indirect home interventions. *Evidence Report Technology Assessment Summary* 2001; **24** (suppl): 1–32.

23   Australian Government. *Multidisciplinary Case Conferencing Items*. http://www.health.gov.au/epc/caseconf.htm (last checked 4 June 2004).

24   Yellowlees P. Government relations, government regulations: jumping through the hoops. *Journal of Telemedicine and Telecare* 2002; **8** (suppl. 3): 83–85.

▶ 4

Telecardiology in Canada and Australia

John Finley and Robert Justo

Introduction

Specialized paediatric services, such as paediatric cardiology, are typically based in tertiary care centres. Because such services are not available in general hospitals or in sparsely populated areas, many tertiary paediatric institutions provide outreach services. These include external clinics for non-urgent consultations and electrocardiogram (ECG) transmission services for the interpretation of paediatric ECGs. Before the 1990s, it was necessary to transfer urgent cases to a tertiary paediatric centre for diagnosis and treatment. Transportation of seriously ill children inevitably implies risk, delay in treatment (possibly exacerbated by weather conditions) and expense. In some cases, transportation may be unnecessary because the condition, when diagnosed, could have been treated at the regional hospital. An alternative to patient transport is the transmission of echocardiograms. Such a service, if it could be made reliable and affordable, would have many benefits (see Box 4.1).

Box 4.1. Case report

It is 03:00 in midwinter in a regional newborn unit – a five-hour drive from a children's hospital. A full-term newborn with meconium staining has respiratory distress and an oxygen saturation of 80% despite 100% oxygen administration. On examination, the baby has good pulses, normal precordial activity and no murmur. The neonatologist is concerned about the possibility of congenital heart disease. The neonatologist contacts the on-call paediatric cardiologist at the children's hospital to request transmission of an echocardiogram on the infant. An adult sonographer is called in to perform the imaging, which is transmitted in real time to the paediatric cardiologist, who guides the study and provides the diagnosis. The scan shows normal cardiac anatomy and function, systemic right ventricular pressures, a patent ductus arteriosus and patent foramen ovale with bidirectional shunting. The paediatric cardiologist suggests that the cyanosis is due to persistent pulmonary hypertension and suggests a treatment plan of 100% oxygen, correction of the acidosis and, if hypoxia persists, administration of prostaglandins. Transport of the infant to a tertiary centre is not necessary.

Comment
Exclusion of congenital heart disease was essential in this scenario. In the absence of local expertise to reliably diagnose cyanotic congenital heart disease, such as transposition of the great vessels, an echocardiographic transmission facility linked to paediatric cardiology expertise allowed safe and rapid diagnosis. Treatment took place at the local hospital, avoiding transport of the infant and its associated risks, especially in winter.

In 1987, the first real-time echocardiographic image transmission facilities were established between regional hospitals and tertiary paediatric facilities in Atlantic Canada.[1] This allowed urgent diagnostic outreach services to be provided. Data transmission in this service is via broadband video links at approximately 45 Mbit/s. Other services around the world have employed various forms of telecommunication, usually at lower bandwidths. A common technique is the use of compressed digital images, sent either by ISDN transmission lines or by Internet Protocol over a computer network. Reported experience with ISDN varies from 128 kbit/s to 1.5–2.0 Mbit/s.[2-5] Studies by Houston *et al* and Finley *et al* have suggested that a bandwidth of at least 384 kbit/s is essential for adequate diagnostic accuracy, and that even higher bandwidths are desirable if available.[6,7]

Atlantic Canada

As high-speed echocardiographic transmission has been used in Atlantic Canada for more than 15 years, the experience represents that of a mature telemedicine network.

Facilities

Echocardiographic transmission facilities were installed for one referring site in December 1987, with the network gradually expanding to seven referring sites and one receiving site in Halifax, Nova Scotia (Fig. 4.1). Operating costs are covered by the budgets of the referring hospitals. Transmissions use broadband (45 Mbit/s) fibre-optic video circuits owned and operated by the regional telephone company. Access is provided 24 hours a day on telephone request from a paediatric cardiologist. Broadcast-quality video signals are transmitted at 30 frames per second, as described elsewhere.[8]

Our indications for echocardiography transmissions include known or suspected heart disease in an infant or child who cannot wait for the next quarterly visit to that centre by a paediatric cardiologist from the Izaak Walton Killam Children's Heart Centre in Halifax. Indications thus include urgent cases and scheduled follow-up of cases of Kawasaki disease or postoperative congenital heart disease. For urgent cases, transmission follows discussion between the referring paediatrician and the receiving paediatric cardiologist. Transmissions are in real time, with the image from the echocardiography machine at the transmitting hospital being seen simultaneously on a monitor in Halifax (Fig. 4.2). A simultaneous telephone call allows conversation between the receiving paediatric cardiologist and the sonographer performing the study. This allows the cardiologist to direct the study while viewing the images in real time. The completeness and quality of the study is assessed as it proceeds, with the diagnosis being provided directly to the transmitting physician at completion.

Continuous prospective evaluation of the network is carried out with a checklist of items to evaluate image quality, transmission problems, diagnostic completeness, diagnosis and whether or not patient transfer was avoided.

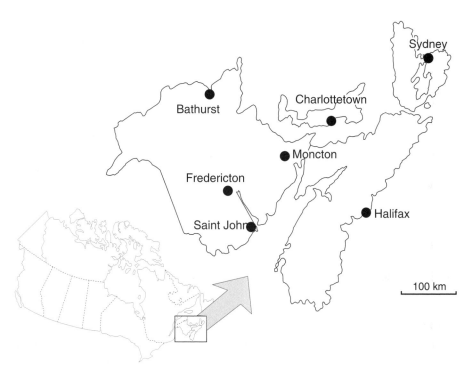

Fig. 4.1. The Canadian Maritime Provinces, showing the centres capable of transmitting echocardiograms to Halifax.

Results

From December 1987 to December 2003, a total of 886 transmissions were performed, with an annual average of about 90 in recent years. During one 24-month period, 135 transmissions were carried out, including 51% urgent examinations of newborns, 22% urgent examinations of older children and 27% scheduled repeat or postoperative studies. Typical diagnoses are shown in Table 4.1. In the 24-month period, 31 of the 135 cases would have been transported if echocardiography information had not been available. Of children who were transported as emergency cases, therapy was often begun during transport on the basis of the diagnosis provided by the transmission.

Because of the high bandwidth used for transmission, no image quality is lost with transmission. Occasionally (<5% of transmissions), connection problems at either end, or poor sedation, have prevented imaging. Mean study duration is less than 20 minutes. Access to transmission lines is provided in less than 20 minutes.

A review of 26 cases, in which repeat studies were performed in person by paediatric echocardiography staff, found no cases of an important discrepancy in diagnosis.[8] In two cases, a patent arterial duct and in three cases pulmonary veins were not clearly seen. Omissions sometimes occur in very brief studies in sick newborns for whom transport to the tertiary centre has already been arranged and repeat imaging will occur in person.

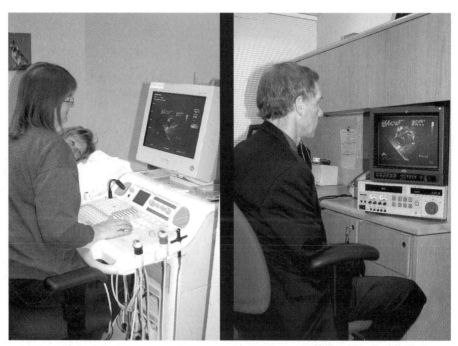

Fig. 4.2. An echocardiogram being performed in the remote centre (left) with simultaneous viewing of transmitted images by the cardiologist in the tertiary paediatric cardiology centre (right).

Table 4.1. Diagnoses of consecutive transmitted echocardiograms during a two-year period in Nova Scotia

Diagnosis	Number
Ventricular septal defect	21
Patent ductus arteriosus	17
Pericardial effusion	17
Kawasaki disease	13
Aortic stenosis	9
Pulmonary stenosis	8
Atrial septal defect	7
Complex	7
Transposition	5
Other (includes five normal echocardiograms)	31
Total	**135**

Economics

Costs and savings have been reviewed in detail elsewhere.[8] Avoidance of air transport resulted in cost savings of approximately Can$8500 per flight. Aircraft were usually assigned to other emergencies. Family savings, which usually involve travel and overnight expenses, were considerable, especially when considering lost income.

Queensland

The experience in Queensland over the last three years represents that of a developing telemedicine network. Queensland is a large state with a population of 3.5 million. An extensive telemedicine service has been developed throughout the state, with low-bandwidth 128 kbit/s transmission facilities now installed at about 250 healthcare sites. Transmission uses compressed digital images via ISDN lines. As part of a paediatric telehealth project established in 2000 (see Chapter 3), the ISDN lines to two centres in Queensland were upgraded, which allowed transmission of paediatric cardiac echocardiograms at a bandwidth of 384 kbit/s.[9] These centres are 300 km and 1000 km from the tertiary paediatric cardiac service in Brisbane (see Fig. 3.1) and only one centre was serviced with paediatric outreach clinics when the project started. Outreach clinics started at the second centre in 2003. Thus, the indication for use of telecardiology services varied between centres, with one centre using the service for elective consultations and the second for urgent and semi-urgent indications.

Facilities

All consultations are conducted in real time with commercially available videoconferencing equipment. Simultaneous audio and video transmission requires ISDN lines at a bandwidth of 384 kbit/s. The advantage of this mode of transmission is that direct concurrent communication can occur between the peripheral ultrasonographer, paediatrician, family and the paediatric cardiologist in the tertiary referral centre. At a bandwidth of 384 kbit/s, the quality of the echocardiographic images shows some minor degradation, but the image quality is, in general, adequate to make an accurate diagnosis. Cardiac scanning is performed at both peripheral centres with an ultrasound machine (ATL HDI Sonos 5000) using standard 3, 5 and 7 MHz probes. The local sonographer, with the guidance of a paediatric cardiologist at the tertiary centre, is able to obtain standard paediatric cardiac diagnostic images. Direct real-time communication between the cardiologist and sonographers allows ongoing education of sonographers and medical staff at the peripheral centre.

Results

From November 2000 until February 2004, a total of 106 paediatric cardiac teleconsultations were performed. Of these, 72 cardiac teleconsultations performed between May 2001 and February 2004 were reviewed to assess the value of the technique. The median age of patients at time of consultation was three months (range 1 day–17 years). Of the children assessed, 11 (15%) had had previous cardiac assessments and five (7%) had more than one teleconsultation. The diagnoses made at the time of the videoconference are listed in Table 4.2.

Overall, 16% of the teleconsultations requested were classified as urgent and were performed on the same day. All infants in this group were aged under one month. Forty percent of teleconsultations were semi-urgent, with assessment of the child occurring within 24 hours of the request being received. The remaining cases were planned

Table 4.2. Diagnoses in Queensland during a 33-month review period

Diagnosis	Number
Normal	25
Septal defects (VSD, ASD, AVSD)*	13
Valve lesions (aortic, pulmonary stenosis)	10
Persistent pulmonary hypertension	6
Patent ductus arteriosus	4
Coarctation	3
Tetralogy of Fallot	2
Other	9
Total	**72**

*VSD, ventricular septal defect; ASD, atrial septal defect; AVSD, atrioventricular septal defect.

elective consultations. At the time of teleconsultation, 7% of the cardiac echocardiographic assessments were felt to be of poor quality – because of either poor image transmission quality or uncooperativeness of the patient. These patients were suggested for further review by a paediatric cardiologist during a subsequent visit to the peripheral centre.

Most patients assessed in this manner could be managed in the peripheral centre. Sixty-five (90%) patients continued local follow-up with the paediatrician or visiting paediatric cardiologist in the peripheral centre and did not need transfer to the tertiary centre. One patient (1%) required urgent transfer to the tertiary cardiac centre. This infant was diagnosed with severe coarctation of the aorta and a large ventricular septal defect. He was transferred to the tertiary centre on a prostaglandin infusion, and subsequent careful echocardiographic examination showed that he had an interrupted aortic arch. This was repaired surgically with success.[10] The remaining six children (9%) had significant cardiac lesions, which were initially managed locally, with subsequent elective transfer at the appropriate time for either surgical or interventional treatment.

Seventeen (24%) of this cohort of patients subsequently had echocardiography performed on site or in the tertiary centre by a paediatric cardiologist. No major discrepancies were detected in the diagnoses made. The only medically different diagnosis was in the infant transferred to the tertiary centre, where the diagnosis was changed from coarctation of the aorta to interruption of the aortic arch. This change in diagnosis did not significantly affect the patient's initial management and care.

Echocardiographic transmission for paediatric cardiology

The experience in Canada, Australia and elsewhere has shown the benefits of echocardiographic transmission for provision of paediatric cardiology services. Transmission at satisfactory bandwidths allows rapid access to diagnostic services and is accurate and cost-effective. Unnecessary transport of sick children can be avoided, thus reducing both risks and costs.

Additional benefits from an echocardiographic transmission service have included improved communication among paediatric care providers, with a resulting greater sense of community, and educational benefits. The rapid provision of accurate diagnostic information directly to the neonatologist or paediatrician in a regional hospital can provide very useful reinforcement of their clinical assessment. For the sonographers who produce the images at remote sites, each transmission provides a tutorial, with constant commentary by the cardiologist supervising the study. We have seen a rapid improvement in paediatric sonographic skills in the centres in our networks. Finally, the availability of telemedicine for follow-up studies in patients discharged from a tertiary centre has the potential for enabling earlier discharge to distant locations, while ensuring safe follow-up without the need to travel.

In Queensland, the establishment of 384 kbit/s echocardiographic transmission resulted in the development of a new peripheral clinic at the second referral site as the usefulness of paediatric cardiology services became apparent. Although echo transmission at 384 kbit/s could be used for routine clinical review or screening, the reduced image quality made it unsuitable for replacing peripheral clinics. The effectiveness of paediatric cardiac teleconsultation has led to a long-term plan to increase the number of centres in Queensland in which this service can be provided. Videoconferencing via ISDN is also ideal for other consultative services to patients and medical staff, and this service will be progressively increased as resources become available.

Although the considerable costs of urgent air transport can be potentially avoided, as shown in the experience in Atlantic Canada,[8] the net savings will be influenced by telemedicine equipment and staffing costs, and the patient workload.[11,12]

Teleconsultation

Since the mid-1990s, the availability of ISDN videoconferencing in paediatric hospitals in Canada has made feasible consultation between specialists and families across considerable distances. Building on the successful experiences with telepsychiatry for children, particularly in Australia,[13] Canadian paediatric institutions began to explore the use of videoconferencing for family interviews and counselling for a variety of medical conditions.

Although Canadian paediatric cardiologists have not rapidly embraced videoconferencing for family interviews, it has been used effectively in at least two centres: the Centre Hospitalier de l'Université Laval (CHUL) in Quebec City and the Izaak Walton Killam Health Centre in Halifax, Nova Scotia. In Quebec, videoconferencing is an integral part of their system for echocardiographic transmission. This allows face-to-face discussion between cardiologist and parents while diagnosing the child, providing effective communication of the medical information. It also builds confidence between the parents and the cardiologist at a time of considerable emotional distress.[4]

In Halifax, ISDN videoconferencing has been used in non-urgent settings for two selected groups of patients and families. The first group includes families whose children have already been assessed and are scheduled for a surgical or catheterization procedure. The aim is to give procedural information face-to-face in the 2–3 weeks before the procedure. The second group includes families with children with supraventricular tachycardia or syncope not previously seen by a paediatric cardiologist. These are children for whom electrocardiographic information is available, as well as a careful history and physical examination by a local paediatrician, who have no anatomical heart disease. For both groups, the aim of teleconsultation is to substitute videoconferencing for in-person consultation.

For pre-procedural counselling, the interview personnel at the paediatric hospital include a cardiac nurse, a child social worker and possibly the surgeon. A coordinator joins the family at the referring hospital. For patients with arrhythmia or syncope, the interview includes the cardiologist and the telemedicine coordinator.

A recent survey of providers and parents involved approximately 30 tele-consultations.[14] The duration of the teleconsultation was similar to an office visit. Either the cardiologist or nurse explained the procedure at the beginning of the session. Most families felt that after the first few minutes of adjustment the teleconsultation was 'as good as in person', and they appreciated avoiding travel and loss of work time. Families also indicated that advance knowledge of the procedure allowed more time for discussion in the family and, thus, time to assimilate the information.

Cardiologists also felt that these interviews were as good as face-to-face ones and that they were able to counsel the family adequately and to make appropriate treatment decisions in the case of arrhythmias. Problems that did arise included some difficulty with background noise at the referring sites where rooms were not well soundproofed and the extra time required to schedule videoconferences at two centres.

Videoconferences for case discussion

Regular meetings of cardiologists, surgeons and intensivists are an essential part of patient management in paediatric cardiac surgery. For cardiologists who practice in a non-surgical centre, it is highly desirable to attend cardio-surgical meetings of the centre to which they refer their patients for surgery. The use of videoconferencing has enabled attendance at these meetings in several regions of Canada, including:

▶ the western provinces of Alberta, Saskatchewan and Manitoba, where surgery is referred to Edmonton, Alberta

▶ the Atlantic provinces, where two centres collaborate

▶ Ontario and Quebec, where there are collaborative networks.

Each conference allows display of echocardiographic and angiographic images from all sites. In addition to facilitating case discussions, such conferences build a strong sense of community in wide geographical areas.

Telemedicine for professional education

In 1998–2000, a pilot project took place among the six paediatric cardiology residency training programmes in Canada to provide monthly training videoconferences for trainees in all centres.[15] These videoconferences used expert teachers from all programmes, acquainted residents with tele-education and provided some exposure to personnel in all programmes across the country. In this way, trainees in all programmes had access to expertise from programmes across the country. The pilot project was very well received by trainees, although certain adjustments by both residents and presenters were needed for videoconferencing. The success of this pilot project led to the expansion of the concept to include paediatric cardiac centres without training programmes, and monthly videoconferences are now held among 12 centres as national paediatric cardiology grand rounds. In addition to their educational value, the rounds increase contact between centres and build a greater sense of community.

Tele-auscultation

The prevalence of heart disease is about 1% in children. One of the main physical signs of heart disease is a heart murmur. Unfortunately for the physician trying to diagnose disease, non-pathological murmurs are extremely common in children, being present in perhaps 50% or more of all children.[16] The distinction between normal and abnormal murmurs can be made by well-trained physicians, but it is a difficult skill that many family physicians and paediatricians are unable to master satisfactorily. Accordingly, many normal children are referred to paediatric cardiologists or for diagnostic tests such as echocardiography – referrals that are avoidable. Although a diagnosis should result from referral, the expense becomes a burden to the individual or the state health insurance system. Furthermore, if patients live in a rural area, they must be referred to a specialist, usually in an urban area, so there are considerable expenses, eg in travel and lost earnings. Avoidable consultations also occupy specialist time that could be better used in treating truly ill children.

The expenses of travel and a face-to-face consultation could potentially be avoided if an accurate recording of a heart murmur could be made in a rural health centre and transmitted electronically to a cardiologist for assessment. Successful trials of such facilities have recently been reported. A Norwegian study recorded heart sounds from 47 children aged 2 months to 10 years with either no murmur, an innocent murmur or a pathological murmur (based on the echocardiographic diagnosis).[17] The authors made multiple recordings of sounds from each patient with an electronic stethoscope, digitized the sounds and sent the resulting wave files by email to another location for review by four cardiologists. Sensitivity and specificity were 90% and 98%, respectively; 93% of cases with a pathological murmur were identified and 87% of cases with a benign murmur. There were five false negatives, which included three children with moderate pulmonary stenosis and two with moderate aortic stenosis.

An American study examined auscultation findings in 76 children of mean age 10 years.[18] A cardiologist examined the children directly with an acoustic stethoscope, while another listened remotely to the sounds transmitted via telephone lines by modem. The agreement between acoustic and remote auscultation was considered satisfactory ($\kappa = 0.63$) for identifying presence and absence of pathology, for using echocardiography as standard and for innocent and certain pathological murmurs. For some abnormal murmurs and all heart sounds, however, agreement was considered unsatisfactory ($\kappa < 0.60$). Agreement was improved with remote examiners of greater experience and with children older than five years.

Further studies will be needed to refine and determine the clinical importance of these techniques.

Future developments

In many countries, telemedicine has become an integral part of day-to-day clinical and educational activity in paediatric cardiac centres. The ability to provide services at a distance has allowed centralisation of these services, while lessening the need for families to travel for care. For clinical conferences and educational presentations, videoconferencing can now be regarded as an essential component of tertiary paediatric cardiac care.

Future applications of telemedicine in paediatric cardiology practice will depend on clinical trials (eg with tele-auscultation noted above) and on technological advances. Intra-operative video and echocardiograms are currently being transmitted in some centres to other locations for viewing procedures in order to obtain advice from experts.[19] As has been shown for surgical procedures, mentoring certain procedures can be provided at a distance using telemedicine video links.[20]

The current dependence of much videoconferencing on ISDN telecommunication, or similar connections, is likely to change with the gradual development of secure, wide-band IP networks that will allow videoconferencing at a guaranteed image quality on desktop computers rather than in studios. The development of broadband wireless communications linked with handheld computers should enable more mobile access to medical data as well as images. Whether or not this will have a significant effect on cardiac care remains to be explored.

References

1   Finley JP, Human DG, Nanton MA, et al. Echocardiography by telephone – evaluation of pediatric heart disease at a distance. *American Journal of Cardiology* 1989; **63**: 1475–1477.
2   Sobczyk WL, Solinger RE, Rees AH, Elbl F. Transtelephonic echocardiography: successful use in a tertiary pediatric referral center. *Journal of Pediatrics* 1993; **122**: S84–S88.
3   Alboliras ET, Berdusis K, Fisher J, *et al*. Transmission of the full-length echocardiographic images over ISDN for diagnosing congenital heart disease. *Telemedicine Journal* 1996; **2**: 251–258.
4   Cloutier A, Boucher J, Guay JM, Houde C, Delisle G. Neonatal echocardiography transmission: experience of a direct echocardiography line between a referral centre and a tertiary care centre. *Canadian Journal of Cardiology* 1995; **11** (suppl. E): 107.

5   Casey F, Brown D, Craig BG, Rogers J, Mulholland HC. Diagnosis of neonatal congenital heart defects by remote consultation using a low-cost telemedicine link. *Journal of Telemedicine and Telecare* 1996; **2**: 165-9.

6   Houston A, McLeod K, Richens T, et al. Assessment of the quality of neonatal echocardiographic images transmitted by ISDN telephone lines. *Heart* 1999; **82**: 222-5.

7   Finley JP, Justo R, Loane M, Wootton R. The effect of bandwidth on the quality of transmitted pediatric echocardiograms. *Journal of the American Society of Echocardiography* 2004; **17**: 227–30.

8   Finley JP, Sharratt GP, Nanton MA, et al. Paediatric echocardiography by telemedicine – nine year's experience. *Journal of Telemedicine and Telecare* 1997; **3**: 200–4.

9   Smith AC, Isles A, McCrossin R, *et al*. The point of referral barrier - a factor in the success of telehealth, *Journal of Telemedicine and Telecare* 2001;**7** (suppl. 2): 75–78.

10   Smith AC, Williams M, Justo R. The multidisciplinary management of a paediatric cardiac emergency. *Journal of Telemedicine and Telecare* 2002; **8**: 112-4.

11   Sicotte C, Lehoux P, van Doesburg N, Cardinal G, LeblancY. A cost-effectiveness analysis of interactive paediatric cardiology. *Journal of Telemedicine and Telecare* 2004; **10**: 78-83.

12   Persaud DD, Jreige S, Skedgel C, *et al*. An incremental cost analysis of telehealth programmes in Nova Scotia: a societal perspective. *Journal of Telemedicine and Telecare* (in press).

13   Gelber H. The experience of the Royal Children's Hospital Mental Health Service videoconferencing project. *Journal of Telemedicine and Telecare* 1998:**4** (suppl. 1): 71-3.

14   Finley J, Sharratt G, Chen R, et al. Impact of telemedicine on pediatric cardiology practice 1987-2001. *Cardiology in the Young* 2001; **11** (suppl. 1): 110.

15   Finley JP, Beland MJ, Boutin C, *et al*. A national network for the tele-education of Canadian residents in pediatric cardiology. *Cardiology in the Young* 2001; **11**: 526–31.

16   Danford DA. Clinical and basic laboratory assessment of children for possible congenital heart disease. *Current Opinions in Pediatrics* 2000; **12**: 487–91.

17   Dahl LB, Hasvold P, Arild E, Hasvold T. Heart murmurs recorded by a sensor based electronic stethoscope and e-mailed for remote assessment. *Archives of Diseases in Childhood* 2002; **87**: 297–301.

18   Belmont JM, Mattioli LF. Accuracy of analog telephonic stethoscopy for pediatric telecardiology. *Pediatrics* 2003; **112**: 780–6.

19   Cloutier A. Perspectives of telemedicine for per operative assistance. *Canadian Journal of Cardiology* 2002; **18** (suppl. B): 196.

20   Marescaux J, Rubino F. Telesurgery, telementoring, virtual surgery and telerobotics. *Current Urology Reports* 2003; **4**: 109–113.

▶ 5

The Applications of Telehealth in Medical Genetics

Tina Babineau and Mark D Ludman

Introduction

Medical genetic services involve several different healthcare activities, including the diagnosis, treatment and management of patients and their families who are affected with, or at risk of, a potentially inheritable condition. One important part of the genetic consultation is the process of genetic counselling, which can be defined as 'the process by which patients or relatives at risk of a disorder that may be hereditary are advised of the consequences of the disorder, the probability of developing or transmitting it and of the ways in which this may be prevented, avoided or ameliorated.'[1] As most of the genetic consultation generally is centred on a dialogue and exchange of information between the healthcare provider and the family, genetics is one of the specialties of medicine in which provision of services by telehealth can be considered.

The Maritime Medical Genetics Service (MMGS) is located in Halifax, Nova Scotia, in eastern Canada, and is housed at the Izaak Walton Killam (IWK) Health Centre. This hospital serves as a tertiary care centre for children's and women's health in Maritime Canada, which includes the three provinces of Nova Scotia, New Brunswick and Prince Edward Island. The MMGS is the region's only genetic service, delivering care to a population of roughly 2 million people spread over an area of 135 000 km^2. The furthest point from Halifax is approximately 900 km or a 7.5-hour drive away.

Travel by MMGS personnel to provide outreach clinics has become increasingly difficult over the past five years. A significant increase in referrals, which was not matched with an increase in human resources, made it impossible for MMGS staff to provide services in cities as far as 700 km away. Patients who were referred for a genetic consultation were asked to travel to Halifax to meet in person with their care providers. For some families, the complexities of travel and the burden of its cost were too great, and they opted not to pursue genetic services in the hope that eventaully outreach clinics would resume.

Over time, it became apparent that for some patients, a telephone discussion could provide a satisfactory means by which the necessary information could be obtained. However, the loss of non-verbal visual cues was felt by the geneticists and genetic counsellors. There was growing concern from the care providers that they were unable to appropriately assess the patient's level of concern regarding the family history. There were also concerns that complex explanations about difficult genetic concepts were not being grasped entirely as the ability to use diagrams had been lost.

The Children's Telehealth Network (Fig. 5.1) has been in operation since 1996. The network allows videoconferencing and the transmission of medical data. The network comprises 63 systems in 46 healthcare facilities across Nova Scotia, New Brunswick and Prince Edward Island. The network in Nova Scotia is part of the Department of Health's Telehealth Network (NSTHN). The equipment used in the NSTHN includes telehealth carts and room-based videoconferencing systems, based on standard PC technology (Fig. 5.2). They are connected at 384 kbit/s using ISDN lines. Detailed technical specifications can be found on the NSTHN website.[2]

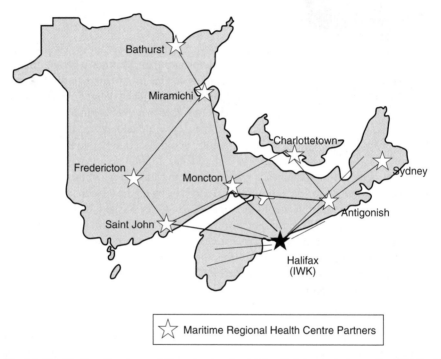

Fig. 5.1. The Maritime Provinces of Canada, showing telehealth linkages between the IWK Health Centre, where the Maritime Medical Genetics Service is located, and remote, regional healthcare centres.

Pilot project in cancer genetics

In the summer of 2000, the question of how the telehealth network could potentially be used by our service was investigated. We carried out a pilot project to evaluate patient satisfaction with the system. The project involved healthy women with a family history of breast and/or ovarian cancer who were coming for their first genetics appointment. Nine patients were seen in telehealth consultations and 10 in face-to-face visits. The women were all from within a 200 km radius of Halifax and had the option to have one support person present. The same genetic counsellor provided information for all

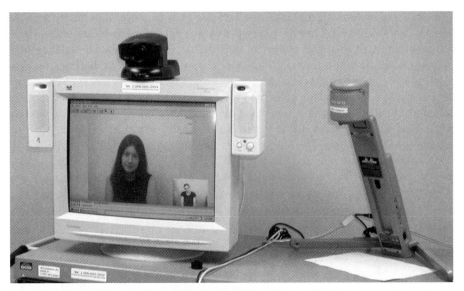

Fig. 5.2. Telehealth equipment used in telegenetics consultations. The document camera for transmitting images from printed pages is at the right.

the patients seen in the study. The participants were asked to complete a questionnaire about demographics, travel expenses accrued and any technical difficulties encountered. The questionnaire included 20 questions, using a five-point Likert scale, to determine comfort level, communication, comprehension and satisfaction with the visit.

The demographics were not significantly different between groups. The travel distance was an average of 54 km for the telehealth group and 107 km for the face-to-face group. Two women in each group required time off work to attend the meeting, and none required an overnight stay. Technical difficulties were few, but included problems connecting to the remote site, poor sound quality, poor picture quality and lack of staff organization at the remote site. The comfort level for both groups was high (4.4–4.8) with regard to using computers, having support staff in the room and being video-recorded. The comfort level at the beginning of the session was lower in the telehealth group (4.3) but had increased by the end of the session (4.9).

Patients were very satisfied with the level of communication they had before and during the appointment (4.8–5.0), such as the organization of the appointment, being able to express concerns and feeling that the concerns were understood and addressed. They also felt their comprehension of the information discussed was good (4.6–4.9). The satisfaction of both groups of patients was very good. Not all of the telehealth patients were convinced that they had received the same level of care as their face-to-face counterparts (4.8) but all overwhelmingly preferred telehealth (5.0). Open-ended narrative evaluations were requested from each person participating in the process. One patient stated: 'It was kind of awkward at first, but in just a few minutes you forgot about it and it feels as if you were really there discussing everything with them. It's unbelievable. Very nice, thank you!'

Gattas *et al* reported findings that echoed those from our pilot study.[3] They reported no obvious difference between patients seen by videoconference or face-to-face. Patients found that communication was easy, the room was comfortable and they were satisfied with the clinic format. They noted a few issues that we have also had to contend with, including the difficulty of fitting multiple family members on the screen and allowing a close enough resolution to visualize facial features and gestures. An additional benefit of telehealth was that it removed the intimidation some patients feel in hospital settings or when first meeting a healthcare provider. In our region, the equipment at remote sites is still located in hospital settings and this added benefit cannot therefore be realized. In a paper by Karp *et al*, it was pointed out that several factors were important in ensuring a good comfort level for the patient.[4] These included the presence of a nursing case manager, orienting patients to the system before the consultation, increasing comfort with technology and using a high-quality system.

The success of our pilot project prompted us to begin trials in other types of cases. By the end of May 2003, 4% of our patients had been seen by telehealth (Table 5.1). The types of cases considered most appropriate for telehealth were those related to cancer genetic counselling, as well as general adult genetic counselling cases for which a physical examination was not required. In several prenatal genetic counselling cases, the patients already had to travel to our centre for ultrasound examination and therefore were seen at the same time in person. Patients to be seen for follow-up of their inherited metabolic diseases were thought to be another group worth considering for teleconsultation.

Table 5.1. Types of cases seen in the pilot trial and method of consultation from 1 January 1 2001 to 31 May 2003

Type of case	Total cases	Method of consultation		
		In person (IWK Health Centre)	Telephone	Telehealth (% total cases)
General	643	509	97	37 (5.8)
Paediatric	517	509	5	3 (0.06)
Prenatal	499	436	50	13 (0.03)
Metabolic	388	380	1	7 (0.02)
Cancer	246	182	24	40 (0.16)
Total	**2293**	**2016**	**177**	**100 (4.4)**

Discussions after prenatal diagnosis

The identification of abnormalities by prenatal ultrasound or through other prenatal diagnosis procedures is a highly stressful experience for a family. This is compounded when, for example, a Francophone couple has to travel for seven hours into an unfamiliar Anglophone city in the middle of a winter storm to have access to a genetic consultation. (This could have been the case for one of our families from New

Brunswick, where 32% of the population has French as their first language.) However, telehealth made the experience very different, by allowing care closer to home.

When a fetus is identified as having a chromosomal abnormality on karyotype obtained by amniocentesis, the parents want as much information as soon as possible. In most cases, explaining complex chromosome anomalies by telephone is almost impossible. Our telehealth system is equipped with a document camera (see Fig. 5.2), which can transmit an image from the printed page. Explaining chromosome structure becomes much easier when one is able to show a picture of 'the little stick-like structures'. It also allows the counsellor to draw any image that may help in the patient's understanding of the situation while speaking with them. While taking a family history, it is also possible to show them the image of the pedigree when requiring clarification, for example, of relationships.

The system has the potential to record any session on VHS videotape. However, any recording would become part of the hospital record and it would then be the responsibility of the health records department to ensure confidentiality and privacy. Our medical-legal advisors felt that it would be best not to offer a recording to the patient because of the impossibility of ensuring confidentiality of a record that is not kept in the institution.

Huntington disease

Huntington disease predictive testing has been one of the most extensively evaluated areas of genetic testing. A specific framework for counselling and testing has been set in place and is followed by genetic groups across the world.[5,6] A number of visits with geneticists and/or genetic counsellors, as well as an evaluation by a neurologist, form part of this four-month-long process. When patients attend a session to receive the results of genetic testing, they usually have a 50% chance of hearing that they will develop a fatal neurological illness for which there is no treatment or a 50% chance of hearing that they will escape the disease.

Traditional views of medicine lead us to believe that it is necessary to see people in person to provide the most appropriate support in these sorts of circumstances. In cases where a person heard devastating news in such a session and then had to drive up to seven hours to get back to their community, we did not feel that we were providing the best care to the family. Our protocol for predictive testing for Huntington disease has become much more flexible and adaptable in order to allow the most appropriate framework of support for our patients. We require our first meeting to be face-to-face so that staff members feel more comfortable that we have had a chance to evaluate properly any mild physical signs of the condition. A face-to-face meeting also allows us to get a sense of how the patient is preparing for the results.

If they prefer, patients can then have their second visit and their result session by videoconferencing. Families are able to have any relatives or friends present for the session to support them. Local family doctors are welcome to attend with their patients and, when necessary, additional local support from counsellors or social workers involved in the patient's care is encouraged, so that they gain a full understanding of the implications that this disease can have for a family.

To date, this method has been successful and it has been welcomed by families. The healthcare workers involved in these sessions describe feelings of being solely providers of good or bad news and not the support people they want to be for the patients. The connection and relationship developed with someone on a video screen is quite different from that resulting from a face-to-face encounter. Nevertheless, patients show as much satisfaction from a telehealth session, leading us to hypothesize that the lack of connection is felt most by the healthcare provider and that patients do not require this type of relationship to feel that they have had adequate care.

This feeling was echoed by Gray et al.[7] They reported that all patients who participated in their pilot study of telegenetics in cancer were satisfied with the service. In their experience, however, the general satisfaction reported by patients was greater than that of health professionals. In fact, patients felt that the telegenetics consultation was not different or preferable to the usual face-to-face interaction, although the genetics nurses reported that it was very different and much worse. This seems to illustrate that effective rapport between patient and consultant definitely influenced the level of satisfaction with the use of videoconferencing.

Haemochromatosis group counselling

Hereditary haemochromatosis (HH) is an extremely common autosomal recessive disease that presents with iron overload. The estimated carrier rate for our population is 1 in 10. One in 400 people is affected by the disorder. Treatment with frequent phlebotomies to reduce the levels of iron in the body is quite successful. As this is such a common condition, each person identified as being affected leads to many other family members being at risk of having the same condition.

Over 200 referrals for genetic counselling about HH have been received by the MMGS since 1999. As HH is a treatable condition and most people are already obtaining care by the time they are referred to us, each was triaged as a non-urgent patient. This meant that with our limited resources, these patients might have to wait for years for access to the genetic counselling they needed.

In order to best address this patient population, we decided to arrange for a public information forum, inviting all patients then on our waiting list and their family members. Letters were sent inviting them to attend either a group, face-to-face session in Halifax or a session at one of the seven participating telehealth sites in the Maritimes. Ninety-seven people attended our first session: 70 in person and 27 at remote sites. The presentation included talks by a haematologist, a hepatologist, a geneticist and a genetic counsellor, as well as time for questions. Satisfaction surveys were provided, and feedback was very positive. Summary consultation letters were sent to each of the physicians who had referred patients to review the contents of the session.

All healthcare providers involved viewed the session as successful, and it has become an annual event. It allows many patients to be seen at once and allows involvement of family members who eventually would have been referred as well. In addition, patients can obtain information from many specialists at once and can ask any questions at the time or by calling the genetic counsellor after the session. The limitations primarily are related to the amount of time spent coordinating the session and arranging for patients to attend. It is also difficult to register and bill for each individual who attends the session. Finally, confidentiality cannot be ensured, as each person attending will suspect that others are there for the same reason. In our experience, patients are much less concerned about this issue than healthcare providers. For example, one man openly discussed his results in order to obtain advice from the haematologist.

Paediatric diagnosis by telehealth

The MMGS has not attempted to provide consultations where a physical examination would be required to provide diagnosis. This was mainly for reasons of cost. In order to obtain satisfactory views of patients with sufficient resolution to evaluate subtle dysmorphic features, each remote site would need to be equipped with an expensive handheld examination camera (about US$4000). These cameras are small and allow views of various areas of the body, such as behind the ears or under the feet. They also provide much finer detail than can be achieved with an ordinary room camera. Minor skin anomalies seen in tuberous sclerosis, for example, would be readily visible using a handheld examination camera.

As well as being expensive, a high-resolution camera needs someone who is familiar with its operation and what a genetic physical examination entails. Therefore, a physician with a special interest in genetics would need to be identified and trained for each site at which we intended to provide physical examinations by telehealth. Given the small populations in each region, and therefore the low frequency of consultations at any site, it would be difficult for collaborating physicians to develop and maintain the necessary expertise. More and more sites in our region, however, are now obtaining high-resolution cameras for other uses, such as teledermatology, so we will reconsider the position in due course.

Several genetic groups, such as those in the states of Maine and Florida, have developed the use of telehealth for genetic diagnosis in the past few years and have had great success. In Florida, diagnoses of mild Brachman–de Lange syndrome, familial velo-cardiofacial syndrome, neurofibromatosis, osteogenesis imperfecta, familial joint hypermobility sequence and Russell–Silver syndrome have been achieved through telehealth (Heather Stalker, personal communication). In Maine, the use of telemedicine was felt to allow care provision to patients who would not have otherwise had access to the service.[5] They offered consultations both for diagnostic purposes and counselling. The main negative perception from the perspective of the local care providers was related to unfamiliarity with technology. It was unclear from the abstract how much education and training the onsite care providers were given. The authors also stated that the quality of the dysmorphology examination largely depended on the training of the onsite care provider and the patient's willingness to cooperate.

National grand rounds

Many syndromes or conditions seen by genetics providers are very rare, affecting sometimes as few as 1 in 500 000 people. Therefore, some geneticists will only see a patient with a particular diagnosis once in their career. In addition, given the number of potential genetic diagnoses, it is not uncommon to come across a patient who clearly has some form of genetic disease but be unable to name the diagnosis. Consultation with other geneticists then becomes crucial to pool the collective experience of others in the hope that someone else has had a patient presenting with similar findings.

One well-established means for seeking assistance in reaching a diagnosis of genetic conditions or consultation regarding management, for example, of rare metabolic diseases, is to use email distribution lists (list-servs), such as Skeldys, Clingen-L, Metab-L and lists maintained by the National Society of Genetic Counsellors. Telemedicine has also been used successfully for remote review and consultation of karyotypes and cytogenetic analyses.[8]

In order to facilitate consultations with colleagues, twice-yearly nationwide Canadian genetic telehealth meetings have been organized. Each participating centre was given the opportunity to bring any cases that required additional suggestions or ideas to the groups for discussion. Everyone benefited greatly from either hearing new ideas of paths to investigate for their patients or confirming, as they had thought, that they had exhausted the possibilities and would have to accept this case as undiagnosed. Unfortunately, once again, coordination of these sessions became a great burden to the group who originally started the process and it was not continued. It was, however, an excellent example of the use of telehealth and its potential for improving the exchange of expertise in medical specialties with relatively small numbers of practitioners.

Learning experiences

Patients are somewhat intimidated by the technology at the start of a videoconference. It is important to spend some time explaining the fact that the system is completely secure and ensuring that they begin to forget that they are talking through a machine. It takes some time to get used to the few seconds of lag in discussions, and it is important to ensure that there are breaks in your discourse during which patients can interrupt to ask questions. It is also helpful to position the cameras to show close-up views of your face and the patient's, in order not to lose the facial expressions that are useful in non-verbal communication. This may not be possible in situations in which several family members attend the session. It may be worth asking the telehealth technician at the remote site to attend and provide close-up views of each of the people who will be speaking.

Satisfaction surveys of the patients seen by telehealth are invariably encouraging. Most patients are grateful for the opportunity to use this novel method of healthcare delivery. They view the loss of personal contact as a small price to pay for obtaining care closer to home. Healthcare providers, however, often feel the sessions are less successful when provided by telehealth. Again, it may be that there is a need to feel a connection to the patient to justify the role of caregiver.

Technology is imperfect, and problems will invariably arise. A bad connection can make the difference between a satisfying session and one that leaves all parties frustrated and promising never to repeat the experience. In one situation where we were to provide very difficult results to a family, the video image was lost from the start of the session. Having waited a long time to hear this information, the family chose to continue with audio exclusively – only to also lose the audio immediately after sharing the results. This was an important lesson learned, and it prompted a new line on our consent form that informs patients that the session will need to be rescheduled if the equipment malfunctions.

Liability is an important concern in medicine and is also important in teleconsultations. Several national and international committees have investigated the best way of ensuring that adequate processes are followed to protect the patients and the healthcare providers. This requires a separate consent form to be signed by the patient, stating that they agree to a consultation in this fashion and understand that their confidentiality is not jeopardized. In Canada, the provinces regulate the licensure of healthcare providers. In providing interprovincial consultations by telehealth, it was discovered that physicians had to obtain licensure in each province in which they intend to hold consultations. Funding and reimbursement issues can also be a limitation in situations where third party payment for a telehealth consultation is not available and such a service is not considered a 'covered benefit'.

Conclusion

The development of telehealth has allowed more flexibility and accessibility of genetic services in our region. To date, telegenetics has been used mostly in sessions in which physical examinations are not required. Telehealth has allowed us to develop new methods of healthcare delivery by providing multi-site group sessions for genetic counselling in common conditions. It also made us question conventional wisdom about methods of service delivery.

Patients who have participated in telehealth sessions have not reported dissatisfaction with the means used to provide clinical information. In most cases, even if technical difficulties required several reconnections to the remote site, patients invariably reported being relieved that they did not need to travel as far to access the information. Patients also reported the same level of satisfaction with the information received by telehealth as those seen in person. An evaluation form is given to each patient undergoing a telehealth visit to ensure that any concerns or issues can be followed up and prevented in other cases.

There are some drawbacks to telehealth. It is not possible to develop the same personal connection with families, and there are limitations about performing physical examinations. The coordination of telehealth visits is time consuming and creates logistical problems when blood sampling is required and specimens must be sent to another site. The use of the equipment requires technical expertise and is limited by space and available technology at the remote site. In addition, long sessions can be quite expensive, because the system requires three ISDN line connections. Furthermore, reimbursement for the service may be limited.

Nevertheless, telehealth has allowed a reduction of cost for families, a reduction of the time required for travel and improved health outcomes by allowing care closer to home. In essence, the use of telehealth supports Canada's Health Act, which mandates equal access to care for all Canadians.

Acknowledgements

We thank Heather Hogg, Sharon Goobie and Dr Teresa Costa for their work on the initial pilot study. We are also grateful to Patricia Steele for her development and coordination of the haemochromatosis group sessions, and to Chris Anne Ingram, Angie Davidson and Melanie McInnes for their support.

Further information

College of Physicians and Surgeons of Nova Scotia. Guidelines for the Provision of Telemedicine Services. http://www.cpsns.ns.ca/telemedicine_guidelines.htm (last checked 9 August 2004).

Nova Scotia Telehealth Network. http://www.gov.ns.ca/health/telehealth/default.htm (last checked 9 August 2004).

National Society of Genetic Counselors, Inc. http://www.nsgc.org/index.asp (last checked 9 August 2004).

References

1   Harper PS. *Practical Genetic Counselling*, 5th edn. Boston: Butterworth Heinemann, 1998.
2   Nova Scotia telehealth equipment. http://www.gov.ns.ca/health/telehealth/equipment.htm (last checked 9 August 2004).
3   Gattas MR, MacMillan JC, Meinecke I, Loane M, Wootton R. Telemedicine and clinical genetics: establishing a successful service. *Journal of Telemedicine and Telecare* 2001; **7** (suppl. 2): 68–70.
4   Karp WB, Grigsby RK, McSwiggan-Hardin M, *et al*. Use of telemedicine for children with special healthcare needs. *Pediatrics* 2000; **105**: 843–847.
5   Smith R, Lea D, Ellingwood S, Schulberger S. Using telemedicine to provide clinical genetics services and genetics education in Maine: results of three year-pilot trial. *American Journal of Human Genetics* 2003; **73**: S29(24).
6   Simpson SA, Harding AE. Predictive testing for Huntington's disease: after the gene. The United Kingdom Huntington's Disease Prediction Consortium. *Journal of Medical Genetics* 1993; **30**: 1036–1038.
7   Gray J, Brain K, Iredale R, *et al*. A pilot study of telegenetics. *Journal of Telemedicine and Telecare* 2000; **6**: 245–247.
8   Meck JM, Munshi G, Plempel J, Amato S, Macedonia C. Cytogenetic analysis using telemedicine consultation: an improved means of providing expert cross-coverage. *Genetics in Medicine* 1999; **1**: 328–331.

▶6

Telemedicine in Advanced Fetal Diagnosis and Therapy

Fung Yee Chan and Barbara Soong

Introduction

As medical care becomes highly specialized, the dissemination of knowledge and skills from super-specialists becomes increasingly difficult. Fetal medicine is a subspecialty in obstetrics in which the wellbeing of a fetus is assessed while in utero, with interventions performed during pregnancy to maximize a favourable outcome. This highly specialized field has emerged as a result of new knowledge in fetal physiology and pathology, and developments in clinical management following the availability of new diagnostic techniques and treatments.

Obstetric ultrasound is now an essential tool in the assessment of fetal problems and wellbeing. Although randomized controlled trials have shown that routine ultrasound screening in pregnancy can reduce perinatal mortality in selected centres,[1] the performance of ultrasound in the diagnosis and assessment of fetal anomalies varies enormously between tertiary referral centres and general units.[2-4] The scarcity of tertiary referral centres, the anxiety and stress created by delay in referrals for equivocal findings, the disruption to family dynamics and the costs of travel often inhibit referral.

Tertiary referral fetal diagnostic centres are scarce, with most being sited in capital cities. Even fewer can perform the most advanced form of fetal therapeutic procedures, such as operative fetoscopy.[5] This is a new surgical approach for the correction of birth defects in utero that uses combined ultrasound and endoscopic imaging. Only a few centres worldwide offer this form of fetal therapy. Traditional apprentice learning in surgery requires the continuous presence of specialized experts. As the incidence of surgically correctable fetal diseases is low, expertise and training opportunities are limited. In this chapter we summarize our experience with telemedicine for advanced fetal diagnosis and therapy.

Real-time tertiary fetal ultrasound and diagnosis

Obstetric ultrasound is now an indispensable tool in the assessment of fetal problems and wellbeing[6] When a fetal anomaly is suspected, accurate diagnosis and prognostication are essential before management options can be discussed with the parents. The families require accurate, unequivocal information and a high standard of compassionate, professional care during these times of crisis. Referral to a tertiary referral unit with a multi-disciplinary team of specialists, such as maternal fetal medicine subspecialists, neonatologists, paediatric cardiologists, neonatal surgeons, geneticists and genetic counsellors, is usually indicated.

Australia is a large continent. Queensland covers an area of over 1.7 million km^2 and accounts for nearly 25% of the total land area of the Australian continent. It has 50 000 births per year, 40 000 of which occur in the central and southern zones of the State, which are served by two major tertiary obstetric hospitals, both of which are located in the state capital of Brisbane. There are approximately 10 000 births in the North Queensland region each year, but there are no accredited fetal medicine specialists outside the Brisbane metropolitan area.

Traditionally, patients with problems in North Queensland have either flown in personally or had their videotapes sent to Brisbane to be assessed. A pregnant mother in a rural area may need to drive for 3–4 hours to a provincial centre, followed by a flight to the capital city. An overnight stay in the city is often required before multiple consultations can be accomplished. The costs of air travel, and the disruption to family dynamics, pose extra problems during these times of intense emotional stress. Videotape review is also problematic, as there is no instantaneous feedback to the sonographer, and the tape may not have detailed all the ultrasound views necessary to make a definitive diagnosis. There is also a delay in response to the consultation, which is often unacceptable to patients during this stressful period of uncertain health of their fetuses.

Tele-ultrasound in North Queensland

Telemedicine involves the delivery of healthcare at a distance, by combining telecommunications and medical expertise. It should be an ideal tool in Australia to help bridge the healthcare gap between the country and the city, as well as to improve access to medical education and enhance the quality of care. In 1997, a pilot tele-ultrasound perinatal consultation service was planned between the Kirwan Hospital for Women – the major referral centre in North Queensland – and the Mater Mothers' Hospital in Brisbane.

The project was initiated by clinicians from both centres, who had direct and extensive experience in dealing with complex perinatal consultations. Technical advice was sought from many parties, including the information technologists from the two hospitals involved. Two project officers (one for each hospital) were recruited to assist in the coordination and smooth running of the project. At least four clinicians and two sonographers from each hospital were involved during the clinical phase of the project.

Technology

In view of the sensitivities in dealing with possible anomalies in fetuses, and the significance of obtaining all information on a fetus during the ultrasound examination, we decided to use real-time video transmission. This means that the clinician can direct the sonographers at the remote site to obtain all the information needed using videoconferencing. The specialist can interpret the findings and then assist in the counselling of women and families on subsequent management. This real-time interaction was one of the most important factors in the success of the project. Real-time work involves the simultaneous availability of both parties, is obviously harder to organize and may be more expensive. However, it improves communication between the two sites, assists in education and training of staff at the remote site, and reduces the risk of liability, which may arise in a store-and-forward transmission approach, when some vital information may have been missed in the pre-recorded examination.

One barrier to telemedicine is the running cost, especially if high bandwidths are required. The transmission of medical imaging information involves high volumes of data. In general, the transmission of still images does not pose major problems, as the slight delay in transmission is usually acceptable. The transmission of real-time moving ultrasound images, however, imposes a technical challenge. Bandwidths as high as 2 Mbit/s have been used in obstetric ultrasound,[7] and near-broadcast-quality video has been transmitted at 45 Mbit/s in paediatric echocardiography.[8] The cost of such high-bandwidth transmission, however, would inhibit the introduction of such services to remote areas, which are, in fact, those most in need. There have been reports in the literature of the use of lower bandwidths such as 384 kbit/s in obstetric ultrasound,[9,10] and even 128 kbit/s in paediatric echocardiography.[11,12] On the other hand, Wootton *et al* found that the diagnostic accuracy with fetal ultrasound transmission at 384 kbit/s was marginally worse than at 1920 kbit/s.[13] The optimum bandwidth for satisfactory transmission of real-time ultrasound images in pregnancy thus remains unclear.

Pilot study

We performed a pilot study to assess the technology required for accurate diagnosis by real-time fetal tele-ultrasound consultation.[14] Randomized blinded comparisons are the 'gold standard' for the most rigorous scientific evaluations. We therefore used randomized blinded assessments to evaluate the different components in the transmission. We also made use of a standard video recording with a pre-agreed scoring protocol, in which the maximum score was 'image quality as good as the original videotape'. This is important, because assessment of image quality is a subjective process. By setting a gold standard, and by using a total of 30 anatomical landmarks, the average scores from each clinician for each of the systems tested were found to follow a normal distribution, allowing statistical analysis with parametric methods.

The pilot study was divided into three phases.[14]

► In *Phase I*, three experienced clinicians evaluated the quality of ultrasound images transmitted at various bandwidths (internally looped back in Brisbane) using a standard ultrasound video recording with eight commercially available codecs at random.

► The two codecs that performed best proceeded to *Phase 2*, where a live link operating at up to 2 Mbit/s was set up between Brisbane and Townsville (1500 km apart). Testing with the standard videotape was performed at seven different bandwidths played at random to four clinicians (who were blinded to the equipment and bandwidths used).

▶ In *Phase 3*, the optimum line rates for transmission were determined, and testing was then performed using these line rates for fetuses with various anomalies.

The results showed significant differences of performance according to bandwidths used ($p < 0.0001$) but not according to observers ($p > 0.36$). The performances could be grouped into three levels: at level I (256 kbit/s), the performance was significantly worse than at level II (384, 512 or 768 kbit/s), which was in turn worse than at level III (1, 1.5 or 2 Mbit/s). However, in each level, the performance of one bandwidth was not significantly different from the others. The most cost-effective rates were therefore determined to be 384 kbit/s and 1 Mbit/s.[14]

Clinical evaluation

To evaluate the clinical value of our tele-ultrasound consultation service, patients who required tertiary ultrasound consultations were recruited from north Queensland. Clinicians from the referral site established an initial diagnosis and management plan. The patients travelled from their primary site of referral to the Kirwan Hospital at Townsville, which is equipped with modern ultrasound equipment and staffed with qualified sonographers (Fig. 6.1). Standard ISDN lines were used to transmit the real-time ultrasound images to the maternal fetal medicine subspecialists in Brisbane – 1500 km away. The ultrasound examination was completed under the direction of the subspecialist (Fig. 6.2). The subspecialist explained the findings to the patient at the end of the session, and discussed the diagnosis and management plans with the clinicians involved. Any diagnosis and management variations were classified into minor and major following agreement by the two teams of clinicians involved. The clinicians and patients in Townsville rated the value of the consultation, and the subspecialists rated the confidence of their diagnoses on five-point scales. Pregnancy outcomes were obtained and the data analysed.

We have already reported the results of our first 24 clinical consultations over a three-month period.[15] Results from the subsequent 100 consultations were similar and have been separately reported.[16] The major indications for referral were:

▶ complex fetal problems such as twin complications or multiple fetal anomalies (43%)

▶ detailed assessment for high-risk patients (19%)

▶ isolated fetal anomalies (17%)

▶ evaluation of markers for anomalies (13%)

▶ assessment of growth restriction or fetal wellbeing in the third trimester (8%).

Effect of consultation on diagnosis and management

The clinicians from both teams reviewed the cases at six-month intervals and rated the effect of teleconsultation on clinical diagnosis and management. Overall, the consul-

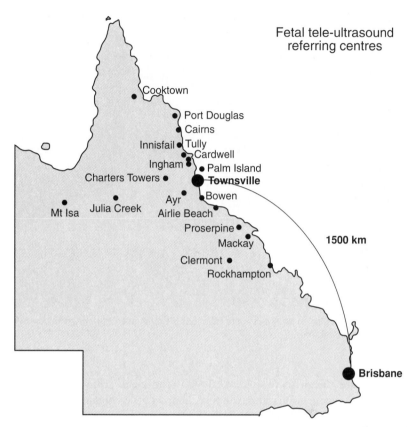

Fig. 6.1. Tele-ultrasound consultation link between Townsville and Brisbane (1500 km apart) and the referral sites around Townsville.

tations resulted in some modifications to the clinical diagnosis in 41% of the cases and modifications to the management plan in 40% of the cases – about half of which were minor variations. It is important to point out that most of the variations were from the initial diagnosis at referral from the primary obstetric site and do not necessarily reflect the performance of the team at the Kirwan Hospital. In fact, most of the 'major' variations in management were in preventing the physical transfer of the patients to Brisbane and the 'minor' variations related to reduced frequency of subsequent monitoring.[16]

Accuracy of diagnosis

Ninety tele-ultrasound consultations were performed for the first 71 patients. Ninety percent of the patients have been delivered, and outcome data have been received on all but one pregnancy. All significant anomalies and diagnoses have been confirmed.[16]

Evaluation by clinicians

The referring clinicians at the Kirwan Hospital rated the usefulness of the tele-consultations on a five-point scale. Overall, the scores were 4 in 25% of cases and 5 in

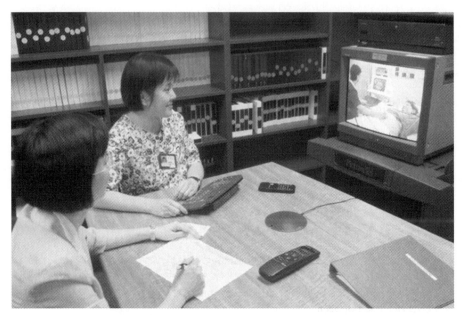

Fig. 6.2. A teleconsultation in progress – the ultrasound examination performed in Townsville is being viewed live in Brisbane.

75% of the cases (mean score 4.7, SD 0.44).[15] The mean score when there were diagnostic or management variations, either alone or in combination, was 4.8 (SD 0.31), while the mean score when there were no variations was 4.7 (SD 0.49).[15] The maternal fetal medicine subspecialists at the Mater Hospital rated their confidence in making diagnoses using telemedicine on a five-point scale. The scores were 4 in 54% of the instances and 5 in 47%, indicating that they were confident or very confident (mean score 4.2, SD 0.43).[15]

Evaluation by patients

Of the 24 clinical consultations performed during the course of the pilot project, a total of 20 feedback forms were sent back by the patients. The results showed that 75% of the women had not used videoconferencing before. Two women participated in the study on two occasions. One woman had used videoconferencing before in the course of her work. Of all the women, 95% felt satisfied that they had had the videoconferencing process clearly explained to them. Before the consultation, 80% felt very positive or positive about seeing a medical specialist in Brisbane, whereas 20% indicated that they felt neutral. During the videoconference, 100% strongly agreed or agreed that they felt comfortable with the specialist in Brisbane. Ninety-five percent of the women strongly agreed or agreed when asked if their privacy and confidentiality were maintained during the videoconference, and 95% indicated that they would recommend videoconferencing to others.[15]

Cost evaluation

A crude estimate of the net cost of real-time tele-ultrasound consultation can be made by balancing the transmission costs for the consultations against the cost of patient transfer should tele-consultation not be available. During the project, the referring clinicians were asked to indicate what method of consultation they would have resorted to if the telemedicine link had not been available. Of the first 71 patients seen (90 consultations), the referring clinicians would have physically referred 24 to Brisbane. For the other patients, they would have either sent their videotapes for review or telephoned for opinions. After the tele-ultrasound consultations, seven patients still had to be transferred to Brisbane for intervention.

Assuming that all patients travelled alone to Brisbane (in fact most of them travel with their partners), the cost of the airfares saved for the 17 patients was A$13 000. The average duration of each tele-ultrasound consultation for these patients was 37 minutes. The transmission bandwidth was 384 kbit/s in 95% of the consultations. The average transmission cost per teleconsultation was calculated to be A$74. The total transmission cost for the 71 patients (90 consultations) therefore amounted to A$6660. The tele-ultrasound service thus resulted in a net saving of A$6340 and at the same time enabled more than four times the number of consultations to be carried out than if the service had not been available.[16]

These are only crude estimates. The costs ignore the initial set-up and equipment costs and the costs of the clinicians' time. On the other hand, there are also reductions in anxiety and social costs to the families involved by the availability of teleconsultations. In addition, the value of support and education to remote clinicians is real, although hard to quantify.

Conclusions

The project showed that tertiary real-time fetal ultrasound consultation by telemedicine is not only technically feasible, it is also welcomed by the clinicians and patients involved. It also contributes to diagnostic and management differences and seems to be an effective strategy for bridging the healthcare gap between country and city.[16]

Fetal endoscopic telesurgery

Operative fetoscopy is a new surgical approach for the correction of birth defects in utero using combined ultrasound and endoscopic imaging.[5,17] One of the most frequently performed fetoscopic operations is laser coagulation of placental anastomoses for twin-to-twin transfusion syndrome (TTTS). This is a severe disorder that affects 10–15% of monochorionic (identical) twins. Unbalanced shifting of blood from one twin to the other through shared placental cotyledons typically results in severe growth restriction, oliguria and anhydramnios of the donor and polyhydramnios and heart failure of the recipient by mid-pregnancy. If left untreated, the perinatal mortality approaches 90%. Conventional treatment with serial amnioreduction improves survival rates to 60%, but with long-term neurological complication rates of 20–25%.[18,19] Endoscopic laser coagulation of the placental anastomoses stops the process. In experienced hands, survival rates are up to 80%, with much reduced neurological complications.[20,21]

Until recently, fetoscopic laser surgery has only been available in a few centres worldwide (Figs 6.3 and 6.4). Most of the active centres are in Europe and the US, with little experience in the Asia Pacific region. The learning curve is long. In a large report of 200 consecutive fetoscopic laser surgeries over a 4.5-year period,[20] the performance of the first 73 surgeries was compared with the subsequent 127. The overall survival improved from 61% to 68%, and the proportion of pregnancies from which both babies survived improved from 42% to 54%.[20]

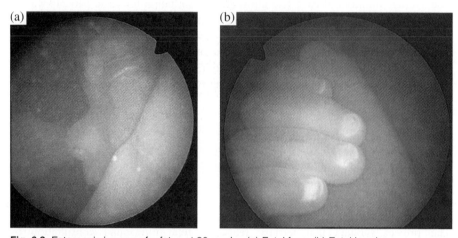

Fig. 6.3. Fetoscopic images of a fetus at 20 weeks. (a) Fetal face. (b) Fetal hand.

Ideal surgical apprentice learning would require the continuous presence of specialists. As the incidence of surgically correctable fetal diseases is low, expertise and training opportunities are limited, especially when the expert lives on a different continent. With our successful experience of using telemedicine for fetal ultrasound diagnosis and counselling,[14–16] we explored the possibility of using telemedicine to assist in the introduction of fetoscopic laser surgery to Australia.

Personnel

Two clinical teams were involved. The novice team was based at the Mater Centre for Maternal Fetal Medicine in Brisbane, and the expert team was based at the Florida Institute for Fetal Diagnosis and Therapy in the US. The clinical teams met and agreed a clinical protocol. Many other teams were involved, including technical staff from the information systems departments of both hospitals, the videoconferencing company involved (Sony-Ericsson) and the telecommunication carriers on both sides of the Pacific.

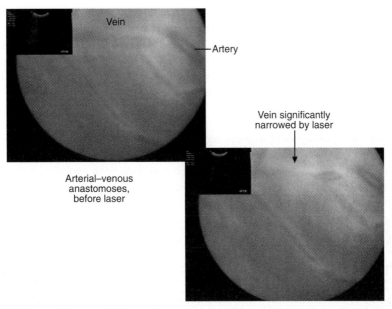

Fig. 6.4. Fetoscopic image of fetal arterial–venous (AV) anastomoses sealed by laser energy.

Legal advice was also sought. The major perceived problem was the possible medicolegal risk involved with telementoring. Although the risk of observing surgery performed by the expert via telemedicine was small, the medicolegal risk for the reverse, while low, was considered prohibitive for full insurance cover. After much negotiation, it was decided that the telesurgery link would only operate live when the expert was performing surgery. The novice would operate independently, with the procedure being video-recorded for discussion with the expert after the operation for opinions.

Technology assessment

Type of transmission

Much telemedicine and videoconferencing work around the world is currently carried out with Integrated Services Digital Network (ISDN) connections, which have proven to be very reliable. They are relatively costly, however, and they are still limited to larger centres in which ISDN access is available. For clinical purposes, multiple ISDN lines, from 384 kbit/s to 2 Mbit/s, have been shown to be necessary.[7,14] The cost of an intercontinental ISDN link is prohibitive for most clinical applications. The rapid evolution of technology, however, has brought the Internet to most parts of the world and the cost of using Internet Protocol (IP) networks is reducing rapidly. Most of the newer videoconferencing equipment can operate on either ISDN or IP networks. We have previously shown in a randomized controlled study that the quality of real-time ultrasound images transmitted by IP networks is slightly lower than with an ISDN link but still clinically adequate.[22] We therefore decided to use an IP connection for the project.

A dedicated international IP connection was established between the two sites (sponsored by AAPT, a local telecommunications carrier). The Brisbane Hospital had a 2 Mbit/s connection and the hospital in Florida had a 1.5 Mbit/s connection. A permanent virtual circuit (PVC) with a Committed Information Rate (CIR) of 512 kbit/s interconnected the sites. The connections at both ends terminated with a 10-base T ethernet port for the videoconferencing equipment.[23]

Equipment and bandwidth

Standard commercial videoconferencing equipment was used (PCS 1600P, Sony). The equipment (sponsored by Ericsson/Sony) was connected to the IP link at each site. Image quality was assessed by randomized comparison with an ISDN link using a standardized videotape viewed by experienced observers blinded to the bandwidth of transmission. This confirmed our previous findings – that the image quality of an IP link is comparable to that of an ISDN link at similar bandwidths.[22]

Technical problems

In practice, the major technical problem was coordinating the many parties involved to work simultaneously, especially as there is a 15-hour time difference between Brisbane and Florida. This was the first time that an IP link had been used for clinical work across such distances, and experience was limited. The major technical issue encountered, which required the coordination of all parties to resolve, was the need for the whole link to be configured from end to end as a simultaneous two-way path (full duplex). If this was not achieved, one-way video and poor quality sound resulted.

Other issues, which had been expected to cause difficulties, did not. For instance, a round-trip delay between Brisbane and Florida of 250–300 ms presented no problems to users or equipment. Small levels of IP packet loss proved tolerable, with the equipment providing automatic compensation. Sound quality proved to be excellent.[23]

The videoconferencing equipment was capable of requesting priority quality of service on the network. Tests showed that the use of this feature had no effect on the transmitted video or sound quality. It should be noted that the use of a dedicated link meant that no other data traffic that could interfere with the video and audio transmission was present.[23]

Clinical evaluation

Quality of transmission

Live surgery performed at Florida was transmitted and viewed at Brisbane. Over a one-year period, 20 surgical procedures were observed. The Brisbane team rated the quality of transmission with a seven-point scale (1 = poor, 7 = excellent). The mean audio quality was rated as 4.8 (SD 0.9), and the mean video quality was rated as 5.5 (SD 1.0). An additional mobile microphone was installed to improve the sound.

Usefulness of transmission

The Brisbane team rated the educational value, as well as the overall usefulness of each case, with a seven-point scale (1 = poor, 7 = excellent). The mean score was 5.7

(SD 1.0) for educational value and 5.8 (SD 0.8) for the overall rating, which suggested that the Brisbane team highly valued the usefulness of the transmission.

Local results of fetoscopic laser surgery

The Brisbane team has performed 19 fetoscopic laser surgeries to date, and 14 of the patients have delivered. The overall survival is 21/28 (75%). At least one baby has survived in 11 pregnancies (79%), and both babies have survived in 10 pregnancies (71%). The median gestation of delivery was 31.5 weeks. The median length of extension of gestation of pregnancy after surgery was 8.5 weeks.[23] These results are comparable with those from experienced centres that have performed over 100 laser surgeries.[20,21]

The number of fetoscopic surgeries performed by the novice Brisbane team is still small (19 pregnancies). Our preliminary results (75% overall survival and 71% of pregnancies with survival of both babies), however, suggest that the learning period has been shortened markedly. This may not be entirely attributable to the telesurgery link. Both surgical operators of the Brisbane team visited Florida before the system came into operation and watched live surgeries. The Florida team also visited Brisbane, and close professional relationships between the two teams were established. Nevertheless, both surgeons in the novice team felt that having the chance to observe operations performed by an expert through the telemedicine link improved their confidence.[23]

Conclusions

This project showed that image transmission via an IP link is satisfactory for clinical purposes. Telemedicine seemed to facilitate the clinicians' education and allowed them to achieve good clinical results quickly. As in other telemedicine applications, good cooperation between the parties was essential to success. Telemedicine is a powerful tool to allow the delivery of highly specialized medical care, as well as a very useful educational tool to accelerate learning for the novice surgeon.[24-28] The excellent education and support received from the expert team in our project no doubt contributed to its success. Nonetheless, telemedicine cannot replace local expertise, which must be competent to deal with any local emergencies or complications that may arise.

The future

The rapid evolution of technology should make telemedicine more affordable and easy to use in future. The two applications described in this chapter involve advanced fetal diagnosis and therapy, and so real-time interaction and relatively high bandwidth for transmission are needed. For less advanced fetal diagnostic applications, store-and-forward techniques can be used. We are investigating the use of compressed video clips, coupled with the use of portable ultrasound machines, for remote consultation.[29] This will enable ultrasound consultation to be carried out at really remote sites, where dial-up access to the Internet may suffice. Another new ultrasound technology, three-dimensional imaging, is especially suited to telemedicine application, as a whole volume of ultrasound data can be acquired in a single sweep and transmitted offline for subsequent interpretation. The remote expert can then cut and review any plane of data as required. Current three-dimensional ultrasound machines are relatively expensive, however, and the volumes of data produced are large and cumbersome. It is likely that exchange of three-dimensional volume data will take place only between tertiary referral centres until the technology improves.

We have shown that telemedicine can assist in fetal therapeutic procedures by improving education of novice surgeons. Telemedicine can also be used in other aspects of fetal therapy. Examples include communication between the referral site and the treatment centre to enable appropriate selection of cases for treatment, accurate timing of referral and subsequent follow-up of patients after the treatment procedure. In addition, telemedicine can be used between treatment centres around the world to standardize the methods of treatment and to develop common protocols for research. In fact, there are numerous applications. Obviously, there are also many barriers to telemedicine. In our experience, technical problems can almost always be surmounted. Geographical boundaries can also be overcome, but the problems with medicolegal risks, cost and remuneration, and certain other human factors, may represent the biggest hurdles to the widespread implementation of telemedicine.

References

1   Saari-Kemppainen A, Karjalainen O, Ylostalo P, Heinonen OP. Ultrasound screening and perinatal mortality: controlled trial of systematic one-stage screening in pregnancy. The Helsinki Ultrasound Trial. *Lancet* 1990; **336**: 387–391

2   Ewigman BG, Crane JP, Frigoletto FD, *et al.* Effect of prenatal ultrasound screening on perinatal outcome. RADIUS Study Group. *New England Journal of Medicine* 1993; **329**: 821–827.

3   Neilson JP. Ultrasound for fetal assessment in early pregnancy. *Cochrane Database Systematic Reviews* 2000: CD000182.

4   Wong SF, Chan FY, Welsh A, *et al.* Outcome of a routine ultrasound screening program in a tertiary center in Australia. *International Journal of Gynecology and Obstetrics* 2004; **87**: 153–4.

5   Quintero RA, Morales WJ. Operative fetoscopy: a new frontier in fetal medicine. *Contemporary Obstetrics/Gynecology* 1999; **April 15**: 45–68.

6   Neilson JP, Alfirevic Z. Doppler ultrasound for fetal assessment in high risk pregnancies. *Cochrane Database Systematic Reviews* 2000: CD000073.

7   Fisk NM, Sepulveda W, Drysdale K. Fetal telemedicine: six month pilot of real-time ultrasound and video consultation between the Isle of Wight and London. *British Journal of Obstetrics and Gynaecology* 1996; **103**: 1092–1095.

8   Finley JP, Sharratt GP, Nanton MA, *et al.* Paediatric echocardiography by telemedicine – nine years' experience. *Journal of Telemedicine and Telecare* 1997; **3**: 200–4.

9   Malone FD, Nores JA, Athanassiou A, *et al.* Validation of fetal telemedicine as a new obstetric imaging technique. *American Journal of Obstetrics and Gynecology* 1997; **177**: 626–631.

10 Malone FD, Athanassiou A, Nores J, D'Alton ME. Effect of ISDN bandwidth on image quality for telemedicine transmission of obstetric ultrasonography. *Telemedicine Journal* 1998; **4**: 161–165.

11 Alboliras ET, Berdusis K, Fisher J, *et al.* Transmission of full-length echocardiographic images over ISDN for diagnosing congenital heart disease. *Telemedicine Journal* 1996; **2**: 251–258.

12 Casey F, Brown D, Craig BG, *et al.* Diagnosis of neonatal congenital heart defects by remote consultation using a low-cost telemedicine link. *Journal of Telemedicine and Telecare* 1996; **2**: 165–169.

13 Wootton R, Dornan J, Fisk NM, *et al.* The effect of transmission bandwidth on diagnostic accuracy in remote fetal ultrasound scanning. *Journal of Telemedicine and Telecare* 1997; **3**: 209–214.

14 Chan FY, Whitehall J, Hayes L, *et al*. Minimum requirements for remote realtime fetal tele-ultrasound consultation. *Journal of Telemedicine and Telecare* 1999; **5**: 171–176.

15 Chan FY, Soong B, Lessing K, *et al*. Clinical value of real-time tertiary fetal ultrasound consultation by telemedicine: preliminary evaluation. *Telemedicine Journal* 2000; **6**: 237–242.

16 Chan FY, Soong B, Watson D, Whitehall J. Realtime fetal ultrasound by telemedicine in Queensland. A successful venture? *Journal of Telemedicine and Telecare* 2001; **7** (suppl. 2): 7–11.

17 Chan FY, Borzi P, Cincotta R, *et al*. Limb constriction as a complication of intra-uterine vesico-amniotic shunt: fetoscopic release. *Fetal Diagnosis and Therapy* 2002; **17**: 315–320.

18 Mari G, Roberts A, Detti L, *et al*. Perinatal morbidity and mortality rates in severe twin-twin transfusion syndrome: results of the International Amnioreduction Registry. *American Journal of Obstetrics and Gynecology* 2001; **185**: 708–715.

19 Cincotta RB, Gray PH, Phythian G, *et al*. Long term outcome of twin-twin transfusion syndrome. *Archives of Disease in Childhood. Fetal and Neonatal Edition* 2000; **83**: F171–F176.

20 Hecher K, Diehl W, Zikulnig L, *et al*. Endoscopic laser coagulation of placental anastomoses in 200 pregnancies with severe mid-trimester twin-to-twin transfusion syndrome. *European Journal of Obstetrics, Gynecology, and Reproductive Biology* 2000; **92**: 135–139.

21 Quintero RA, Dickinson JE, Morales WJ, *et al*. Stage-based treatment of twin-twin transfusion syndrome. *American Journal of Obstetrics and Gynecology* 2003; **188**: 1333–1340.

22 Chan FY, Taylor A, Soong B, *et al*. Randomized comparison of the quality of realtime fetal ultrasound images transmitted by ISDN and by IP videoconferencing. *Journal of Telemedicine and Telecare* 2002; **8**: 91–96.

23 Chan FY, Soong B, Taylor A, *et al*. Fetal endoscopic telesurgery using an Internet Protocol connection: clinical and technical challenges. *Journal of Telemedicine and Telecare* 2003; **9** (suppl. 2): 12–14.

24 Allen D, Bowersox J, Jones GG. Telesurgery. Telepresence. Telementoring. Telerobotics. *Telemedicine Today* 1997; **5**: 18–20, 25

25 Angelini L, Papaspyropoulos VV. Telesurgery. *Ultrasound in Medicine and Biology* 2000; **26** (suppl. 1): 45–47.

26 Marescaux J, Soler L, Mutter D, *et al*. Virtual university applied to telesurgery: from teleeducation to telemanipulation. *Studies in Health Technology and Informatics* 2000; **70**: 195–201.

27 Marescaux J, Rubino F. Telesurgery, telementoring, virtual surgery, and telerobotics. *Current Urology Reports* 2003; **4**: 109–113.

28 Quintero RA, Munoz H, Pommer R, *et al*. Operative fetoscopy via telesurgery. *Ultrasound in Obstetrics and Gynecology* 2002; **20**: 390–391.

29 Begg L, Chan FY, Edie G, *et al*. Minimum acceptable standards for digital compression of a fetal ultrasound video-clip. *Journal of Telemedicine and Telecare* 2001; **7** (suppl. 2): 88–90.

▶7

Child and Adolescent Telepsychiatry

Jean Starling and David Dossetor

Introduction

Rural and remote communities across the world often have high levels of social and economic disadvantage.[1] Indicators of poor community health, such as high rates of infant mortality, accidents and injury, are also more common in remote regions.[2] Suicide rates are higher, particularly in young men in rural areas.[3] Despite this high clinical need, access to healthcare is poor. This can be due to staff shortages or the logistical difficulties of providing services for sparse populations across large areas, complicated by hostile climates and poor public transport. Isolated areas also tend to have high staff turnover and difficulty employing enough senior clinicians. Even if staffing is adequate, there is not likely to be a network of professional colleagues to provide clinical discussion and support.

Even populations with adequate numbers of general clinicians may lack access to expertise for less common conditions such as psychotic disorders in childhood, anorexia nervosa, intellectual disability or autism. The expertise in these disorders tends to be clustered in specialty services located in large urban hubs. It is not surprising, therefore, that remote and disadvantaged areas such as the Australian outback or the Canadian far north have been among the first to develop telepsychiatry services.

Example telepsychiatry service

The Child and Adolescent Psychological Telemedicine Outreach Service (CAPTOS) started as a pilot programme from the Department of Psychological Medicine at the Children's Hospital in New South Wales, Australia, to Dubbo and Bourke in the western part of the state. The pilot trial ran from December 1996 to July 1997 and during that time there were 72 videoconferencing interviews with 54 patients. Although only 24% of families returned the questionnaire, they reported a high level of satisfaction with the service.[4] This study showed that an acceptable service could be provided entirely via videoconferencing, where previously telemedicine consultations had been used as a supplement to direct face-to-face contact and only for a triaging interview or follow-up appointments.

After evaluation of the pilot programme, the New South Wales Health Department funded staff and equipment so that the CAPTOS Service could be extended from the

Children's Hospital at Westmead to all of remote and rural New South Wales (except for the southern area). This service was evaluated between September 1999 and September 2000 inclusive.[5] Data were collected from 136 consultations and included information on symptom severity, service satisfaction and ease of use of technology. These measures have been described in detail in several papers.[4-6]

The mean age of the young people seen was 12 years (range 4–23 years). Sixty-five percent were boys, and 28% had safety or 'at-risk' issues. The most common diagnostic group was the behavioural disorders (37%), followed by depression (16%), anxiety disorders (13%) and developmental disorders (7%) (Fig. 7.1).[6] Both rural clinicians and rural families had high levels of satisfaction with the service: 96% of families and 99% of rural clinicians rated the quality of service as good or excellent, were very or mostly satisfied with the services they required and felt that they received the service that they wanted (Table 7.1).

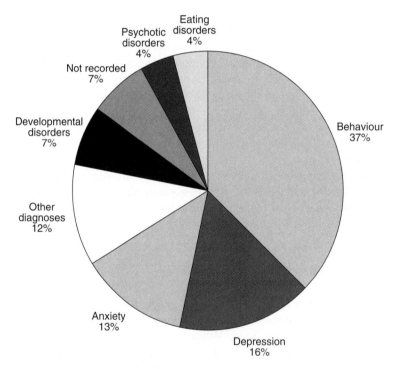

Fig. 7.1. Diagnoses made at consultation.

Perhaps surprisingly, the rural families and clinicians found that the equipment was easy to use and did not interfere with the consultation. Less than half of the hospital clinicians found the equipment easy to use, although most felt that it was still possible to perform an adequate consultation. They had concerns about the sound and picture

Table 7.1. Satisfaction with the service

Question	Family	Rural clinician
Quality of service good or excellent	78/81 (96%)	102/103 (99%)
Received the service they wanted	80/83 (96%)	102/103 (99%)
Very or mostly satisfied with the service received	80/83 (96%)	102/103 (99%)
Would be inconvenient or very inconvenient to attend a face-to-face consultation	66/82 (80%)	85/96 (89%)

Table 7.2. Satisfaction with the technology

Question	Rural family	Rural clinician	CHW* clinician
Good or excellent ease of using equipment	77/79 (97%)	87/100 (87%)	65/136 (48%)
The equipment interfered with the consultation slightly or not at all	77/79 (97%)	95/101 (94%)	118/136 (87%)
The sound quality was good or excellent	77/79 (97%)	87/101 (86%)	36/136 (26%)
The visual quality was good or excellent	75/79 (95%)	80/101 (79%)	19/136 (14%)
The overall quality of the videolink was good or excellent	76/79 (96%)	88/101 (87%)	25/136 (18%)
Telepsychiatry is almost as good or as good as a face-to-face consultation	77/79 (97%)	92/101 (91%)	22/136 (16%)

*CHW, Children's Hospital at Westmead.

quality (Table 7.2). An example of technical difficulties was that sometimes there was a need to continue an interview by telephone when the video link lost sound.

As the telepsychiatry service developed, however, it became clear that there were other limitations to the mental health services provided to rural families. For the telepsychiatry service to work, rural clinicians were expected to prepare case summaries, sit in on consultations and implement treatment recommendations. At times, this proved difficult. Rural clinicians had various levels of clinical skills. They did not always have the experience needed to implement specific treatment programmes. Some were new graduates and needed a high level of supervision that was often not available close to their workplace. However, it was possible to use the CAPTOS equipment to provide other supervision and training. Further services offered from the CAPTOS hub site now include professional supervision by nurses, clinical psychologists and social workers, and family therapy training.[6,7]

The CAPTOS service now has permanent funding from the New South Wales Health Department and has the capacity to provide telepsychiatry clinics to 41 towns spread across all eight rural and remote areas of New South Wales. Some towns have regular and continuing services. Others have been able to find visiting psychiatrists and so use the service less. There are currently six to eight half-day clinics conducted routinely each week, with additional psychology, social work and family therapy supervision sessions. Approximately 280 children and families were seen in 2003. The service is limited to New South Wales, as Australian legislation has separate medical registration for each state.

Other examples

The Royal Children's Hospital in Melbourne, Victoria, started their telepsychiatry service with a pilot programme in 1995. This was evaluated and found to be an effective clinical tool.[8] This led to telepsychiatry being incorporated into the routine service, with a total of 587 videoconferences being carried out in the five-year period up to December 2001.[9]

This service not only provides telepsychiatry assessments and professional support but is also used as part of the inpatient service. Pre-admission assessments were carried out by videoconference. Videoconferencing was also used throughout the admission to enable rural mental health workers to remain involved, and even for rural parents to participate in family meetings. After discharge, telepsychiatry enabled ongoing follow-up and continuity of care.

Several key principles were identified as essential to move from a pilot/research phase into a routine clinical service. These include running the service as a collaborative partnership with the rural Child and Adolescent Mental Health Service (CAMHS), involving consumers to improve the user-friendliness of the service and constantly broadening clinical applications as needed by the users. It was also stressed that technology should only be used where it is helpful and should never replace face-to-face contact where this is possible. Finally, a commitment to ongoing evaluation is essential.

The University of Kansas has a long-standing child and adolescent telepsychiatry service between their university clinic and a rural community mental health centre. This service offers routine and crisis assessments and has been able to offer good quality services to severely disturbed children.[10] Several other services have also been trialled in many other parts of the world, but the literature contains limited documentation.

Models of child and adolescent telepsychiatry

Direct patient care

The assessment/consultation model is the most commonly used model in child telepsychiatry. A rural mental health clinician (who may be a mental health nurse, social worker, psychologist or indigenous mental health worker) refers their client to the hub clinician (who is often a psychiatrist but may also be a clinical psychologist, social worker, family therapist or other specialist mental health clinician). The rural clinician establishes and sits in on the session, usually making active contributions. A diagnosis, formulation and treatment are discussed during the session, and a summary and recommendations are documented for the rural clinician. There can be reviews as needed as treatment progresses.

An alternative is the provision of treatment model. In this model, the telemedicine clinician provides direct care to the child and adolescent or family. This is usually after an initial face-to-face consultation or episode of treatment, for example, to provide follow-up after an admission. Although this model is common in adult psychiatry, it is less suitable for children and adolescents for several reasons. Practically, young people are less able to operate equipment or understand that it cannot be used as a toy (although this is not confined to young people – one of the authors had difficulty using equipment at a rural community health centre after the local community had re-tuned the large-screen TV so that they could have a party and watch an international football match together). Providing therapy via a screen requires a client with a high level of cooperation and almost adult levels of cognitive functioning. A rural clinician is needed to support a child or adolescent and explain what is happening; see Case Example 1.

Box 7.1. Case Example 1: Rebecca

Rebecca, a 14-year-old girl with a two-year history of a severe eating disorder, who lived in a rural town eight hours away from the CAPTOS service, was repeatedly hospitalized for re-feeding and relapsed each time she returned home. Towards the end of her last admission, the eating disorders family therapist liaised with the CAPTOS psychiatrist and the rural mental health service so that the specialist team could continue to provide weekly intensive family therapy via videoconferencing. This was in collaboration with the ongoing medical monitoring and individual counselling that the local service had been able to offer previously. With the intensive family therapy, Rebecca and her family were able to continue treatment at home with local support, preventing frequent readmissions.

Case conferencing and clinical case discussion

Case conferences and discussions are the second most common form of service offered in child and adolescent telepsychiatry after direct clinical consultation. A rural clinician may feel that they have a good grasp of a case but need a few extra ideas. It is also useful where the family or young person is unwilling to be seen at a telepsychiatry consultation. See Case Examples 2 and 3 (Boxes 7.2 and 7.3).

Box 7.2. Case Example 2: Brayden

Brayden, a seven-year-old boy, was repeatedly taken by his mother to tertiary paediatric services, requesting drugs, despite living 11 hours away from these services. She had removed him from school, saying that his needs were not being met, and refused to be seen by her local CAMHS team. The CAPTOS service met her request to see a child psychiatrist but insisted on local team involvement. She agreed to this because of her wish to see a psychiatrist from a tertiary paediatric setting.

A videoconference was held with the rural psychologist and school counsellor to set up an assessment plan. The school had been extremely concerned that Brayden had significant intellectual and behavioural problems but were unable to assess him, as he was not attending school. He was found to have an IQ of 54, which led to his placement in a special class with learning and behavioural support. A year after the conference, he continues to attend school regularly, his behaviour has improved and he is on much less medication. The CAPTOS involvement supported the local services and enabled them to implement treatment.

Box 7.3. Case Example 3: Keely

Keely was a 14-year-old girl with a two-year history of out-of-control behaviour and psychotic symptoms. She had previously been hospitalized in a local adult unit, but she and her family had found this very distressing and insisted on early discharge. She refused assessment by the local mental health team or a telepsychiatry session. A telepsychiatry case conference was held with the child psychiatrist at the hub site, the rural mental health team and the rural indigenous mental health workers. Enough information was gained to be clear that she had a severe psychosis and needed treatment for her own safety. A second session was organized with her mother and her aunt, and they agreed on a treatment plan. A bed was organized in a metropolitan adolescent unit, safe transport was booked (she lived 10 hours by road from the city) and accommodation was organized so her family could support her during the admission. When all this was ready, the local general practitioner visited and certified her for involuntary hospitalization. After three weeks in hospital, her symptoms settled and she was discharged, remaining cooperative with treatment 12 months later.

Clinical supervision/professional training

Access to high-quality, appropriate supervision is essential not just for good clinical practice but also for professional accreditation. In Australia, mental health professionals such as psychologists and psychiatry registrars cannot receive full registration and professional recognition without mandatory supervision. This prevents them from being employed in isolated areas. The CAPTOS Service has provided supervision for psychology registration via telemedicine, supplemented with one or two rural visits by the supervisor and hub visits by the rural clinician.

The same methods can be used for more specific forms of training. For example, family therapy skills are generally taught with a mixture of didactic teaching and clinical supervision. Telemedicine links can be used for both with good effect. The model that the authors use involves a hub clinician meeting face to face with a rural group for introductory teaching, then regular telemedicine links for tutorials and supervision of the group. This finally becomes the rural clinical group providing peer group supervision, with diminishing support from the hub clinician.

Evaluations of child and adolescent telepsychiatry

A summary of the studies that have evaluated child and adolescent telepsychiatry can be found in a thorough review by Pesamaa et al.[11] The best quality evidence for evaluating any treatment comes from randomized controlled trials (RCT). Only two RCTs of child and adolescent telepsychiatry have been published to date. Most studies are case series or single case reports. There is a need for further studies in all the areas detailed below, especially outcome studies and economic evaluations.

Service satisfaction

Patient satisfaction

Four studies that describe parental satisfaction with videoconferencing have been published; two of these also assessed the satisfaction of participating children. Two of the four have been described above, as evaluations of the New South Wales CAPTOS service, which assessed only parental satisfaction.[4,5] The others described services in Kentucky and Newfoundland and investigated satisfaction of both the parent and the child.[12,13] There were generally high levels of satisfaction with the service in both children and their families. There were some concerns, however, about the service being less personal and missing some information, particularly non-verbal communications such as facial expressions. Most preferred videoconferencing to travelling long distances to see a psychiatrist.

Clinician satisfaction

Several studies have reported on rural staff satisfaction with videoconferencing in child and adolescent mental health. The four studies above plus several others have reported that clinicians find videoconferencing useful for clinical consultations, teaching and professional supervision.[8-10,12] The rural workers were able to access specialized knowledge and felt less professionally isolated.

Outcome evaluations

Clinical

As yet, only two published RCTs have looked at outcomes of videoconferencing or treatment. The first RCT, of 23 patients, found that diagnosis and treatment recommendations were similar in 96% of consultations performed by both a videoconference and a face-to-face interview.[14] This study did not look at treatment. The second study found that face-to-face sessions and videoconferencing were equally effective in treating two groups of children aged 8–14 years with depression;[15] however, the treatment groups were relatively small (each of 28).

Other studies have been single case reports that describe the successful treatment of depression and behavioural disorders.[16-18] Although these reports suggest that treatment via videoconferencing is feasible, more trials are needed to provide good data on effectiveness.

Economic

An economic evaluation of a service can be performed in several possible ways. The simplest is to compare the costs of two comparable services, presuming that they are both equally effective. For child and adolescent telepsychiatry, the costs of a telemedicine link can be compared either with the cost of a visiting child psychiatrist (although often the telepsychiatry service is used because there is no visiting psychiatrist) or with the expenses of a family travelling to the nearest available psychiatrist. Three studies have made some provisional calculations of assumed costs and found that telemedicine was less costly.[4,13,19]

More complicated economic evaluations measure the cost of an intervention against its effectiveness. This requires good data on comparative effectiveness, ie an RCT, and so is not yet possible in child and adolescent telepsychiatry.

Techniques for successful consultation

Successful techniques in telepsychiatry for children and adolescents are not very different from those for telepsychiatry in adults, or for real-time telemedicine generally.

Obtain adequate background information

To be most successful, telepsychiatry consultations need careful preparation. The rural clinician should write a case summary, attaching reports from the school and other treating professionals such as paediatricians, with specific questions for the psychiatrist to answer. This serves several purposes. It enables the psychiatrist to focus on crucial areas and not ask again for information that is already known. It also helps the rural clinician put their thoughts together before the consultation and clarify issues.

Use additional interview techniques

Telepsychiatry is a novel experience for most families, and it is important to explain the process to them and acknowledge that it may seem weird. Often young people and children have little difficulty with the concept. They are used to many forms of technology, including the Internet and mobile phones that take photos, so a doctor on the television who interacts with them is not so surprising.

Once the assessment has started, it is important to modify the usual face-to-face interview style. Most information at interview is gained from non-verbal communications, including facial expressions, small movements and body posture. Although the verbal content alone provides the history, it is not adequate to assess emotions or mental state. This is particularly true when a family is seen. The way the family members interact with each other is not seen as well over a video link. Similarly, the family sees less of the body language of the clinician. To help gain rapport, it is important for the clinician to exaggerate gestures and facial expressions. Language needs to be simplified, short sentences work better and it is important to ask only one question at a time. This is similar to working with an interpreter, where verbal padding or unnecessary statements can interfere with understanding. There needs to be less reliance on non-verbal cues, although great concentration is required not to miss any of the subtle signs that you may see. At times, it may be necessary to ask directly about possible non-verbal cues. For example, you may be concerned that the young person being interviewed is becoming distressed and withdrawing from you. If they do not respond, you could ask the rural clinician to enquire if the young person has been upset by your question.

At times, to clarify what is happening, the hub clinician can also manage the rural camera remotely and 'zoom in' on the client or couple central to the interview, enabling a close look at facial expressions or interactions when cued to do so.

Develop partnerships with rural areas

Telepsychiatry consultations are most successful if the consultant has some knowledge of the rural area and the available services. This can slowly develop via the teleconsultations, but it is more quickly and accurately developed with regular visits. It is helpful to know, for example, that the one local high school is short-staffed or under stress – not just for background information but also to help with rapport. If you are able to ask a young person a relevant local question, it helps gain rapport. Knowledge of local services and their areas of expertise helps the hub clinician to make appropriate treatment suggestions as well. For example, intensive specialized cognitive behavioural therapy (CBT) may be the accepted, evidence-based treatment for a condition, but if only a junior mental health nurse and a GP are available, then either the treatment skill will need to be taught to them or a different, more practical option suggested.

In longstanding telepsychiatry partnerships, the hub clinician will become a senior member of the team. One of the authors, who has been consulting to a rural area for seven years, is now by far the longest serving team member. He provides essential continuity as well as his child psychiatry skills.

Potential pitfalls of child and adolescent telepsychiatry

As in other areas of telemedicine, telepsychiatry has a number of potential problems.

Limitations of telepsychiatry

In telemedicine, the best possible picture and sound quality are needed, especially for interviews with several people. The ISDN lines (we use three lines, giving a bandwidth of 384 kbit/s) provide a good picture, although at times there are still technical difficulties, with the picture freezing or sound difficulties. These problems can be minimized by staff training and regular maintenance of equipment but can never be avoided completely.

There are also patients and families for whom the technology is distressing or unsuitable; however, these occur less commonly than might be predicted. For example, patients with possible paranoia could in theory be distressed by a consultation via a television screen. In practice, this is very rare and is only seen in those who are acutely unwell. In our service, there was also some concern about rural indigenous families' acceptance of the technology. However, when we started consultations this was not a problem. Some of the rural indigenous health workers suggested that these families, who often had a history of children in previous generations being removed from their care after contact with health services, in fact preferred the 'city specialist' to be a safe distance from them.

Legal and ethical considerations

Telemedicine, like any other treatment, requires a patient's informed consent. We do this with a written consent form. This allows families to consider what is involved before the session and discuss their concerns with the rural clinician.

It is also essential both to maintain patient confidentiality and to demonstrate this to the patient in consultations. Some patients are concerned that the sessions could be video-recorded. In the New South Wales services, the State Government has mandated that this should not be done – even with patient consent. We find that this reassures families. It is also important that no one observes the sessions without the patients' or families' consent. If a large room is being used, there may be observers who cannot be seen on the screen, but it is essential that they are introduced and permission gained for them to be there.

Another essential issue to consider is lines of responsibility – or who is responsible for the day-to-day care of the patient. This is easier where consultations are carried out with a rural clinician, who then knows what has been said and is also part of a treatment team that can provide ongoing care. It is also helpful to provide the rural primary medical practitioner with as much information as possible (with patient consent). If there is no local clinician at the session, the hub clinician has responsibility for follow-up, which can work for arranged appointments but can lead to difficulties in a crisis situation.

Future directions

Child and adolescent telepsychiatry has become an essential part of many remote and rural mental health services, with good evidence that the technology is acceptable to rural families and clinicians. It is also clear that successful services work best as an ongoing partnership between specialized hub services and the rural teams. They require an ongoing commitment not only from the partners but also from those responsible for the delivery of mental healthcare to rural and remote communities. Providing the infrastructure and maintaining it in working order requires a major commitment from service providers, whether or not they are government or other services.

It is also clear that there are major gaps in our knowledge about the clinical effectiveness and comparative costs of child and adolescent telepsychiatry services. Evaluation and research must continue in these essential areas if we are to make a good case for the ongoing expansion of telepsychiatry services.

Further information

Wootton R, Yellowlees P, McLaren P, eds. *Telepsychiatry and e-Mental Health.* London: Royal Society of Medicine Press, 2003.

Royal Australian and New Zealand College of Psychiatry. *Telepsychiatry Position Statement* (includes guidelines, clinical responsibility, technology). See http://www.ranzcp.org/publicarea/posstate.asp (last checked 3 August 2004).

References

1 Rey JM. The mental health of young Australians. *Medical Journal of Australia* 2001; **174**: 380–1.

2 NSW Health. *Young People's Health: Our Future.* See http://www.health.nsw.gov.au/living/youth.html (last checked 3 August 2004).

3 Dudley MJ, Kelk NJ, Florio TM, *et al.* Suicide among young Australians, 1964-1993: an interstate comparison of metropolitan and rural trends. *Medical Journal of Australia* 1998; **169**: 77–80.

4 Dossetor DR, Nunn KP, Fairley M, Eggleton D. A child and adolescent outreach service for rural New South Wales: a telemedicine pilot study. *Journal of Paediatrics and Child Health* 1999; **35**: 525–529.

5 Kopel H, Nunn K, Dossetor D. Evaluating satisfaction with a child and adolescent psychological telemedicine outreach service. *Journal of Telemedicine and Telecare* 2001; **7** (suppl. 2): 35–40.

6 Starling J, Rosina R, Nunn K, Dossetor D. Child and adolescent telepsychiatry in New South Wales: moving beyond clinical consultation. *Australasian Psychiatry* 2003; **11** (suppl. 11): 117–119.

7 Rosina R, Starling J, Nunn K, *et al.* Telenursing: clinical nurse consultancy for rural paediatric nurses. *Journal of Telemedicine and Telecare* 2002; **8** (suppl. 3): 48–49.

8 Gelber H, Alexander M. An evaluation of an Australian videoconferencing project for child and adolescent telepsychiatry. *Journal of Telemedicine and Telecare* 1999; **5** (suppl. 1): 21–23.

9 Gelber H, Starling J. Telemedicine for child and adolescent psychiatry. In: Wootton R, Yellowlees P, McLaren P, eds. *Telepsychiatry and e-Mental Health.* London: Royal Society of Medicine Press, 2003: 161–169.

10 Ermer DJ. Experience with a rural telepsychiatry clinic for children and adolescents. *Psychiatric Services* 1999; **50**: 260–261.

11 Pesamaa L, Ebeling H, Kuusimaki ML, *et al.* Videoconferencing in child and adolescent telepsychiatry: a systematic review of the literature. *Journal of Telemedicine and Telecare* 2004; **10**: 187-192.

12 Blackmon L, Kaak O, Ranseen J. Consumer satisfaction with telemedicine child psychiatry consultation in rural Kentucky. *Psychiatric Services* 1997; **48**: 1464–1466.

13 Elford DR, White H, St John K, Maddigan B, Ghandi M, Bowering R. A prospective satisfaction study and cost analysis of a pilot child telepsychiatry service in Newfoundland. *Journal of Telemedicine and Telecare* 2001; **7**: 73–81.

14 Elford R, White H, Bowering R, *et al.* A randomized controlled trial of child psychiatric assessments conducted using videoconferencing. *Journal of Telemedicine and Telecare* 2000; **6**: 73–82.

15 Nelson EL, Barnard M, Cain S. Treating childhood depression over videoconferencing. *Telemedicine Journal and e-Health* 2003; **9**: 49–55

16 Alessi N. Telepsychiatric care of a depressed adolescent. *Journal of the American Academy of Child and Adolescent Psychiatry* 2002; **41**: 894–895.

17 Hilty DM, Sison JI, Nesbitt TS, Hales RE. Telepsychiatric consultation for ADHD in the primary care setting. *Journal of the American Academy of Child and Adolescent Psychiatry* 2000; **39**: 15–16.

18 Rendon M. Telepsychiatric treatment of a schoolchild. *Journal of Telemedicine and Telecare* 1998; **4**: 179–182.

19 Mitchell J, Robinson P, Seiboth C, Koszegi B. An evaluation of a network for professional development in child and adolescent mental health in rural and remote communities. *Journal of Telemedicine and Telecare* 2000; **6**: 158–162.

▶**8**

Diabetes and Telemedicine

Jennifer Batch and Anthony C Smith

Introduction

Diabetes is a common medical problem that affects children, young people and adults. The World Health Organization defines diabetes mellitus as a metabolic disorder of multiple aetiologies, characterized by chronic hyperglycaemia with disturbances of carbohydrate, fat and protein metabolism resulting from defects in insulin secretion, action or both. Diabetes mellitus can be classified into a range of subtypes, the most common being type 1 and type 2 diabetes. Type 1 (previously known as insulin-dependent diabetes mellitus, IDDM) is the most common endocrine disorder in childhood and adolescence. Half of the cases of type 1 diabetes are diagnosed in children aged under 16 years. Type 2 diabetes (previously known as non-insulin-dependent diabetes mellitus, NIDDM) occurs more commonly in adults, although rates of type 2 diagnosis in children and young people are escalating in association with the epidemic of paediatric and adolescent obesity.

The principles of management of diabetes mellitus of all aetiologies involve strategies to optimize metabolic (glycaemic) control. The aims are to achieve normal psychosocial adjustment, best possible glycaemic control and normal growth and development. It is also desirable to develop individualized diabetes management plans that incorporate the particular needs of the child or adolescent and the family. The Diabetes Control and Complications Trial showed unequivocally that intensive diabetes treatment reduced the risk of diabetes complications including retinopathy, nephropathy and neuropathy and has provided the impetus for exploring ways to improve diabetes management.[1]

The management of type 1 diabetes in children and young people includes initial and ongoing diabetes education, a home management plan and periodic diabetes team review. Home management includes blood glucose monitoring, insulin dose adjustment and injections, an integrated nutritional approach with dietary adherence, and appropriate healthy exercise. Optimum management of diabetes thus requires home-based intervention with considerable dependence on self-care or care administered by parents and other caregivers.

Every child with type 1 diabetes, including those from rural and remote areas, deserves the right to have access to the best medical management. Children and adolescents with diabetes should have access to care from a multidisciplinary team trained in childhood and adolescent diabetes.[2,3] This training should involve:

▶ the patient and their family

▶ a paediatric endocrinologist or physician trained in the care of children and adolescents with diabetes

▶ a diabetes educator

▶ a dietician

▶ a psychologist/social worker.

Care provided by a specialized diabetes multidisciplinary team has been shown to result in fewer days in hospital, higher levels of diabetes self care practices, decreased re-admission rates, better glycaemic control and delayed development of complications.[4-6] In rural and remote areas with low population density and small numbers of children and adolescents with diabetes, it may not be possible to provide a local multidisciplinary team. In these situations, care may be successfully provided by a local paediatrician/physician with access to resources, and support and advice from a tertiary diabetes centre via outreach clinics or telemedicine.

Why is telemedicine appropriate for diabetes management?

Telemedicine is the delivery of healthcare and the exchange of healthcare information across distances, with the 'common thread for all telemedicine applications being that a client of some kind (eg a patient or healthcare worker) obtains an opinion from someone with more expertise in the relevant field, when the parties are separated in space, in time or both'.[7] Diabetes care is a complex task shared by a large number of different professionals over the years, such as physicians, nurses, dieticians, podiatrists, laboratory personnel, pharmacists and others. Gathering and sharing information and performing long-term analysis are crucial for long-term outcome. In several situations, consultation with other professionals is necessary, and up-to-date data, using digital media and instant online connections, are often beneficial both for professionals and patients. The goal of information technology is to provide valuable support to enhance diabetes management. In this respect, telemedicine offers a platform for standard documentation, improved quality control and evaluation of diabetes services generally. Telemedicine can also improve preventive actions. Patient education, a fundamental part of diabetes self-care, will also use new media more in the future.

Telemedicine in its various forms is thus well suited to diabetes management, as, in many ways, the cornerstone of diabetes management is an emphasis on home-based self-care, supported by the diabetes health professional team, with a limited and intermittent requirement for face-to-face contact. Self-management is crucial to obtaining the best metabolic control that will prevent the microvascular complications of the disease. It requires continuing training and education of the patient. Support by the diabetes healthcare team can take many forms, including telephone contact, fax transmission of home blood glucose monitoring with feedback and the use of email.

New and emerging forms of telemedicine for diabetes include the use of websites for patients, families and health professionals and the delivery of clinical care by videoconferencing. The use of each of these forms of telemedicine in diabetes management is reviewed briefly below.

Established forms of telemedicine in diabetes management

Computer interfacing and data management with blood glucose monitors are increasingly common in the management of diabetes. Combining such technology with some form of telemedicine provides an opportunity for enhanced diabetes self-management and improved metabolic control (eg 'Computerising your meter' at http://www.childrenwithdiabetes.com/d_06_150.htm).

Telephone

Telephone counselling and advice given by diabetologists, diabetes educators, dieticians and other health professionals to patients and families for routine and urgent diabetes issues has formed the cornerstone of outpatient management between formal review appointments for patients with newly diagnosed and established diabetes. A wide range of issues may be covered, including insulin dose adjustments, management of hypoglycaemia and sick days, and variations to daily routines and their subsequent effect on diabetes. Proactive telephone contact from diabetes nurse educators and other health professionals has also been shown to have a beneficial effect on metabolic control, dietary prescription and blood glucose testing adherence.[8] Telephone management of patients on intensified therapy has been investigated to assess the potential for time and cost savings. Biermann *et al* concluded that telephone management of insulin-requiring diabetic patients is a cost-saving and time-saving procedure for the patients and results in metabolic control comparable to that of conventional management.[9] Wojcicki *et al* used telemedicine in a three-year study of pregnant women and reported improvements in the control group;[10] however, they did not present any economic data.

The importance of developments in technology and its effect on diabetes management has been recognized by governments, with projects such as the M2DM project funded by the European Commission to investigate the potential of novel telemedicine services in diabetes management[11] and the Telematic management of Insulin Dependent Diabetes Mellitus (T-IDDM) project investigating the feasibility of telemedicine in the management of young patients with type 1 diabetes.[12] Daily remote telephone monitoring of indigent adults with type 2 diabetes has shown benefits, including reduced use of emergency room and admission time, fewer routine diabetes reviews, improved quality of life and enhanced self-management behaviours.[13]

Fax

As fax transmission has become common in workplaces and homes, many patients and families send blood glucose recordings to diabetes educators and diabetologists for advice about changes to insulin doses between regular review appointments or as a follow-up after changes to the management regimen made at a review appointment.[14]

Email

Email has been used in various forms to enhance diabetes management or provide information to patients, families and healthcare providers. In some instances, families relay details of home blood glucose measurements via email attachments and receive email feedback in a manner analogous to the use of the fax.[15] Another use of email has been reported, in which a proposed change to a diabetes regimen was emailed to the treating physician to confirm or modify before the patient was offered the proposed modification to their regimen.[16] Recently, Chase *et al* reported the use of modem transmission of glucose values in lieu of a routine clinic visit.[17] They found that electronic transmission of blood glucose levels and other diabetes data every two weeks in lieu of a clinic visit resulted in a similar level of glucose control and incidence of acute complications as did standard care.

New forms of telemedicine in diabetes management

The Internet provides a powerful vehicle for the interchange of information and advice in its many forms. Some of these are discussed briefly below.

Discussion forums

Online communication is one of the principal forms of communication for many young people. Iafusco *et al* reported preliminary results using an online chat room moderated by a paediatric diabetologist as an adjunct to the teaching tools generally used in their clinic in the education of young people with type 1 diabetes.[18] They reported the use of this chatline by 43 patients (age range 11–25 years, disease duration 0.1–15 years). During chatline sessions, patients used a nickname that also identified their sex. Meetings took place weekly, lasted 90 minutes and covered a topic voted on at the beginning of the session. The topics covered included anxiety about future management and interpersonal and social relationships. Online messages were keyed in, with the discussion recorded by the moderator and subsequently evaluated by a psychologist. Preliminary results reported an improvement in metabolic control, improved capacity for self-management and improved adherence with management. Studies are underway to investigate the longer-term effectiveness of this form of telemedicine.

Web-based self-management programmes

To achieve home management of diabetes, patients with diabetes and their families need to be educated and to make appropriate insulin dose adjustments using acquired knowledge and an understanding of insulin action or validated algorithms.[19–21] Despite education and a good understanding of insulin action, however, patients may remain reluctant to take the responsibility of increasing or decreasing their insulin dose.

Boukhors *et al* reported on the use of an Internet-delivered computer program designed to store blood glucose recordings, analyse the data and make specific recommendations for adjusting insulin doses to assist patients to improve their diabetes management.[22] The results of this study showed that there were no serious adverse effects associated with the use of the computer program by the patient to adjust their insulin doses to achieve and maintain near normoglycaemia. Furthermore, improved knowledge of the disease was highly appreciated by the study participants. Cavan *et al* also reported on use of the Internet to optimize self-management of type 1 diabetes.[23] They developed a structured patient education program that used the Diasnet computer model to display and manipulate patient data.[24] They experienced limited uptake of the system, with problems including lack of user-friendly entry screens and difficulties entering data manually while being connected to the Internet. They suggested that future development could be directed to facilitating automated data collection by download from a blood glucose meter or from a mobile phone. McKay *et al* reported on use of the Internet to provide a support service for diabetes self-management.[25] Users included people across a broad age range and duration of diabetes. The most popular areas of the site were the social support conference and diabetes information pages. User ratings showed high satisfaction with the service. The authors concluded that the Internet has great potential for providing support and services for patients with diabetes and other chronic illnesses.

Web-based educational resources

Kim and Ladenson reviewed a range of healthcare websites to identify accurate and relevant consumer information about the diagnosis and treatment of diabetes mellitus.[26] They also reported that tracking surveys show that more than half of all consumers who visit healthcare websites on the Internet are looking for information about specific diseases. Diabetes mellitus has been identified as a common topic of interest among healthcare information seekers. A Google search identified diabetes as one of the most common medical search terms entered by users – second only to cancer in a rank list of specific disorders.

Doctors and other health professionals are often concerned that patients and families may be accessing websites that do not necessarily deliver relevant or reliable information.[27] Similar concerns apply to diabetes-related information on the web. To address this concern, a number of authors and organizations have developed guidelines intended to help Internet users determine the reliability of health information on the net.[28] The Health on the Net Foundation (http://www.hon.ch/HONcode) was launched in early 1996 with the aim of raising the quality of healthcare information available on the Internet (see Chapter 28). It is a self-regulatory, voluntary certification system based on an 'active seal' concept and is primarily intended for healthcare site developers and publishers. It also helps users identify sources of reliable information. Recently, Kusec *et al* reported on the readability of diabetes websites accredited by the Health on the Net Foundation.[29] They found that 87% of the websites reviewed provided information that would be too difficult for the average reader, thus negating the potential benefit of the information to the patient or family.

Web-based material has also been used in a study aimed at improving diabetes education for school staff. As school-aged children are typically unable to assume responsibility for diabetes management decisions, teachers and other school staff have a duty of care to provide appropriate supervision and input into a child's diabetes management while they are under the care of the school. This cannot be achieved without appropriate education. Radjenovic and Wallace reported on the use of a web-based computer system to provide diabetes information.[30] Two groups of teachers were presented with diabetes training material either via paper or online. Participants who used the web-based system had significantly higher knowledge scores and were significantly more satisfied with the training session than those who used paper documents traditionally used for teacher training.

Web-based resources for health professionals

A myriad of information websites are directed towards diabetes health professionals. Many of these are supported by professional organizations and are password protected for members only. They may include information or position statements on a range of topics. Examples of these include web pages for the Australian Diabetes Society (http://www.racp.edu.au/ads/), the Australasian Paediatric Endocrine Group (http://www.racp.edu.au/apeg/) and the American Diabetes Association (http://www.diabetes.org/home.jsp).

Websites designed to assist doctors to deliver evidence-based diabetes care have also been developed. The American Diabetes Association is currently developing a system that will provide answers to clinical scenarios based on real patients on the basis of data derived from clinical trials, epidemiological data and sophisticated models that can take into account such things as the physiological effects of the different combinations of drugs that might be prescribed in an individual patient. The website will use a system called Archimedes – predictive software developed by the Bio-Mathematics Unit of the Care Management Institute at Kaiser Permanente, a California-based, non-profit health maintenance organization (HMO).[31]

Delivery of clinical services

Diabetes clinical services have been delivered to patients either in remote locations or at home, using videophones or standard commercial videoconferencing equipment.

Videophones

Use of home-based videophones has been reported in a study of elderly patients with diabetes.[32] There were few technical problems. The themes discussed included the patient's clinical status, promotion of compliance with drugs and treatment, psychosocial issues, general informal discussion and patient education. Gelfand *et al* also reported the use of telephone, and subsequently videophone, support in the intensive management of five at-risk adolescents with diabetes.[33] Most of the adolescents improved their metabolic control, and all five subjects showed a reduction in glycosylated haemoglobin during the three months of the study. The authors concluded that the use of telehealth facilitated the treatment of adolescents with poor glycaemic control.

Videoconferencing

Videoconferencing has been shown to be feasible in the delivery of specialist diabetes medical services, in diabetes education and for screening for diabetic retinopathy. Videoconferencing has also been reported as an alternative to physical outreach specialist diabetes services.[34,35] Malasanos reported the use of videoconferencing instead of quarterly outreach clinics in 44 children and young people.[34] Animated diabetes education was made available online to patients, and mental health telemedicine services were provided to children with poorly controlled diabetes. In severely affected children, there was a significant reduction in glycosylated haemoglobin and a reduction in waiting time for appointments. In addition, ophthalmology services were delivered at the recommended intervals in most patients. There was also a reduction in hospitalizations after implementation of the project, with an associated reduction in emergency room visits. More than 90% of the patients were satisfied with the service and wished to continue with telemedical delivery of their diabetes care. After online education, there was an improvement in patients' test scores. There were also considerable cost savings from the study.

We have used videoconferencing to deliver specialist diabetes services in Queensland, a large decentralized state, where patients with diabetes are often isolated in regional and remote areas.[35] In the first 28 months of the study, 160 patient consultations were performed in routine telepaediatric clinics, as urgent cases or as cases that needed additional management between routine clinics. Further details are discussed below.

Columbia University College of Physicians and Surgeons is currently undertaking a large project to study how telemedicine can improve diabetes care. In the study, 1500 diabetic patients will be randomly selected from impoverished, medically underserved areas. The goal of the study is to evaluate the feasibility, acceptability, effectiveness and cost-effectiveness of telemedicine. The focal point of the intervention is the home telemedicine unit, which provides four functions:[36,37]

▶ videoconferencing over standard telephone lines

▶ electronic transmission for finger-stick glucose and blood pressure readings

▶ secure web-based messaging and clinical data review

▶ access to web-based educational materials.

Personal computer-based videoconferencing has also been used to facilitate the transfer of knowledge from the specialist to the generalist in a 12-month study consisting of a network of a diabetes specialist and four general practitioners.[38] In the 12-month period, a total of 154 patients with type 2 diabetes entered the study, and showed an improvement in metabolic and haemodynamic variables. The study showed that therapeutic counselling can be achieved through videoconferencing and suggested that hospital admissions could be reduced and quality of care improved.

Diabetes education has also been successfully delivered via videoconference in both the paediatric and adult arena.[35,39] Smith *et al* reported the use of videoconferencing to provide urgent diabetes education to children and families with newly diagnosed diabetes in remote and rural areas from which the family were unable to travel to received the input from the nearest regional diabetes team.[35] They also reported the use of videoconferencing for diabetes education and upskilling of staff. Izquierdo *et al* compared diabetes education administered through telemedicine with face-to-face education in a group of 56 adults who were randomized to one of the two forms of education.[39] They reported that patient satisfaction was high in the telemedicine group. Diabetes education via telemedicine and in person was equally effective in improving glycaemic control, and both methods were well accepted by patients.

Tele-ophthalmology is a well developed area of telemedicine (see Chapter 13). Tele-ophthalmology has been used as a tool for screening and follow-up of diabetic retinopathy with a nine-field fundus photography system by Shiba and colleagues.[40] They reported that this system was appropriate for screening and follow-up of diabetic retinopathy in adult and adolescent diabetic subjects, especially when applied to telemedicine over the Internet.

Use of telemedicine in diabetes at the Royal Children's Hospital

Telemedicine has been used at three levels in the delivery of specialist diabetes services for children and adolescents by the Department of Endocrinology and Diabetes at the Royal Children's Hospital in Brisbane. These include:

▶ coordination of consultative routine specialist diabetes clinics with regional paediatric diabetes clinics via videoconference

▶ ad-hoc patient consultations for collaborative management during acute presentations and at times of urgent clinical need

▶ delivery of diabetes education to patients and staff throughout the state.

Routine telepaediatric clinics

Telepaediatric services were established as part of a research project at the Royal Children's Hospital. The roles and benefits (including cost-effectiveness) of the telepaediatric service have been examined.[41,42] As part of the project, a telepaediatric service for children with diabetes was arranged between the tertiary facility and two regional hospitals in Queensland. Additional services were also provided to other regional and remote hospitals on a less frequent ad hoc basis.

Smith *et al* reported on a total of 16 routine telepaediatric clinics for children with diabetes held every three months.[35] Each clinic involved members of the specialist staff of the Royal Children's Hospital, including a paediatric diabetologist, diabetes nurse educator, dietician and mental health worker (Fig. 8.1). Staff at the regional site included the referring paediatrician and the regional diabetes educator, dietician and mental health worker.

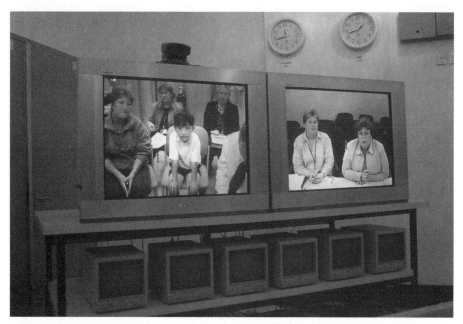

Fig. 8.1 Patient history provided by the regional paediatrician, the patient and family members via videoconference.

At the beginning of each consultation, patient information – such as a brief history of the underlying condition and the patient's height, weight, glycosylated haemoglobin result and current insulin doses – were relayed by the regional paediatrician. Relevant investigation results were faxed before the clinic or viewed via the document camera at the time of the consultation. An examination of injection sites via videoconferencing was also possible (Fig. 8.2). Blood sugar readings recorded by the patient and family could also be viewed via videoconferencing using a document camera (Fig. 8.3). Each clinic involved 2–14 patients (median 6) (Table 8.1). Routine videoconference clinics ran for a median time of 130 minutes (interquartile range 60–240) (Table 8.2).

Non-routine patient consultations

Twenty-five single patient consultations were also reported by Smith *et al.*[35] Most of these patients were not normally seen in routine clinics or required more intensive follow-up to monitor and guide the management of their diabetes. Several of these cases involved the input of more than one paediatric subspecialist, eg paediatric

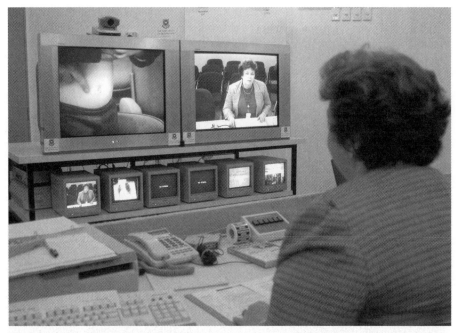

Fig. 8.2 Injection sites being reviewed.

Table 8.1. The three types of telepaediatric sessions

Session type	Sessions	Patients
Routine clinic (>1 patient)	21	135*
Consultation (1 patient)	25	25
Educational	10	0
Total	**56**	**160**

*Median = 6 per clinic; interquartile range = 6–7.

Table 8.2. Videoconference usage (time per session)

Session type	Number	Total time (minutes)	Median time per session (minutes)	Interquartile range
Routine clinic (>1 patient)	21	3210	130	60–240
Consultation (1 patient)	25	1230	45	30–60
Educational	10	640	60	60–60
Total	**56**	**5080**		

diabetologist and paediatric gastroenterologist, plus other members of the tertiary team. Four consultations were for urgent cases of isolated children with newly diagnosed type 1 diabetes, where for social reasons the family were unable to travel to

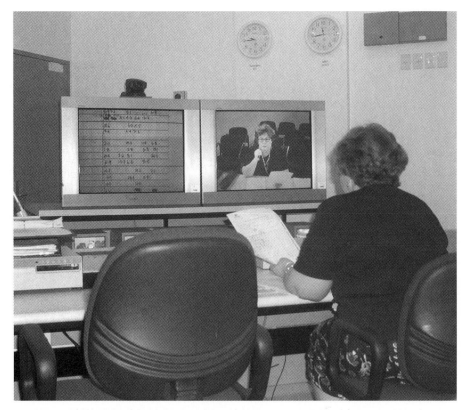

Fig. 8.3 Blood sugar readings being reviewed using the document camera at the remote site.

the nearest regional centre for diabetes stabilization and education (the recommended standard option). Immediate medical advice was given via telephone, and a videoconference consultation involving the patient, family, local clinicians and specialist was arranged.

Diabetes education for patients and staff

Education sessions for four rural or remote children with newly diagnosed diabetes were reported by Smith *et al.*[35] Instead of travelling to the nearest regional or tertiary centre for diabetes education, the diabetes nurse educator and dietician presented a series of teaching modules to the patient and family via videoconference. Videoconference education sessions for regional diabetes health professional staff also took place. Lectures (60 minutes in duration) were given by the diabetologist to the local paediatrician, junior medical staff and nurses. In addition, multipoint lectures were delivered to a network of diabetes educators throughout Queensland by the staff of the Department of Endocrinology and Diabetes. Each of these sessions lasted 90 minutes and was delivered to between 4 and 12 sites (Fig. 8.4).

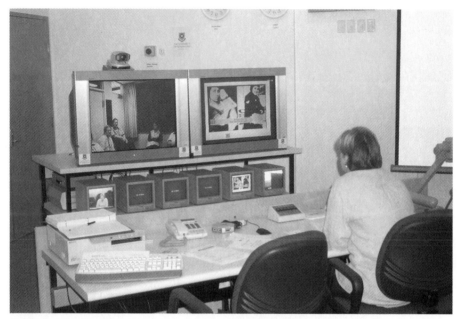

Fig. 8.4 Diabetes nurse educator presenting a lecture by videoconference to staff in a regional hospital.

Case study

S.C. is a 14-year-old girl with type 1 diabetes since the age of 8 years. Coeliac disease was also diagnosed at 10 years of age. She lived with her mother and older brother in a rural town, 5 hours' driving time west of the closest regional paediatric centre and paediatrician and 14 hours from the nearest tertiary diabetes care. Local resources consisted of a small country hospital and a sole local medical officer for the district.

S.C.'s diabetes was characterized by recurrent episodes of life-threatening diabetic ketoacidosis associated with ongoing poor metabolic control and poor adherence to the recommended management regimen. In addition, there was poor compliance with the gluten-free diet for the associated coeliac disease.

A series of multipoint videoconferenced consultations were conducted with the patient, her mother and the local medical officer in the rural hospital, the supervising paediatrician in the regional centre and members of the specialist tertiary diabetes team, including the diabetologist, diabetes educator, dietician and psychologist. One of the consultations also included a paediatric gastroenterologist who counselled the patient and her mother about the need for a gluten-free diet to manage her coeliac disease. Further in-depth sessions were held with the patient, her mother, a local community health nurse and the psychologist from the tertiary centre, during which the complex psychosocial issues underlying the poor metabolic control and adherence were addressed. These sessions continued every two weeks for six months, during which time a gradual improvement in diabetes management was seen, with no further episodes of diabetic ketoacidosis and improved adherence to both the diabetic and gluten-free treatment regimens.

Limitations of telemedicine and diabetes

The limitation of any form of telemedicine is the lack of a direct face-to-face interchange between the patient and the doctor or other health professional. In addition, the ability to perform direct physical examination as part of a medical consultation is lost, and reliance must be placed on the clinician at the remote site.

Despite the obvious practical limitations, however, the use of telemedicine offers exciting new potential ways of improving diabetes care for remote communities or for the individual at home. Merrel (personal communication) recently proposed a set of criteria for assessing whether or not a telemedicine programme is technologically sound. Merrel stated that the elements of a successful telemedicine programme include:

▶ accurate collection of data in a digital format

▶ incorporation of those data into an electronic record that may be transmitted with fidelity

▶ protocols for distant analysis

▶ communication tools to allow effective dialogue among primary managers, patients and consultants.

The application of telemedicine to diabetes could be argued to fulfil all of these criteria.

The future of telemedicine and diabetes

Telemedicine has been used in various forms to improve access to diabetes health professional services. Despite a number of reports of pilot projects in both adult and paediatric diabetes management, at present little evidence shows that telemedical devices or telemedicine guarantee a better long-term outcome or reduce treatment expenses significantly. The challenge for the future is to continue to expand successful pilot programmes and conduct both clinical and health economics research to prove definitively that telemedicine provides sound clinical and economic benefits in diabetes management.

Further information

American Diabetes Association. http://www.diabetes.org (last checked 10 August 2004).
Joslin Diabetes Center. http://www.joslin.harvard.edu (last checked 10 August 2004).

The Diabetes Monitor. http://www.diabetesmonitor.com (last checked 10 August 2004).

Diabetes Portal: Diabetes Living. http://www.diabetesliving.com (last checked 10 August 2004).

Children with diabetes. http://www.childrenwithdiabetes.com (last checked 10 August 2004).

Australian Diabetes Society. http://www.racp.edu.au/ads/ (last checked 10 August 2004).

Australasian Paediatric Endocrine Group. http://www.racp.edu.au/apeg/ (last checked 10 August 2004).

Juvenile Diabetes Research Foundation International. http://www.jdrf.org (last checked 10 August 2004).

Juvenile Diabetes Foundation of Australia. http://www.jdrf.org.au (last checked 10 August 2004).

Diabetes Australia. http://www.diabetesaustralia.com.au (last checked 10 August 2004).

References

1 Diabetes Control and Complications Trial Research Group. The effect of intensive treatment of diabetes on the development and progression of long-term complications in insulin-dependent diabetes mellitus. *New England Journal of Medicine* 1993; **329**: 977–986.

2 International Society for Paediatric and Adolescent Diabetes. *ISPAD Consensus Guidelines for the Management of Type 1 Diabetes Mellitus in Children and Adolescents.* Netherlands: Medforum; 2000. http://www.medforum.nl/ispad_consensus_guidelines.htm (last checked 14 August 2004).

3 American Diabetes Association. Standards of medical care for patients with diabetes mellitus. *Diabetes Care* 2003; **26** (suppl. 1): 33–50.

4 Bloomfield S, Farquhar JW. Is a specialist paediatric diabetic clinic better? *Archives of Disease in Childhood* 1990; **65**: 139–140.

5 Zgibor JC, Songer TJ, Kelsey SF, *et al.* The association of diabetes specialist care with health care practices and glycemic control in patients with type 1 diabetes: a cross-sectional analysis from the Pittsburgh epidemiology of diabetes complications study. *Diabetes Care* 2000; **23**: 472–476.

6 Zgibor JC, Songer TJ, Kelsey SF, *et al.* Influence of health care providers on the development of diabetes complications: long-term follow-up from the Pittsburgh Epidemiology of Diabetes Complications Study. *Diabetes Care* 2002; **25**: 1584–1590.

7 Craig J. Introduction. In *Introduction to Telemedicine.* Craig J, Wootton R, eds. London: Royal Society of Medicine Press; 1999.

8 Kim HS, Oh JA. Adherence to diabetes control recommendations: impact of nurse telephone calls. *Journal of Advanced Nursing* 2003; **44**: 256–261.

9 Biermann E, Dietrich W, Rihl J, Standl E. Are there time and cost savings by using telemanagement for patients on intensified insulin therapy? A randomised, controlled trial. *Computer Methods and Programs in Biomedicine* 2002; **69**: 137–146.

10 Wojcicki JM, Ladyzynski P, Krzymien J, *et al.* What we can really expect from telemedicine in intensive diabetes treatment: results from 3-year study on type 1 pregnant diabetic women. *Diabetes Technology and Therapeutics* 2001; **3**: 581–589.

11 Bellazzi R, Arcelloni M, Bensa G, *et al.* Design, methods, and evaluation directions of a multi-access service for the management of diabetes mellitus patients. *Diabetes Technology and Therapeutics* 2003; **5**: 621–629.

12 d'Annunzio G, Bellazzi R, Larizza C, *et al.* Telemedicine in the management of young patients with type 1 diabetes mellitus: a follow-up study. *Acta Bio-medica de L'Ateneo Parmense* 2003; **74** (suppl. 1): 49–55.

13   Cherry JC, Moffatt TP, Rodriguez C, Dryden K. Diabetes disease management program for an indigent population empowered by telemedicine technology. *Diabetes Technology and Therapeutics* 2002; **4**: 783–791.

14   Bailey TS. How to communicate home blood glucose monitoring more effectively: a low-tech fax solution to a common diabetes data management dilemma. *Clinical Diabetes* 1999; **17**: 85–86.

15   Perlemuter L, Yomotov B. Feasibility and usefulness of dedicated software and e-mail for self-monitoring blood glucose in treating diabetes. *Diabetic Medicine* 2002; **19**: 697–703.

16   Henault RG, Eugenio KR, Kelliher AF, *et al.* Transmitting clinical recommendations for diabetes care via e-mail. *American Journal of Health-System Pharmacy* 2002; **59**: 2166–2169.

17   Chase HP, Pearson JA, Wightman C, *et al.* Modem transmission of glucose values reduces the costs and need for clinic visits. *Diabetes Care* 2003; **26**: 1475–1479.

18   Iafusco D, Ingenito N, Prisco F. The chatline as a communication and educational tool in adolescents with insulin-dependent diabetes: preliminary observations. *Diabetes Care* 2000; **23**:1853.

19   Lehmann ED, Deutsch T, Carson ER, Sonksen PH. AIDA: an interactive diabetes advisor. *Computer Methods and Programs in Biomedicine* 1994; **41**: 183–203.

20   Lehmann ED. Why people download the freeware AIDA v4.3a diabetes software program: a proof-of-concept semi-automated analysis. *Diabetes Technology and Therapeutics* 2003; **5**: 477–490.

21   Lehmann ED. Who is downloading the free AIDA v4.3a interactive educational diabetes software? A 1-year survey of 3864 downloads. *Diabetes Technology and Therapeutics* 2003; **5**: 879–890.

22   Boukhors Y, Rabasa-Lhoret R, Langelier H, *et al.* The use of information technology for the management of intensive insulin therapy in type 1 diabetes mellitus. *Diabetes and Metabolism* 2003; **29**: 619–627.

23   Cavan DA, Everett J, Plougmann S, Hejlesen OK. Use of the Internet to optimize self-management of type 1 diabetes: preliminary experience with DiasNet. *Journal of Telemedicine and Telecare* 2003; **9** (suppl. 1): 50–52.

24   Hejlesen OK, Andreassen S, Hovorka R, Cavan DA. DIAS – the diabetes advisory system: an outline of the system and the evaluation results obtained so far. *Computer Methods and Programs in Biomedicine* 1997; **54**: 49–58.

25   McKay HG, Feil EG, Glasgow RE, Brown JE. Feasibility and use of an internet support service for diabetes self-management. *Diabetes Educator* 1998; **24**: 174–179.

26   Kim MI, Ladenson PW. Hot topic: diabetes on the internet: resources for patients *Journal of Clinical Endocrinology and Metabolism* 2002; **87**: 3523–3526.

27   Berland GK, Elliott MN, Morales LS, *et al.* Health information on the internet: accessibility, quality and readability in English and Spanish. *Journal of the American Medical Association* 2001; **285**: 2612–2621.

28   Fallis D, Fricke M. Indicators of accuracy of consumer health information on the Internet: a study of indicators relating to information for managing fever in children in the home. *Journal of the American Medical Informatics Association* 2002; **9**: 73–79.

29   Kusec S, Brborovic O, Schillinger D. Diabetes websites accredited by the Health On the Net Foundation Code of Conduct: readable or not? *Studies in Health Technology and Informatics* 2003; **95**: 655–660.

30   Radjenovic D, Wallace FL. Computer-based remote diabetes education for school personnel. *Diabetes Technology and Therapeutics* 2001; **3**: 601–607.

31   Pirisi A. Can a supercomputer help doctors manage patients? American Diabetes Association hopes online computer consultant will improve diabetes care. *Lancet* 2003; **362**: 452–453.

32   Demiris G, Speedie S, Finkelstein S, Harris I. Communication patterns and technical quality of virtual visits in home care. *Journal of Telemedicine and Telecare* 2003; **9**: 210–215.

33   Gelfand K, Geffken G, Halsey-Lyda M, *et al.* Intensive telehealth management of five at-risk adolescents with diabetes. *Journal of Telemedicine and Telecare* 2003; **9**: 117–121.

34   Malasanos T. The Florida initiative in telehealth and education. *Journal of Telemedicine and Telecare* 2003; **9** (suppl. 2): 87.

35   Smith AC, Batch J, Lang E, Wootton R. The use of online health techniques to assist with the delivery of specialist paediatric diabetes services in Queensland. *Journal of Telemedicine and Telecare* 2003; **9** (suppl. 2): 54–57.

36   Starren J, Hripcsak G, Sengupta S, *et al.* Columbia University's Informatics for Diabetes Education and Telemedicine (IDEATel) Project: technical implementation. *Journal of the American Medical Informatics Association* 2002; **9**: 25–36.

37   Shea S, Starren J, Weinstock RS, *et al.* Columbia University's Informatics for Diabetes Education and Telemedicine (IDEATel) Project: rationale and design. *Journal of the American Medical Informatics Association* 2002; **9**: 49–62.

38   Abrahamian H, Schueller A, Mauler H, *et al.* Transfer of knowledge from the specialist to the generalist by videoconferencing: effect on diabetes care. *Journal of Telemedicine and Telecare* 2002; **8**: 350–355.

39   Izquierdo RE, Knudson PE, Meyer S, *et al.* A comparison of diabetes education administered through telemedicine versus in person. *Diabetes Care* 2003; **26**: 1002–1007.

40   Shiba T, Yamamoto T, Seki U, *et al.* Screening and follow-up of diabetic retinopathy using a new mosaic 9-field fundus photography system. *Diabetes Research and Clinical Practice.* 2002; **55**: 49–59.

41   Smith AC, Isles A, McCrossin R, *et al.* The point-of-referral barrier – a factor in the success of telehealth. *Journal of Telemedicine and Telecare* 2001; **7** (suppl. 2): 75–78.

42   Smith AC, Williams M, Van der Westhuyzen J, *et al.* A comparison of telepaediatric activity at two regional hospitals in Queensland. *Journal of Telemedicine and Telecare* 2002; **8** (suppl. 3): 58–62.

▶9

Telemedicine Applications in the Management of Asthma

Michael J Romano

Introduction

In many ways, asthma is the perfect application for telemedicine. Asthma affects a large number of people. The prevalence of asthma in Australia is 14.7% and in the US 10.9%.[1] Several studies have shown that asthma care provided by specialists results in better outcomes than care provided by non-specialists.[2,3] Finally, the diagnosis and management of asthma relies heavily on symptom history and measurements of lung function. The physical examination consists primarily of auscultation and inspection – techniques that are easily accomplished with telemedicine – and electronic transmission of pulmonary function measures is also possible.

Telemedicine provides the potential to provide care shown to improve clinical outcomes to a large population with a high prevalence of disease. This chapter reviews the key components of asthma care and highlights how they have been applied via telemedicine.

Comprehensive asthma care

A number of national and international guidelines for the diagnosis and management of asthma have been published, including the Global Initiative for Asthma, the National Expert Panel Report 2 (US) and the National Asthma Handbook 2002 (Australia). These documents are remarkably similar in the key aspects of long-term asthma control, which include patient education on avoiding asthma triggers, symptom recognition and long-term management strategies; establishing an individual plan for managing a patient's asthma; measurement of lung function; and regular follow-up care. Certain of these components – such as education, symptom recognition and regular follow-up care – are not unique to asthma, and it is reasonable to generalize their feasibility from successes with other traditional targets of disease management such as diabetes or hypertension. Other components, including individualized treatment plans, training in and maintenance of inhaler technique, and measurement of lung function, are specific to asthma care.

Measurement of lung function is a potentially important application of telemedicine. Relatively few general practitioners have ready access to spirometry in their offices or are skilled in the subtleties of interpreting the data obtained. The feasibility of obtaining spirometry data in a patient's home and transmitting the information to a central site has been shown using telephone lines,[4] personal computers[5] and an early-generation handheld computer.[6] A key issue with peak flow monitoring and spirometry is that they are effort-dependent manoeuvres. Obtaining maximum effort, particularly with children, frequently needs coaching. Finkelstein *et al* showed the validity of home spirometry in a small number of adults.[7] No data have been published about the validity of home pulmonary function measures in children. There should be no particular obstacle, however, as observation of effort and coaching could be provided through a real-time video and audio link.

Current guidelines in the US recommend inhaled corticosteroids (ICS) as the preferred first-line treatment in persistent asthma.[8] Instruction in the appropriate use of metered dose inhalers (MDIs) and dry powder inhalers is essential to their successful use. Patients frequently report never having received instructions or are seen to be using them incorrectly. Bynum *et al* studied the effect of telemedicine compared with written instruction on eight discrete steps for correct MDI technique in a group of rural school students.[9] Compared to the group receiving written instruction, the telemedicine instruction group achieved higher scores immediately after training and better maintained these skills at a 2–4-week follow-up visit.

Comprehensive care models

There are few descriptions of comprehensive care models of asthma delivered via telemedicine. Chan *et al* evaluated a hybrid asthma care delivery model combining periodic face-to-face evaluations by a paediatric respiratory physician and twice-weekly evaluations of inhaler technique, peak flow meter utilization and symptom diary review.[10] The data were transmitted with a store-and-forward technique. Patients were randomized to receive their asthma education in person or via an educational website. The authors found no differences in clinically important markers of asthma care. Peak flow rate as a percentage of personal best increased in both groups to a similar extent, as did inhaler technique scores, and there were no differences in caregiver or patient quality of life scores between groups. A disadvantage of this model was that it required patients to come to the clinic to receive the medical component of their care.

We have evaluated the feasibility of providing all aspects of medical care via telemedicine.[11] Seventeen schoolchildren in rural West Texas were followed for 24 weeks in a school-based health clinic (SBHC). All participants already had access to primary care paediatrics on site in the SBHC. The school nurse received specific training on the National Institutes for Health (NIH) guidelines,[12] spirometry, peak flow and inhaler technique, and in obtaining targeted symptom histories. The school nurse provided onsite training and retraining in inhaler and peak flow meter usage, as necessary, and encouraged completion of symptom diaries (Fig. 9.1). Participants were given a vinyl mattress and pillow wraps. After a face-to-face evaluation with the study's physician at study entry, patients were evaluated via a telemedicine link from the clinic at 4, 12 and 24 weeks. Before each visit, the school nurse obtained a symptom history and drug record, and reviewed the patient's inhaler technique and spirometry. The medical component of each follow-up visit included a review of these data, including visual inspection of the spirometry flow–volume loops, auscultation of the lungs and inspection of the nasal mucosa. Ongoing education was provided by the physician during the telemedicine evaluations and offline by the school nurse.

The participants showed significant improvements in clinically important measures of asthma management, including an 83% increase in mean number of symptom-free days and a 44% reduction in mean daily symptom scores. Significant improvements in quality of life were reported by caregivers and patients at study completion. These improvements were seen in a population that already had access to primary care paediatrics and showed the role of telemedicine to deliver specialty asthma care.

Using telemedicine to enhance compliance

Compliance with prescribed treatment plans is an essential step in the effective management of any chronic disease, including asthma. Several concepts have been proposed as a means of enhancing compliance, including patient education and simplification of treatment regimens and reminder systems. Reminder systems typically involve telephone or postal contact. Several reviews have suggested some improvement in clinic attendance with appointment reminders but variable results in terms of drug adherence.[13,14] Telemedicine, in its broadest sense, would obviously include web-based interventions as well as paging and wireless communication modes. Finkelstein *et al* provided preliminary data showing that a comprehensive asthma care model using a handheld device linked to a central computer with nurse support enhances compliance.[15] Erickson has described a non-randomized pilot study evaluating the effect of a series of patient-specific messages related to asthma care delivered to their pagers.[16] Clinically meaningful increases in compliance with oral and inhaled drug usage were found over the 30-day study period.

Moving towards effective primary care

Despite the existence of national and international practice guidelines, incorporation of these guidelines into general practice remains low. A full discussion of the factors that affect incorporation of practice guidelines is beyond the scope of this chapter. Two recent articles summarize factors that affect adoption of clinical guidelines in general and in asthma specifically.[17,18] Physician compliance with practice guidelines can be described as encompassing three steps: knowledge of the relevant guidelines, acceptance of the guidelines leading to a change in physician attitude and a resultant change in physician behaviour. Strategies to enhance provider compliance must recognize that internal and external constraints may limit provider compliance with guidelines, even though there is acceptance of the guidelines 'in theory'.

Telemedicine may provide opportunities to enhance compliance with national asthma guidelines at multiple points. Certainly, education about guidelines can be

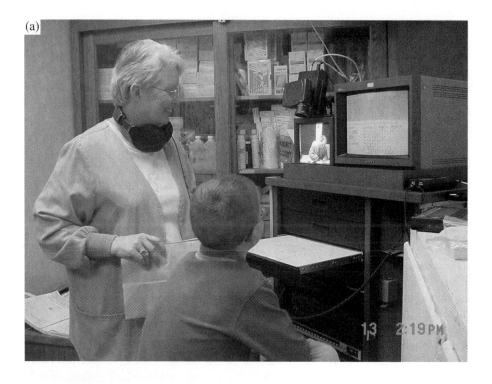

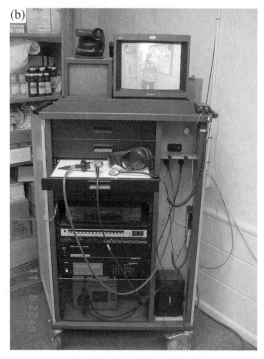

Fig. 9.1 (a) School nurse in the Hart School health clinic demonstrating the telemedicine system to a patient. (b) The telemedicine equipment, including otoscope and stethoscope.

provided via telemedicine. Enhancing acceptance of guidelines is somewhat more challenging, as it is clear that providers differ in how they react to new information and incorporate it into their practice.[19] In this respect, telemedicine may provide an opportunity to model general practitioners' behaviour by allowing them to 'sit in' with the specialist during a consultation The specialist may serve as a mentor, via telemedicine, to the generalist. Telemedicine could conceivably remove some external barriers to adoption of national asthma guidelines. Training in and periodic validation of inhaler technique could be accomplished via telemedicine with a dedicated, well-trained, centrally located nurse, pharmacist or respiratory therapist, thereby removing one obstacle to general practitioner prescription of inhaled corticosteroids as a first-line therapy.

Research opportunities in asthma telemedicine

Telephone delivery of educational voice messages showed efficacy across a wide spectrum of content delivery methods.[14] Children and young adults are very accepting of electronic communication, including email, voice mail and instant messaging. The widespread familiarity with and availability of these communication formats provides opportunities to improve patient education and training and enhance compliance. Can automated email, instant messaging or wireless transmissions to a personal data assistant reminding a patient to take their drugs improve compliance and outcomes? Ultimately, long-term, large-scale, outcome-based studies will be needed to define the role of telemedicine in the care of patients with asthma.[20]

Conclusion

Asthma represents a unique opportunity to employ telemedicine. The challenges of attacking disease with high prevalence, significant morbidity and a wide age spectrum are balanced by the availability of highly effective, relatively straightforward treatment options. The successful use of telemedicine is likely to involve multiple strategies based on individual assessments of barriers to current best practice and then application of telemedicine based on the local needs of both provider and patient.

References

1 Masoli M, Fabian D, Holt S, Beasley R. *Global Burden of Asthma*. http://www.ginasthma.com (last checked 8 June 2004).
2 Asthma care specialists improve outcomes. *Healthcare Benchmarks* 1999; **6**: 76–78.
3 Diette GB, Skinner EA, Nguyen TT, *et al*. Comparison of quality of care by specialist and generalist physicians as usual source of asthma care for children. *Pediatrics* 2001; **108**: 432–437.
4 Bruderman I, Abboud S. Telespirometry: novel system for home monitoring of asthmatic patients. *Telemedicine Journal* 1997; **3**: 127–133.
5 Steel S, Lock S, Johnson N, *et al*. A feasibility study of remote monitoring of asthmatic patients. *Journal of Telemedicine and Telecare* 2002; **8**: 290–296.

6   Finkelstein J, Hripcsak G, Cabrera M. Telematic system for monitoring of asthma severity in patients' homes. *Medinfo* 1998; **9**: 272–276.

7   Finkelstein J, Cabrera MR, Hripcsak G. Internet-based home asthma telemonitoring: can patients handle the technology? *Chest* 2000; **117**: 148–155.

8   *The NAEPP Expert Panel Report: Guidelines for the Diagnosis and Management of Asthma – Update on Selected Topics 2002 (EPR – Update 2002).* Bethesda, MD: National Heart, Lung, and Blood Institute; 2002. National Institutes of Health Publication no. 02-5075.

9   Bynum A, Hopkins D, Thomas A, *et al.* The effect of telepharmacy counseling on metered-dose inhaler technique among adolescents with asthma in rural Arkansas. *Telemedicine Journal and e-Health* 2001; **7**: 207–217.

10   Chan DS, Callahan CW, Sheets SJ, *et al.* An Internet-based store-and-forward video home telehealth system for improving asthma outcomes in children. *American Journal of Health-System Pharmacy* 2003; **60**: 1976–1981.

11   Romano MJ, Hernandez J, Gaylor A, *et al.* Improvement in asthma symptoms and quality of life in pediatric patients through specialty care delivered via telemedicine. *Telemedicine Journal and e-Health* 2001; **7**: 281–286.

12   *Guidelines for the Diagnosis and Management of Asthma.* Bethesda, MD: National Heart, Lung, and Blood Institute; 1997. National Institutes of Health Publication no. 97-4051.

13   Bennett JW, Glasziou PP. Computerised reminders and feedback in medication management: a systematic review of randomised controlled trials. *Medical Journal of Australia* 2003; **178**: 217–222.

14   Krishna S, Balas EA, Boren SA, Maglaveras N. Patient acceptance of educational voice messages: a review of controlled clinical studies. *Methods of Information in Medicine* 2002; **41**: 360–369.

15   Finkelstein J, O'Connor G, Friedmann RH. Development and implementation of the home asthma telemonitoring (HAT) system to facilitate asthma self-care. *Medinfo* 2001; **10**: 810–814.

16   Erickson SR, Ascione FJ, Kirking DM, Johnson CE. Use of a paging system to improve medication self-management in patients with asthma. *Journal of the American Pharmaceutical Association* 1998; **38**: 767–769.

17   Cabana MD, Rand CS, Powe NR, *et al.* Why don't physicians follow clinical practice guidelines? A framework for improvement. *Journal of the American Medical Association* 1999; **282**: 1458–1465.

18   Cabana MD, Ebel BE, Cooper-Patrick L, *et al.* Barriers pediatricians face when using asthma practice guidelines. *Archives of Pediatrics and Adolescent Medicine* 2000; **154**: 685–693.

19   Wyszewianski L, Green LA. Strategies for changing clinicians' practice patterns. A new perspective. *Journal of Family Practice* 2000; **49**: 461–464.

20   Wainright C, Wootton R. A review of telemedicine and asthma. *Disease Management and Health Outcomes* 2003; **11**: 557–563.

▶10

Post-acute Burns Care for Children

Roy Kimble and Anthony C Smith

Introduction

The only tertiary paediatric burns centre in Queensland, the Stuart Pegg Paediatric Burns Centre (SPPBC), is located in the southeast corner of the state. The centre treats approximately 400 new burns patients per year and there are 1300 outpatient attendances annually. The outpatient department runs a multidisciplinary service that includes burns surgeons, nursing staff, physiotherapists, occupational therapists and social workers. The number and frequency of the outpatient appointments needed for each patient depend on the severity of the injury and treatment requirements. Outpatient follow-up may continue for several years.

Queensland is a large state with a population of about four million people and a land area seven times greater than that of Great Britain. Queensland also has the highest ratio of people living outside the major city of any Australian state. Thus a conventional outpatient appointment will often involve a long journey by road, rail or air. This results in major upheaval for the family concerned in terms of lost wages, absence from school and additional living expenses.[1] It is also costly for the health service, which pays for the travel and accommodation. Not surprisingly, non-attendance because of the inconvenience is common.

The concept of using telemedicine for the delivery of emergency and post-acute care is not new. Some experience has been reported in the literature – but mainly in adult burns telemedicine. This confirms that online communication techniques, such as videoconferencing and email, can be used for a proportion of the long-term management of patients after a burn injury.

Most reports have related to short-term pilot studies. In 1999, an American study reported that videoconferencing could be used to link regional patients with specialists in the burns centre. It was reported, however, that telemedicine consultations were convenient for the patient but more time consuming for the specialists.[2] In a separate American study reported in 2002, the satisfaction of patients and specialists involved in burns telemedicine sessions was reported to be very high, and the methods used were described as appropriate for diagnosis and clinical management.[3]

There seems to be little previous experience of telemedicine for paediatric burns patients.

Telepaediatric burns services

Telepaediatric services for children in Queensland started in November 2000 as part of a university-led research project run by the Centre for Online Health (University of Queensland).[4] The burns team at the SPPBC was encouraged to trial the use of videoconferencing as a method of reviewing patients. As a consequence of this trial, a routine programme of telepaediatric burns clinics has been integrated into the existing outpatient service.

Eligibility

The trial was not designed to deal with the acute phase of treatment for a burns injury. In our experience, patients who are post-acute are best suited for the telepaediatric service, as they require no dressing changes. Children who need minor dressing changes that can be done at home or at the local healthcare facility are also suitable. To be eligible, a patient needs to live at least two hours by road from the tertiary burns centre.

Equipment

Standard commercial videoconferencing equipment is adequate for telepaediatric burns follow-up. The bandwidth for most consultations has been 128 kbit/s because of the restricted number of ISDN lines available in the regional and remote parts of Queensland. Four sites had access to three ISDN lines, allowing a bandwidth of 384 kbit/s. High resolution digital still images are sent occasionally via email for review by the burns team or as a secondary resource during the videoconference.[5] Still photographs can be printed during the videoconference with a colour video printer and stored in the hospital records.

Personnel

In order for the consultation to equate to that performed in the conventional burns clinic, a multidisciplinary team has to be assembled for each videoconference (Fig. 10.1). This includes a burns surgeon, a burns nurse, a physiotherapist and an occupational therapist. It can often be difficult to assemble a full team, but there should be at least a surgeon, nurse and occupational therapist present, with feedback to the other members of the team as necessary. Although social workers are often present in the conventional face-to-face clinic, they have felt unable to participate in group telemedicine sessions, as this would be considered a breach of confidentiality.

At the remote end are the child, the parent(s) and a healthcare worker. The healthcare worker is usually the local occupational therapist or, less often, a nurse. Occasionally a local doctor will attend.

Clinical examination

During each appointment, the staff from the SPPBC discuss with the patient and family any concerns about treatment and progress. They also consult with local staff to decide jointly on the appropriate management, including changes to dressing requirements or the need for follow-up surgery. When connected via videoconference, the camera can

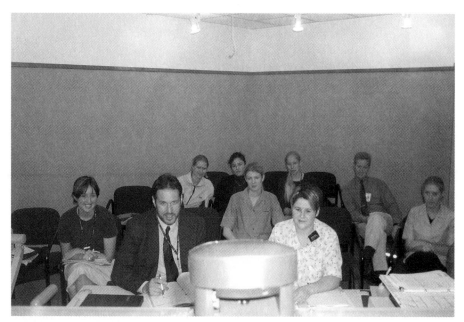

Fig. 10.1. Videoconference session in progress. Telepaediatric consultations are multi-disciplinary and involve medical, nursing and allied health staff.

be used for close up images (Fig. 10.2). Depending on the available bandwidth and the child's ability to remain still, most images obtained are perfectly satisfactory for assessing the condition of the injury. If high-quality images are required, digital images can be sent via email – either before or after the consultation (Fig. 10.3).

Coordination of the clinics

Consultations are held 15 minutes apart, and a clinic may include as many as eight patients from different centres. The coordination of telepaediatric burns consultations is a dual task shared by the telepaediatric service and staff from the SPPBC. The telepaediatric service is responsible for booking the equipment at each of the required sites throughout the state. The coordination of bookings and consultation with regional staff is performed by the burns liaison nurse along with the burns outpatient clerk. This is a critical and demanding role, which can be time-consuming, requiring multiple phone calls to healthcare workers and families. With experience, this has become less arduous, and we have now employed a part-time occupational therapist to coordinate these clinics with the aid of the clinic clerk. Appointments are made at the time of the previous consultation up to one year in advance. A letter to the parents is sent by post and telephone calls are made one month and one week before the appointment to ensure that attendance remains high. The healthcare worker accompanying the family is notified by email one month before the appointment. Clinics are currently held at a rate of five per month, with 2–8 patients seen per clinic.

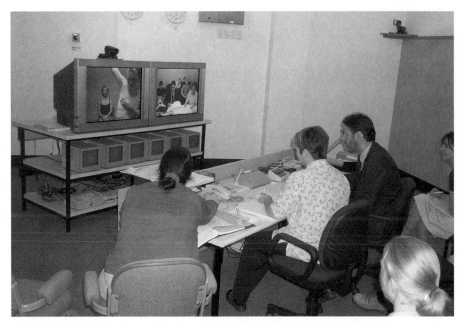

Fig. 10.2. Examination of a burn injury via videoconference.

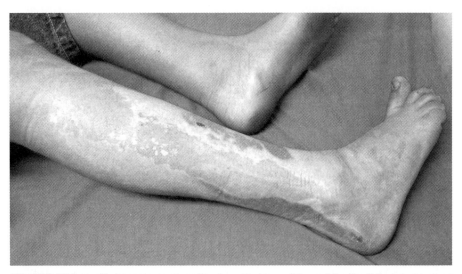

Fig. 10.3. High-quality images are occasionally sent via email to assist with clinical assessment decisions.

Predicted problems

The burns team was originally pessimistic about how a teleconsultation would compare to a conventional face-to-face appointment. The problems that were predicted related to difficulties with the technology at both ends, poor quality images and the obvious inability to examine the children physically. It was also expected to be difficult to get the patient and personnel at both sites to be present at the same time. Even if all these potential problems were solved, the question remained whether or not the service would be acceptable as a means of following-up a paediatric burns patient. We felt we had to answer this question from the perspectives of both clinical reliability and patient satisfaction.

A review of service activity

During the first three years of operation, a total of 293 patient consultations were facilitated via videoconference.[6] Videoconference consultations involved links to 31 regional and remote hospitals situated throughout Queensland (Fig. 10.4). The main application involved routine follow-up for children treated at the centre. Twelve consultations were also performed on an ad hoc basis. The burns team reviewed new burn injuries and provided advice about treatment – or interim management if transfer to the tertiary centre was deemed necessary. Occasionally during the videoconference, the need for surgery was identified. The consultant was then able to discuss this procedure with the child and family and negotiate a timeframe that suited the family. The median distance between the centre and remote site was 640 km (interquartile range 350–1180 km). During the three-year period, a total of 78 hours were spent providing clinical consultations via videoconference. Since the service began, the number of consultations per year has almost tripled from 55 in 2001 to 145 in 2003.[6]

Patient satisfaction (family and patient satisfaction)

To obtain feedback on the service, we performed a patient satisfaction survey. Within one week of a specialist appointment via videoconference, 55 families were contacted and invited to answer a series of questions about their level of satisfaction. The overall feedback was very positive for each of the categories assessed (Table 10.1). Picture and sound quality during the videoconference was adequate, with most of the families agreeing that they could see the specialist easily (95%) and that they had no difficulty hearing the specialist (95%). Ninety-six percent of families agreed that they were able to say everything that they wanted to during the consultation. Very few families (6%) agreed that the videoconference (ie the television camera) made them uncomfortable and even fewer (2%) were worried that others might have been listening during the consultation. Eighty-seven percent of families agreed that the videoconference appointment saved them money and time, and 82% agreed that the videoconference saved them stress. Most families (87%) agreed that they were confident that their child's condition could be sorted out via videoconference.

Is videoconferencing as reliable as a face-to-face consultation?

This question had to be answered to make sure that quality of care was not being compromised. We wanted to compare the agreement of clinical assessments

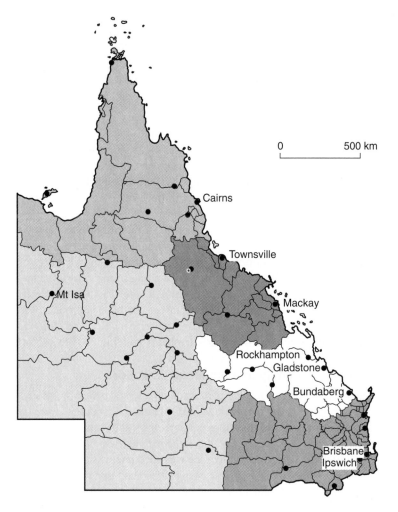

Fig. 10.4. During the first three years, telepaediatric burns services were provided to 31 sites throughout Queensland.

conducted via videoconference with assessments conducted in the conventional manner (face-to-face). A total of 35 children were involved in a research trial, all of whom required an outpatient appointment at the specialist centre for a previous burn injury.[7] A series of three consecutive appointments were facilitated for each child. The first was conducted by a consultant in the outpatients department (face-to-face). The additional appointments were conducted by a second consultant who reviewed the patient via videoconference followed by a review in person. Clinical assessments of scar appearance, scar thickening, contractures, range of motion, activity level, breakdowns and adequacy of the consultation were compared in each

Table 10.1. Satisfaction with consultations conducted via videoconference (n = 55)

Questions	Patient's response (%)					
	Strongly agree	Agree	Neutral	Disagree	Strongly disagree	Don't know
I could see the specialist clearly	67	27	2	2	2	0
I had trouble hearing what was being said	2	4	0	22	73	0
I was able to say what I wanted	58	38	4	0	0	0
I was worried that others may have been listening	0	2	4	33	62	0
The TV camera made me feel uncomfortable	0	5	4	29	62	0
The appointment saved me money	60	27	7	0	0	5
The appointment saved me time	60	27	9	0	0	4
The appointment saved me stress	53	29	13	2	0	0
I was confident that my condition could be sorted out via videoconference	44	44	11	2	0	0
The appointment was not as good as a face-to-face appointment	4	13	35	42	7	0

patient. Levels of agreement were measured first for two independent consultants, both seeing each patient in person, and second for one consultant seeing each patient in person and then seeing the same patient via videoconference. For both groups, the concordance results were almost identical. This study confirmed that the quality of information collected during a videoconference appointment is comparable with that from appointments traditionally conducted in person.[7] Despite the comparable levels of agreement, the consultants reported that the colour of a scar seen by videoconference was difficult to ascertain. In future, colour cards may be a useful resource for clinical assessment.

Conclusions

Telemedicine is a feasible method for the delivery of post-acute burns care. Telemedicine is a useful alternative to face-to-face consultations for outpatient follow-up, although it is accepted that some patients will still need to travel on occasions to the specialist burns centre for surgical intervention and more comprehensive examination. Communication between local clinicians and specialists via videoconference is useful for emergency presentations as it allows provision of interim advice and assessment pending transfer to the tertiary centre. Families involved in a consultation are very satisfied with this method of health service delivery. The quality of information collected during a videoconference appointment is comparable with that from appointments traditionally conducted in person. Our experience has confirmed that videoconferencing is an effective method for the delivery of specialist burns services to clinicians and families living in rural and remote areas of Queensland.

Further information

Australian and New Zealand Burn Association. http://www.anzba.org.au/ (last checked 4 August 2004).

American Burn Association. http://www.ameriburn.org/ (last checked 4 August 2004).

Burns – Journal of the International Society for Burn Injuries. http://www.elsevier.com/wps/find/journaldescription.cws_home/30394/description ?navopenmenu=-2 (last checked 4 August 2004).

Journal of Burn Care and Rehabilitation. Journal of the American Burn Association. http://www.burncarerehab.com/pt/re/jburncr/home.htm;jsessionid=AOZ0j0I7rBl8 gsJNwdtUfrLSHAGKn5zJ5luSpzr4SiqR5BZ6i571!1032750822!- 949856031!9001!-1 (last checked 4 August 2004).

References

1   Smith AC, Youngberry K, Christie F, *et al*. The family costs of attending hospital outpatient appointments via videoconference and in person. *Journal of Telemedicine and Telecare* 2003; **9** (suppl. 2): 58–61.

2   Massman NJ, Dodge JD, Fortman KK, *et al*. Burns follow-up: an innovative application of telemedicine. *Journal of Telemedicine and Telecare* 1999; **5** (suppl. 1): 52–54.

3   Redlick F, Roston B, Gomez M, Fish JS. An initial experience with telemedicine in follow-up burn care. *Journal of Burn Care and Rehabilitation* 2002; **23**: 110–115.

4   Smith AC, Isles A, McCrossin R, *et al*. The point of referral barrier – a factor in the success of telehealth, *Journal of Telemedicine and Telecare* 2001; **7** (suppl. 2): 75–78.

5   Smith AC, Kairl J, Kimble R. Post-acute care for a paediatric burns patient in regional Queensland. *Journal of Telemedicine and Telecare* 2002; **8**: 302–304.

6   Smith AC, Youngberry K, Mill J, *et al*. A review of three years experience using email and videoconferencing for the delivery of post-acute burns care to children in Queensland. *Burns* 2004; **30**: 248–252.

7   Smith AC, Kimble R, Mill J, *et al*. Diagnostic accuracy of and patient satisfaction with telemedicine for the follow-up of paediatric burns patients. *Journal of Telemedicine and Telecare* 2004; **10**: 193–198.

▶11

Telemedicine in Paediatric Surgery

Grant G Miller

Introduction

Although telecommunications have been used in medicine for decades, it was not until the 1980s that advances in telecommunications and information technology made telemedicine practicable. In the 1990s, healthcare administrations began to expand their service delivery using telemedicine. In Saskatchewan, Canada, the provincial government recognized the need for improved healthcare services and enhanced practice support in remote areas of the sparsely populated prairie region. In 1999, they sponsored a one-year pilot project – the Northern Telehealth Network – costing $1.65 million. The telemedicine project was designed to improve service and support to seven northern communities. The network included one university hospital (tertiary care), two regional hospitals (secondary care), three community hospitals (primary care) and two remote nursing stations. The pilot project led to the creation of Telehealth Saskatchewan, with expanded coverage to central and southern parts of the province through the addition of four more sites. All sites are similarly equipped with a mobile workstation designed around a personal computer-based videoconferencing unit (Fig. 11.1). Telecommunication uses ISDN lines at 384 kbit/s or Switch-56 lines at 336 kbit/s. The videoconferencing camera has a 12 times zoom, with autofocus, pan and tilt features.

Initially, the project involved child psychiatry, dermatology, medical/nursing education, patient education, orthopaedic/trauma consultations with radiology support and obstetric consultations with ultrasound support. Subsequently, the list was expanded to include paediatric general surgery. The objectives were to:

▶ improve access to health services and providers for residents of rural and remote areas of the province

▶ enhance rural practice support

▶ improve access to specialists and other healthcare providers

▶ encourage optimum use of specialist personnel and resources in the province

▶ provide continuing education for healthcare providers

▶ provide health information and education to patients and the public

▶ improve patient outcomes through improved access to health services in urgent or emergency cases.

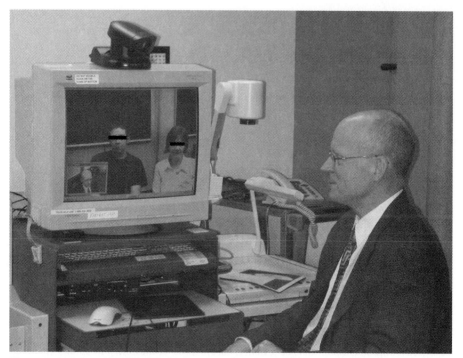

Fig. 11.1. A teleconsultation with a family using a telemedicine mobile workstation.

In paediatric surgery, telemedicine has been used primarily for consulting, including both preoperative assessment and postoperative follow-up. In addition, there has been some more limited experience with telementoring. In other centres, the telemedicine service has been expanded to include teleproctoring and, on a very limited scale, tele-operation.

Teleconsultations

Telemedicine offers a unique opportunity to provide patient-centred care in paediatric surgery. In Saskatchewan, a single paediatric general surgeon serves a population of approximately 1 million people in a vast region. Telemedicine is a natural way of providing patient-centred care. Tertiary paediatric care is focused at one site – a university hospital – that also serves as the primary provider site for the telemedicine network. Teleconsultation clinics for paediatric surgery are conducted one day per month. The surgeon selects patients he deems appropriate for teleconsultation, including follow-up appointments and new consultations, on the basis of information provided by the referring physicians. Families are given the option of being seen in person in the paediatric surgery clinic at the university hospital or by telemedicine at the nearest telemedicine site.

Traditionally, seeing a paediatric surgeon for even minor surgical problems required three visits: one for preoperative assessment, one for operative treatment and one for postoperative reassessment. For caregivers, attendance at these clinic visits can sometimes provide significant challenges in taking time off work, arranging child care and incurring travel and other expenses. For many of the less serious surgical problems, telemedicine can reduce the number of visits that need long distance travel from three to one. Paediatric surgeons are particularly sensitive to the challenges for families and have modified the traditional approach of three visits to try and reduce this burden.

Fitzgerald *et al* reported on their experience without a postoperative follow-up visit for routine paediatric inguinal hernia repairs.[1] They did not have routine follow-up appointments or telephone follow-up. Instead, detailed instructions were provided to families on postoperative discharge, and open access to follow-up was ensured when required. Only 4% of patients who did not have an in-person follow-up appointment wished they had. They concluded that this was as effective as the traditional postoperative clinic visit for patients who had undergone routine inguinal hernia repair. Some surgeons are concerned, however, that without follow-up minor complications might be missed. Furthermore, it is argued that early in a surgeon's career, postoperative clinic visits provide important positive or negative feedback. Practical issues of postoperative care are often discussed, and surgeons can see the results of their work at first hand. Telemedicine provides an alternative method that addresses these issues and is also sensitive to the family needs, particularly where long distances are involved.

Tagge *et al* tried to reduce the traditional three visits to one visit for outpatient paediatric surgical problems in a pilot project.[2] The objective was to improve patient satisfaction and decrease cost for patients with minor surgical problems who had long travel distances to be seen and treated by a paediatric surgeon. They used an initial telephone questionnaire to determine appropriateness for a single visit. Telemedicine provides the opportunity to meet the surgeon, discuss the indications and options for operative treatment, discuss potential complications and expected outcome, begin the consent to treatment process, and carry out preoperative teaching. Although a telephone call might allow the same dialogue, it does not permit the same personal contact or allow both parties to pick up on the non-verbal communication that can be very important in ensuring that the issues discussed are truly understood and that the caregiver is prepared to proceed.

Videoconferencing somewhat restricts the traditional way that physicians evaluate patients. Surgeons who evaluate patients by telemedicine are challenged by a lack of depth perception. However, much as in laparoscopic surgery, surgeons have learned to adapt to the loss of the third dimension. Surgeons have also learned to adapt to the loss of tactile evaluation in laparoscopic surgery. The same challenge is present in clinical consultation by telemedicine. Because they are unable to use percussion and palpation, physicians must rely on a thorough history and on visual examination. Common, relatively minor, surgical problems such as thyroglossal duct cyst (Fig. 11.2) and inguinal hernia (Fig. 11.3) lend themselves to telemedicine assessment. The referring physician often suspects the diagnosis on the basis of the clinical assessment. The history and visual inspection of the problem during teleconsultation are often enough to plan operative treatment. The visual inspection can sometimes be enhanced with the use of a handheld patient assessment camera. This allows the physician to see the area from different angles. Furthermore, the assistance of a skilled nurse at the remote site can be invaluable in demonstrating physical findings, such as the reducibility of an inguinal hernia. With this information, the operative treatment can be scheduled, subject to confirmation by an in-person physical examination on the day of the operation. Using this approach in Saskatchewan, we have had good success and have not had any errors in diagnosis. We have been able to proceed with the planned operative repair as scheduled.

Surgeons, particularly those who treat children, are embracing telemedicine as a way of delivering care. Overall, 63% of 1433 teleconsultations at the Toronto Hospital for Sick Children from 1996–2002 were for surgical problems.[3] However, there are not many reports in the medical literature of telemedicine care in surgical specialties. Endean *et al* compared clinical assessment versus telemedicine assessment by surgeons in patients with vascular problems.[4] Two surgeons were blinded to the other's assessment. One assessed the patient by videoconferencing and the other by standard clinical assessment. They found concordance in 91% of patients regarding their treatment recommendations. They rated their confidence in the telemedicine assessment to the physical examination at 70%, and they concluded that telemedicine

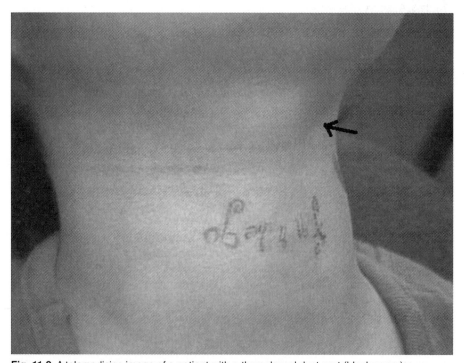

Fig. 11.2. A telemedicine image of a patient with a thyroglossal duct cyst (black arrow).

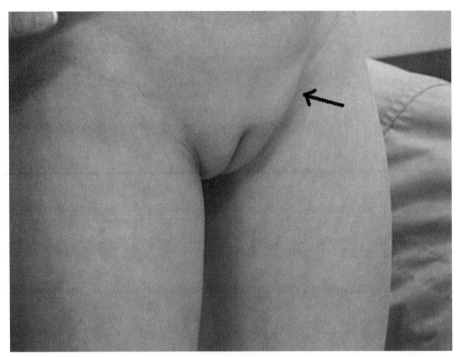

Fig. 11.3. A telemedicine image of a patient with an inguinal hernia (black arrow).

evaluation of vascular patients is as effective as in-person evaluations for a variety of vascular problems. Furthermore, they stressed that important adjuncts to enhance the success of a telemedicine evaluation are physician experience with the technology and the presence of a knowledgeable onsite assistant.

Orthopaedic surgery lends itself to teleconsultation, particularly for fracture management. Emergency nurse practitioners at a minor accident and treatment service in consultation with a hospital-based orthopaedic service were able to save time and prevent the unnecessary transfer of patients to main hospitals.[5] They found the technical quality of most of the consultations to be satisfactory.

Over a 16-month period from January 2000 to April 2001, 45 paediatric patients were seen in the Saskatchewan Paediatric Surgery Telehealth Clinic. The conditions assessed are listed in Table 11.1. We found that the telemedicine consultation often allows more efficient planning of visits to the tertiary healthcare centre. For instance, an infant with a large fluctuant skin-covered neck mass may be suspected of having a cystic hygroma. By seeing the child via telemedicine first, the suspected problem can be discussed with the parents and the appropriate arrangements made for investigations such as ultrasonography or computed tomography under sedation or general anaesthesia. Depending on the availability of resources, these investigations can be performed locally, regionally or coordinated with a clinic visit with the paediatric general surgeon to follow on the same day to discuss the findings and treatment plans.

Table 11.1. Indications for teleconsultation

Reason for referral	Number of patients
Neck masses (eg brachial, thyroglossal duct cyst, cystic hygroma)	14
Inguinal hernia	15
Gastro-oesophageal reflux	6
Other	10
Total	**45**

Patients and caregivers have responded positively to teleconsultations. Harrison *et al* reported that 43 of 45 patients who participated in teleconsultations for a variety of specialties, including paediatrics, otolaryngology and urology, felt that the experience was positive and 84% stated that they would use it again.[6] Dick *et al* reported on participant satisfaction with teleconsultations for a variety of paediatric specialties.[7] They found that 58% felt they were very comfortable with the idea of a teleconsultation before it occurred and 77% after. For the overall experience, 71% expressed complete satisfaction and 94% responded that they would not have preferred to travel to see the specialist. The most significant independent predictors of satisfaction with the experience were perceived comfort of the specialist with seeing the patient by telemedicine, respect for the patient's privacy and comfort with the use of cameras for the examination. In our own experience of teleconsultations for paediatric general surgery, 100% of those surveyed indicated that they would use telemedicine again and 100% indicated that they would recommend it to another person.[8]

Telementoring

Telementoring is a telemedicine technique that involves the remote guidance of a treatment or a procedure where the caregiver has no, or limited, experience of it.[9] This was first reported in 1965 by DeBakey, who transmitted guidance on open heart surgery from the US over a broadband satellite link to surgeons in Europe.[10] In the late 1990s, surgeons began to publish their experiences with telementoring, particularly for laparoscopic procedures being performed by less experienced surgeons at a distance. This typically involves relatively expensive equipment and communication using T1 lines (1.54 Mbit/s), to connect mentoring and operative sites. However, telementoring has also been successful using less sophisticated technology. Successful telementoring has been accomplished internationally, including some experience with mentoring surgeons in lesser industrialized countries. This has been done with personal computer-based systems that use public telephone lines.[11]

We have mainly used telemedicine for mentoring other surgeons performing complex operative procedures. However, we have also used telemedicine to aid physicians at a distance with minor paediatric surgical problems. For example, a five-year-old child with a profound neurodevelopmental defect had a Bard Button Replacement Gastrostomy Device (CR Bard Inc, Billerica, MA US) that became displaced. The family lived in a community 150 km away. The placement of a gastrostomy button is a relatively simple procedure for the experienced clinician but can be intimidating for the inexperienced. The local physician had no experience with such a procedure. In normal circumstances, it would have been necessary to transport the child 150 km to our hospital. With the aid of our telemedicine link, we were able to instruct and successfully guide the local physician through the procedure. Both the child's caregiver and the local physician were very pleased with the use of telemedicine in this instance.

Winnipeg Children's Hospital has also used telementoring to facilitate discharge planning. A small child with extensive burns was to be discharged from the burn unit to their local community hospital. The burn unit nursing staff were able to use telementoring to assist the community hospital nursing staff with burn dressing changes. The patient, family and healthcare providers all benefited from the use of telemedicine.

Teleproctoring

Teleproctoring is the monitoring and evaluation of surgical trainees from a distance and can be used for credentialing purposes and to provide a more uniform standard of care and assessment of skills across hospitals. A caregiver's procedural skills can be assessed and assistance provided for such things as intermittent bladder catheterization, gastrostomy tube changing and tracheostomy tube changing, as well as enterostomal and wound care. This can make assessment of a caregiver's newly acquired skills easier and provide feedback and reassurance to the caregiver. In turn, this benefits the caregiver and can also reduce the frequency of complications and the need for urgent access to hospital care.

In sparsely populated areas such as Saskatchewan, surgical care cannot always be provided by paediatric general surgeons. In these circumstances, general surgeons often provide operative treatment for such routine problems as hypertrophic pyloric stenosis and inguinal hernia repair. Teleproctoring can provide a mechanism whereby a paediatric general surgeon can assist from a distance. This can ensure quality of care and provide important feedback and reassurance to surgeons.

Surgery at a distance

Telesurgery is an exciting development for the technophile surgeon. Robotically mediated telesurgery has made it possible for surgeons to operate while standing at a considerable distance from the operating table without touching or directly seeing the surgical field. This technique is rapidly gaining popularity with the surgical community. The goal is to perform remote procedures on patients with modern surgical skills and thus overcome obstacles of time and distance.

Modern medical robotic telemanipulation systems, such as the da Vinci Surgical System (Intuitive Surgical, Incorporated, Sunnyvale, CA, USA) and the Zeus Surgical

System (Computer Motion, Incorporated, Santa Barbara, CA, USA), allow very precise and controlled movements of surgical instruments guided by a remote surgeon. They have motion scaling and tremor reduction that refine the surgeon's hand movements to enhance the precision of the instruments and reduce trauma to the tissues. Robotic surgical systems have been successfully used to perform telesurgery in both adults and paediatric patients. Usually, this involves the surgeon being in close proximity to the patient. However, in 2001, history was made when a patient in France underwent a laparoscopic cholecystectomy performed by a surgeon in the US using the Zeus robotic system. This required a high-speed network connection with a bandwidth of 10 Mbit/s and a lag time of 155 ms.[12] The da Vinci Surgical System is currently being used in more than 100 hospitals worldwide.

Telepresence surgery is an advanced technique, in which the surgeon directly controls the motion of instruments but also has inputs such as three-dimensional vision, stereophonic sound, tactile and force feedback to create the illusion of actually being present at a remote site. Although there are still many limiting factors, this exciting field has the potential to make surgical expertise available throughout the world, improving patient access and surgical training.

Conclusion

Telemedicine is becoming more readily accessible and affordable, and its various applications are growing rapidly with promising results. It has proved to be very practical and effective in providing patient-centred specialty paediatric care to remote locations. Telemedicine has been reliable for preoperative assessment, preoperative teaching and postoperative follow-up for common surgical problems such as inguinal hernia. It also has utility for the initial assessment of more complex problems, allowing more efficient investigations and planning. Users generally are quite satisfied with the teleconsultation experience and find that it offers savings in time and money. Healthcare providers, as well as patients and their families, have benefited from telementoring and teleproctoring. Telesurgery, although still in its infancy, may be a positive development in providing paediatric surgical care to rural and remote locations.

Further information

American Telemedicine Association. http://www.atmeda.org/. Last checked 12 August 2004

Canadian Surgical Technologies and Advanced Robotics. http://www.c-star.ca/about.aspx (last checked 12 August 2004).

Canadian Society of Telehealth. http://www.cst-sct.org/ (last checked 12 August 2004).

Primer of Robotic and Telerobotic Surgery. Ballantyne GH, Marescaux J, Giulianotti PC. Philadelphia: Lippincott Williams and Wilkins, 2004 (last checked 12 August 2004).

References

1   Khan Y, Fitzgerald P, Walton M. Assessment of the postoperative visit after routine inguinal hernia repair: a prospective randomized trial. *Journal of Pediatric Surgery* 1997; **32**: 892–893.

2   Tagge EP, Hebra A, Overdyk F, *et al.* One-stop surgery: evolving approach to pediatric outpatient surgery. *Journal of Pediatric Surgery* 1999; **34**: 129–132.

3   http://www.sickkids.on.ca/telehealth/default.asp (last checked 1 June 2004).

4   Endean ED, Mallon LI, Minion DJ, *et al.* Telemedicine in vascular surgery: does it work? *American Surgeon* 2001; **67**: 334–340.

5   Tachakra S, Hollingdale J, Uche CU. Evaluation of telemedical orthopaedic specialty support to a minor accident and treatment service. *Journal of Telemedicine and Telecare* 2001; **7**: 27–31.

6   Harrison R, Clayton W, Wallace P. Can telemedicine be used to improve communication between primary and secondary care? *British Medical Journal* 1996; **313**: 1377–1380.

7   Dick PT, Filler R, Pavan A. Participant satisfaction and comfort with multidisciplinary pediatric telemedicine consultations. *Journal of Pediatric Surgery* 1999; **34**: 137–142.

8   Miller GG, Levesque K. Telehealth provides effective pediatric surgery care to remote locations. *Journal of Pediatric Surgery* 2002; **37**: 752–754.

9   Rosser JC, Gabriel N, Herman B, Murayama M. Telementoring and teleproctoring. *World Journal of Surgery* 2001; **25**: 1438–1448.

10 Society of American Gastrointestinal Endoscopic Surgeons. Guidelines for the surgical practice of telemedicine. *Surgical Endoscopy* 2000; **14**: 975–979.

11 Rosser JC Jr, Bell RL, Harnett B, *et al.* Use of mobile low-bandwidth telemedical techniques for extreme telemedicine applications. *Journal of the American College of Surgeons* 1999; **189**: 397–404.

12 Marescaux J, Leroy J, Gagner M, *et al.* Transatlantic robot-assisted telesurgery. *Nature* 2001; **413**: 379–380.

▶12

Telemedicine in Physical and/or Sexual Abuse

Philip O Ozuah, James P Marcin, Deborah Burton and Deborah Stanley

Introduction

The physical and sexual maltreatment of children remain important problems for medical providers all over the world. Children who are victims of physical or sexual abuse need urgent and specialized treatment, including a complete physical and forensic examination. According to the American Academy of Pediatrics:[1] 'Children who have been sexually abused should be evaluated by the pediatrician or mental health provider to assess the need for treatment and to measure the level of parental support. Unfortunately, treatment services for sexually abused children are not universally available'. Appropriate services may not be available for several reasons, including inadequate training of personnel, lack of standardized knowledge and lack of equipment, as well as legal and financial considerations. These problems may be worse in rural and underserved areas.

Past studies have suggested shortcomings in the provision of care to acutely ill and injured children and those presenting to rural hospitals who require evidentiary examination for physical or sexual abuse, or both.[2-7] Rural emergency departments (EDs) may be inadequately equipped to care for paediatric emergencies, inadequately trained for proper evidentiary examinations and underserved with respect to paediatric specialty services.[2,3] Furthermore, personnel working in rural EDs, including physicians, nurses, pharmacists and support staff, may be less experienced in caring for these children. The relative lack of equipment, infrastructure and personnel well versed in delivering specialty care to children may result in delayed or incorrect diagnoses, suboptimal therapies and imperfect medical management.[8-15] As a consequence, acutely injured children and children who need acute evidentiary examinations for physical or sexual abuse, or both, may receive lower quality of care than children who present to large metropolitan hospitals that specialize in paediatric medicine.[6,7,16-18]

Telemedicine has been shown by several centres to be a feasible means of providing specialist consultations for adults and children who present to rural and urban EDs.[19-25] Telemedicine has also been used specifically for child abuse consultations in rural and underserved areas.[23-26] The goals of such work have included providing expertise to less experienced clinicians in rural areas, establishing an approach to peer review and quality assurance in sexual abuse cases, and provision of emotional support for professionals dealing with cases of child maltreatment. Kellogg *et al* identified several problems encountered by existing networks, including difficulties in funding the equipment and reimbursing staff for consultations, inconsistent technical support, poor technical expertise or motivation on the part of clinicians, and lack of network infrastructure.[26] In addition, potential medicolegal problems include licensure exemptions for consulting across state boundaries, the possibility of malpractice, patient confidentiality and security of images transmitted via modem connections, and the liability of the equipment, consulting site and consultant in any criminal proceedings. Kellogg *et al* concluded that teleconsultations offer a unique opportunity to raise the standard of care in child abuse evaluations but that success depends on clinician motivation, appropriate infrastructure, and ongoing funding and technical support.

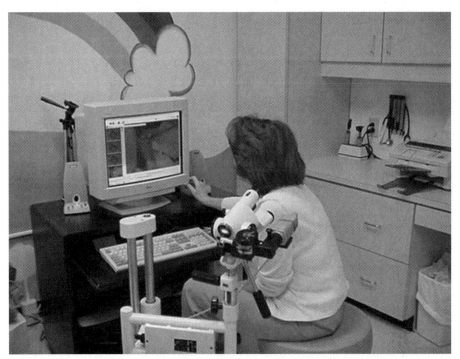

Fig. 12.1. Examination for suspected sexual abuse being carried out by telemedicine.

Case study: California

For children who need acute evidentiary examinations for physical or sexual abuse, or both, the University of California Davis Children's Hospital (UCDCH) critical care physicians and physicians working in the UCDCH Child and Adolescent Abuse Resource and Evaluation (CAARE) Center have established telemedicine links to four rural EDs in northern California. The aim is to provide the rural EDs with paediatric critical care or paediatric child abuse expertise shortly after a child presents with either acute illness or injury, or following acute physical or sexual abuse. When a case occurs, an appropriate consultant is called and a teleconsultation is initiated. This service is available 24 hours per day, seven days per week. The consultants have telemedicine access available at one of eight telemedicine stations at the UCDCH, and some also have telemedicine access from their homes.

Each of the EDs has a wall-mounted telemedicine unit with a flat-screen monitor, which can be pulled over an acute care ED trolley. Videoconferencing uses a T1 connection or three ISDN lines. The telemedicine unit is connected to a colposcope and a video recorder (see Figs. 17.1 and 17.2).

During a telemedicine consultation, the examinations are conducted so that images through the camera or colposcope can be recorded for quality assurance purposes and as court evidence, if necessary. Teleconsultations have so far concerned questions of acute sexual abuse. These consultations have assisted the remote site's physician to decide whether or not there has been acute sexual abuse, which diagnostic and therapeutic measures should be conducted and what the follow-up should entail. Although this programme began only recently, 10 consultations for suspected child mistreatment have been conducted. Approximately 50% of consultations involved live interactive evidentiary examinations, while the rest have addressed quality assurance reviews. There has been a high level of satisfaction with telemedicine.

Case study: Kentucky Chandler

One method of addressing the shortage of services for child victims of alleged sexual abuse is by triaging services through a children's advocacy centre, where all services for sexually abused children are located in one facility (medical forensic examination, law enforcement interviews, prosecuting attorney interviews and social work intervention services, including mental health services). In 1999, the number of child sexual abuse cases in Kentucky was increasing. The cases came from 66 of the 120 counties in rural Kentucky. There were fewer than 20 physicians in the state to provide child sexual abuse clinical examinations, so a physician training programme was established to meet the demand for such medical services in rural Kentucky, particularly in rural Appalachia, where there were health provider shortage areas. A three-year pilot project was funded through a federal grant (Appalachian Regional Commission).[23]

The project was a collaboration between a local non-profit Children's Advocacy Center, an academic medical centre, regional hospitals in the state, primary care clinics and community mental health centres. Several types of technology, including web-based communication and high-bandwidth videoconferencing, allowed case conferencing and training from national experts in child sexual abuse for isolated physicians, nurses and other professionals in rural Appalachia. Physicians in the project received colposcopes, printers and workstations, speakerphones, videophones, video-scan converters, fax machines, back-up power generators, technical assistance and equipment training.

Physicians were able to connect via any convenient computer, whether it was in the office, home or conference hotel room in a remote city. Each month, a two-hour, peer-review case conference was held with a combination of telephone conferencing and web-based Internet Protocol (IP) videoconferencing via an encrypted Internet site. This provided an opportunity for individual physicians to learn through collaborative sharing of each other's problem cases. Physicians were also able to link individually with the expert physician in Lexington for a consultation on a particular case. Alternatively, the expert physician could conference with the physician or the child via an ordinary telephone line using an analogue videophone. Finally, physicians and other health professionals participated in two-hour monthly educational programmes. Videoconferencing connections were established, through videoconferencing equipment located in rural hospitals, primary care clinics and community mental health facilities, through various high-bandwidth telehealth networks in Kentucky and occasionally through analogue videophones, with national experts connected by ISDN.

In three years, 14 rural Kentucky physicians in Appalachian counties received expert training and the proper equipment to perform examinations, while 8 other physicians participated in training programmes. Physicians received 96 hours of free continuing medical education credits by participating in 23 two-hour educational sessions and 25 two-hour peer review case conferences over the three-year period. The evaluation component of the project focused on quality of care, access to services, use and usefulness of technology, use of telemedicine, effect on clinical decision-making and effect on physician behaviour. In the third year of the project, nurses who assisted physicians were also given educational training: 61 nurses participated in the programmes and received free continuing nursing education credits.

During the three-year project, specialists from the department of psychiatry at the University of Kentucky's Chandler Medical Center also used the videoconferencing network to provide 22 two-hour peer-review case conferences and 26 two-hour educational sessions, with free continuing education credits, to enhance training for rural mental health professionals. Participants included social workers, psychologists, therapists, mental retardation developmental delay staff and court-appointed advocates. In addition, some programmes attracted attorneys, school teachers and members of law enforcement groups.

The evaluation showed that the number of counties with access to sexual abuse examinations by a qualified physician increased from 23 counties in the first year to 45 in the second year. There was also an increase in the number of cases reviewed: from 83 cases in the first year to 613 in the third year. Rural health professionals' knowledge of child sexual abuse also increased. Physician participants reported that telemedicine outreach provided more rapid feedback from experts, allowed for peer review of their findings, increased their knowledge about sexual abuse and increased their confidence in performing sexual abuse examinations. Overall, satisfaction with teleconsultation was high.

Conclusion

Several telemedicine programmes have been developed for medical consultations and continuing education in child abuse in rural and underserved areas.[23–26] These initiatives have attempted to provide expertise to less experienced clinicians in rural areas, to establish quality assurance in sexual abuse cases and to provide emotional support for professionals dealing with cases of child maltreatment. Despite some problems, teleconsultations provide a unique opportunity to raise the standard of care in child abuse evaluations. Published reports suggest that the use of telemedicine in these circumstances can improve access to specialty physicians and improve the quality of care while maintaining high levels of user satisfaction.

References

1   Botash AS. Examination for sexual abuse in prepubertal children: an update. *Pediatric Annals* 1997; **26**: 312–319.
2   Athey J, Dean JM, Ball J, *et al.* Ability of hospitals to care for pediatric emergency patients. *Pediatric Emergency Care* 2001; **17**: 170–174.
3   McGillivray D, Nijssen-Jordan C, Kramer MS, *et al.* Critical pediatric equipment availability in Canadian hospital emergency departments. *Annals of Emergency Medicine* 2001; **37**: 371–376.
4   Esposito TJ, Sanddal ND, Dean JM, *et al.* Analysis of preventable pediatric trauma deaths and inappropriate trauma care in Montana. *Journal of Trauma* 1999; **47**: 243–251; discussion 251–243.
5   Moody-Williams JD, Krug S, O'Connor R, *et al.* Practice guidelines and performance measures in emergency medical services for children. *Annals of Emergency Medicine* 2002; **39**: 404–412.
6   Durch J, Lohr KN (eds). *Emergency Medical Services for Children.* Washington, DC: National Academies Press, 1993.
7   Durch JS, Lohr KN. From the Institute of Medicine. *Journal of the American Medical Association* 1993; **270**: 929.
8   Pollack MM, Alexander SR, Clarke N, *et al.* Improved outcomes from tertiary center pediatric intensive care: a statewide comparison of tertiary and nontertiary care facilities. *Critical Care Medicine* 1991; **19**: 150–159.
9   Pollack MM, Getson PR. Pediatric critical care cost containment: combined actuarial and clinical program. *Critical Care Medicine* 1991; **19**: 12–20.
10 Lawrence LL, Brannen SJ. The impact of physician training on child maltreatment reporting: a multi-specialty study. *Military Medicine* 2000; **165**: 607–611.
11 Kronick JB, Frewen TC, Kissoon N, *et al.* Influence of referring physicians on interventions by a pediatric and neonatal critical care transport team. *Pediatric Emergency Care* 1996; **12**: 73–77.
12 Tilford JM, Roberson PK, Lensing S, Fiser DH. Improvement in pediatric critical care outcomes. *Critical Care Medicine* 2000; **28**: 601–603.
13 Tilford JM, Simpson PM, Green JW, *et al.* Volume–outcome relationships in pediatric intensive care units. *Pediatrics* 2000; **106** (2 Pt 1): 289–294.
14 Phibbs CS, Bronstein JM, Buxton E, Phibbs RH. The effects of patient volume and level of care at the hospital of birth on neonatal mortality. *Journal of the American Medical Association* 1996; **276**: 1054–1059.
15 Hampers LC, Trainor JL, Listernick R, *et al.* Setting-based practice variation in the management of simple febrile seizure. *Academic Emergency Medicine* 2000; **7**: 21–27.
16 Seidel JS, Henderson DP, Ward P, *et al.* Pediatric prehospital care in urban and rural areas. *Pediatrics* 1991; **88**: 681–690.
17 Seidel JS, Hornbein M, Yoshiyama K, *et al.* Emergency medical services and the pediatric patient: are the needs being met? *Pediatrics* 1984; **73**: 769–772.
18 Gausche M, Seidel JS, Henderson DP, *et al.* Pediatric deaths and emergency medical services (EMS) in urban and rural areas. *Pediatric Emergency Care* 1989; **5**: 158–162.
19 Lambrecht CJ. Emergency physicians' roles in a clinical telemedicine network. *Annals of Emergency Medicine* 1997; **30**: 670–674.
20 Lambrecht CJ. Telemedicine in trauma care: description of 100 trauma teleconsults. *Telemedicine Journal* 1997; **3**: 265–268.
21 Brennan JA, Kealy JA, Gerardi LH, *et al.* Telemedicine in the emergency department: a randomized controlled trial. *Journal of Telemedicine and Telecare* 1999; **5**: 18–22.
22 Brennan JA, Kealy JA, Gerardi LH, *et al.* A randomized controlled trial of telemedicine in an emergency department. *Journal of Telemedicine and Telecare* 1998; **4** (suppl. 1): 18–20.

23 Burton DC, Stanley D, Ireson CL. Child advocacy outreach: using telehealth to expand child sexual abuse services in rural Kentucky. *Journal of Telemedicine and Telecare* 2002; **8** (suppl. 2): 10–12.

24 Inouye J, Cerny JE, Hollandsworth J, Ettipio A. Child abuse prevention program with POTS-based telehealth: a feasibility project. *Telemedicine Journal and e-Health* 2001; **7**: 325–332.

25 Whitworth JM, Mullins HC, Morse K. Design and implementation of an urban/rural Telehealth Network for the Evaluation of Abused Children: implications for global primary care applications. *Medinfo* 2001; **10** (Pt 1): 863–865.

26 Kellogg ND, Lamb JL, Lukefahr JL. The use of telemedicine in child sexual abuse evaluations. *Child Abuse and Neglect* 2000; **24**: 1601–1612.

►13

Paediatric Tele-ophthalmology

Kanagasingam Yogesan, Sajeesh Kumar, Mei-Ling Tay Kearney, Ian Constable and Beth Hudson

Introduction

The two most common childhood ophthalmic conditions are strabismus (a crossed eye) and amblyopia (a lazy eye). Left untreated, the crossed or lazy eye will never fully develop. A lazy eye can often be corrected by placing a patch over the good eye, thereby forcing the brain to use and increase the strength of the weak partner. One of the other important diseases is retinopathy of prematurity (ROP), which is the leading cause of childhood blindness in the developed world.[1] Early detection of ROP and appropriate treatment can reduce severe vision loss and adverse outcome in infants. Children also suffer the same eye diseases as their adult counterparts, the most common being congenital defects, cataracts, glaucoma and retinal tumours. Treatment of these conditions is managed by paediatric ophthalmologists in consultation with specialists from neuro-ophthalmology, retina, cornea and external disease, glaucoma, and oculoplastics.

The tests and devices available for paediatric eye examination are unique and limited. The small size of the eye and pupil make examination more difficult. Often children are uncomfortable with a bright light shining in their eyes and are uncooperative or hyperactive. A lid speculum is often used under anaesthesia in the paediatric eye clinic.

Apart from fundus examination, evaluation of visual function is also equally important in determining the visual status of the eye. Most of the visual function tests for children are objective in nature of administration. In practice, visual function tests are administered by a trained practitioner.

The development of non-invasive and portable digital fundus cameras and slit lamps has facilitated the use of telemedicine in the diagnosis of anterior lesions and retinal abnormalities in children. Neonatal nurses or medical practitioners can operate the devices to obtain diagnostic quality images. Children who are usually uncomfortable with a table-mounted slit lamp with its chin rest and adjoining gadgets will be more relaxed with the sleek-designed, torch-like portable slit lamps and fundus cameras.

Review of existing studies and trials

A systematic review of the peer-reviewed literature indicates that few studies have specifically addressed paediatric tele-ophthalmology.[2-7] Examination of paediatric eyes with the RetCam fundus camera for ROP and case reports on telemedicine examinations for strabismus have been published.[2-6]

Schwartz *et al* have investigated whether or not ROP can be evaluated and managed by telemedicine.[2] Ten patients with ROP were evaluated face-to-face and remotely. Digital images were obtained using the RetCam fundus camera (Massie Laboratories Inc, CA, USA) and sent to a remote site for evaluation. The authors proposed that telemedicine may be highly accurate as a screening tool. However, it is difficult to draw a firm conclusion from such a small data set.

In another study on ROP from 46 eyes, Yen *et al* indicated that examination with the RetCam camera had low sensitivity due to its technical limitations.[3] It was difficult to capture the peripheral retina in small eyes. A lid speculum was used under topical anaesthesia. The authors recommended using a lid speculum better adapted for the camera system.

Cheug *et al* have evaluated the reliability of assessing strabismus by telemedicine.[4] Altogether, 42 patients aged over 4 years were examined in person by a paediatric ophthalmologist and also by an ophthalmic fellow at a remote site. Telemedicine equipment may allow accurate assessment of eye deviation and eye movements. The authors found that strabismus examination can be performed with a good but not excellent level of reliability with the use of medium bandwidth videoconferencing equipment. The ophthalmologist, using telemedicine equipment, had difficulties in identifying oblique muscle actions and vertical strabismus. The authors also indicated that there was a high patient acceptance and cooperation for telemedicine strabismus evaluation.

Another study by Dawson *et al* indicated that young patients who were unable to sit still were unsuitable for strabismus assessment via telemedicine.[5] An ophthalmologist and an orthoptist saw 30 patients face-to-face; the same patients were then referred to another ophthalmologist by telemedicine link. There was 83% agreement between the face-to-face and telemedicine-based consultations. The authors found that the latent strabismus and micro-movements were difficult to diagnose with a videoconferencing link at a bandwidth of 384 kbit/s.

A study by Helveston *et al* reported that a store-and-forward telemedicine consultation technique that uses digital images and email was an effective means of carrying out consultations for patients with strabismus.[6] This study in Cuba used a digital camera and image transmission by email. Altogether, 50 patients were seen using this method, and there was a high correlation between face-to-face and telemedicine consultations (both were done by the same observer).

Present technologies

In paediatric tele-ophthalmology, the diagnostic performance depends on the technology used for teleconsultation.[8-11] Additional difficulties will be involved when ophthalmic diagnostic devices are used in children. A very important aspect of the paediatric tele-ophthalmological interaction is the use of peripherals at the remote site: direct ophthalmoscopes, retinal cameras and slit lamps must be integrated with the telemedicine system to capture the images needed to be sent to a consultant. As children are usually not co-operative and are uncomfortable with such gadgets and bright lights, non-invasive, portable and handheld devices are preferred (Fig. 13.1).

The RetCam fundus camera has been used in telemedicine studies to image the retina of children. This imaging device is a contact mydriatic fundus camera that provides a 120° field of view of the retina. The camera needs to touch the cornea to image the retina and also needs a lid speculum under anaesthesia. The other devices widely used in the ophthalmic clinics are the slit lamp and ophthalmoscope. It is not generally possible to attach a camera to an ophthalmoscope, but a video or digital camera can be connected to a slit lamp with appropriate adapters to obtain anterior segment images.

Even though two different modes of transmission (store-and-forward and real-time) have been used in paediatric tele-ophthalmology, no reports have compared these modalities. In paediatric tele-ophthalmology, store-and-forward capabilities to capture still images are essential for the following reasons:

▶ higher resolution can be captured with still images than with video images

▶ high-resolution still images can be used to monitor disease progression over the years as the child grows

▶ store-and-forward information does not require immediate, online evaluation by a consultant.

In paediatric work to date, real-time ophthalmology (videoconferencing) has not been a major focus because of the importance of image resolution: video resolution is generally lower than still image resolution. In some subspecialties such as strabismus, however, the history and a dynamic examination such as pupillary and muscular reflex are essential for diagnosis. In one published study, manifest strabismus was safely diagnosed and managed using telemedicine at 128 kbit/s, although 384 kbit/s was preferred because it avoided the need for repeated examination.[5] Latent strabismus and micro-movements were difficult to diagnose using telemedicine, however, even at 384 kbit/s.

Australian paediatric tele-ophthalmology experience

Internet based tele-ophthalmology services (http://www.e-icare.com) have been developed at the Lions Eye Institute (LEI) in Perth. The system stores and transmits patient data to a secure, central database. The information includes demographic data, medical history, ophthalmic images, video and audio. In cooperation with the Department of Health in Western Australia (WA), the LEI has set up a tele-ophthalmology centre at the Carnarvon Rural Health Centre in the Gascoyne Region of WA. This centre provides remote consultation in eye care for children and adults in a region located 900 km from Perth. Travel times to Perth are 1.5 hours by air and 11 hours by road. The region has a population of 6400.

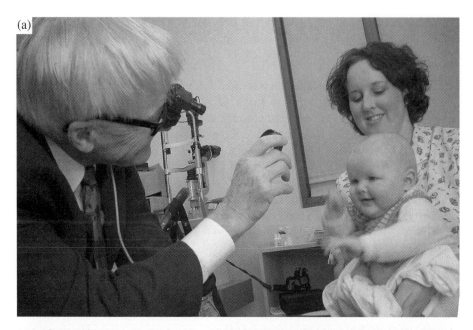

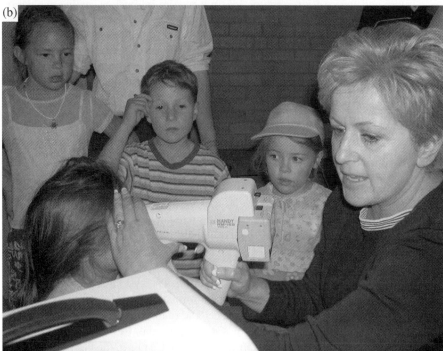

Fig. 13.1. (a) Ophthalmologist trying to see the retina using an ophthalmoscope. (b) Health professional using a digital fundus camera to obtain a fundus image from a child. Photographs provided by Chris Barry from the Lions Eye Institute; patients' permission to use the photographs was obtained.

The service is made available to patients referred by local general practitioners and to patients at community screenings. Emergency cases are also seen. A dedicated tele-ophthalmology protocol is also in place for the web-based eye care consultation.

Children from regional areas have been examined. On average, we have seen two children per month and five adults per week. The child's parents or carer provide details of the child's general medical and eye condition, which includes age at onset of the eye condition, the child's perinatal period, history of previous eye surgery and any family history of eye conditions. The child's best-corrected visual acuities are assessed, where possible with a Snellen chart. Slit-lamp examination of the anterior segment is performed. The fundus is examined by digital photography.

Using the Internet-based system, patients have been screened or consulted for anterior and posterior eye diseases. A trained telehealth coordinator takes retinal photos and external eye pictures with equipment developed by the LEI (Fig. 13.2). The equipment includes a portable digital slit lamp, a portable air-puff tonometer (Keeler Pulsair 3000) and a non-mydriatic digital fundus camera (Canon CR4-45NM; see Fig 13.3 for transmitted images). Captured data were first stored in a computer and then transmitted to a central server. The data were then accessed and diagnosed by a designated specialist ophthalmologist. An automatic email message was sent to the specialist in Perth each time a patient was screened at Carnarvon. The specialist reviewed the data, recorded image quality, diagnosed the eye disease and made recommendations about management and subsequent care. Specialist advice was returned to the Carnarvon healthcare centre in 24 hours. Further services were managed in Carnarvon itself. In case of emergency, services were scheduled (to be done locally or at Perth) according to urgency and severity. In the case of screening and non-emergency cases, a report on the tele-ophthalmology consultation was sent by mail to the patients. Before the web-based consultation, each patient or carer was given an information sheet about the service and a consent form to sign. A specially prepared questionnaire was also sent to all patients or carers, together with a stamped return address envelope. Patient participation was voluntary. No fee was charged.

A tele-ophthalmology protocol was prepared for the web-based consultation. The protocol detailed the consultation criteria, technical and training requirements for those involved. It also specified the rights and responsibilities of the patients, preparation of the patient for consultation, privacy and confidentiality issues, screening, referral or consultation procedures and other relevant information.

Case report

A 3-year-old girl with a six-week history of lumps in the right inner lower eyelid presented at the tele-ophthalmology centre at Carnarvon, Western Australia. The tele-ophthalmology coordinator took the medical history and other details (Fig. 13.4). According to the girl's parents, the child had no history of any external or internal ocular abnormalities. The mother observed that the child had had a sand fight and developed the lumps in her eyelids since that time. The child had been taken to see the

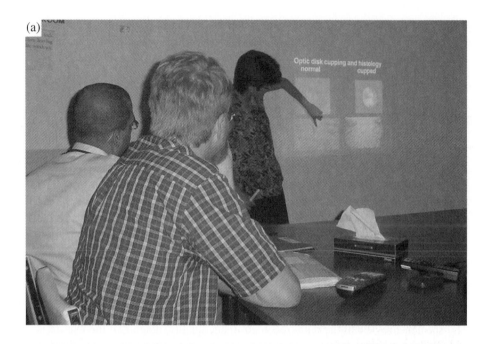

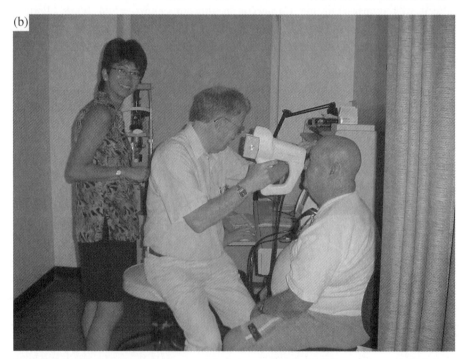

Fig. 13.2. (a) Training programme on ophthalmic conditions. (b) How to use a digital fundus camera. Patient's permission to use the photograph was obtained.

Images (Part 1)	Date: Mar 15 2004
Right Eye:	Left Eye:

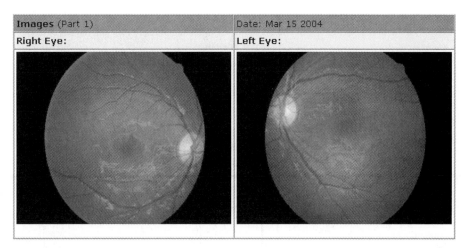

Fig. 13.3. Transmitted retinal images obtained from a fundus camera (CR4-45NM, Canon).

local general practitioner two weeks before who prescribed oral antibiotics and chloromycetin (0.5%) drops and ointment. No improvement of the condition occurred. At the tele-ophthalmology centre, it was decided to consult a specialist ophthalmologist in Perth.

The external examination of the lid was carried out with the hand-held portable digital slit lamp. The child was cooperative during the eye examination. The examination was carried out in accordance with the tele-ophthalmology protocol developed by the LEI. The lids, eye lashes, conjunctiva and cornea were observed with low to medium background illumination and an angle of illumination of 30–35° from the straight-ahead position. The optic section was used primarily to determine the depth or elevation of any defect of the cornea and conjunctiva or for locating the depth of any opacity in the lens of the eye. The slit lamp was then used to scan across the lower lid and lashes, observing the tear meniscus, the lid apposition to the globe and the openings of the meibomian glands.

The child was then informed that the examiner was going to touch her lower eyelid. The examiner placed her index finger close to the patient's lower lash margin and everted the lower lid. The inferior palpebral and bulbar conjunctiva was scanned, looking for elevations, depressions or discolorations. The images from the digital slit lamp were then forwarded to the specialist ophthalmologist in Perth using the Internet. The quality of the images was deemed to be sufficient for a diagnosis by the specialist (Fig. 13.5).

The specialist noted that the presence of three lumps in the lower lid was a little unusual for chalazion and recommended a warm compress and lid massage. The specialist advised that if the treatment did not improve the condition, the child should be sent to Perth for treatment. The child was sent to Perth and fully recovered after treatment by an ophthalmologist.

Personal Details	
	Gender: F
	Date of Birth: 06/04/00
	Screened By:
Referred to Doctor:	

Medical History	

<u>Glaucoma</u>
No data
<u>Diabetic Retinopathy</u>
No data
<u>Anterior Segment Diseases</u>

2003-07-21	Right Eye	Left Eye
Other observations
Please see History		

2003-07-22	Right Eye	Left Eye
Other observations
3 year old child with 6 week history of lumps in R) inner lower eyelid. Had sand fight and mother states has developed from that time. S/B GP 2 weeks ago – oral abs and chlorsig drops and ointment. No improvement.		

Notes	
History / Other notes	
2003-07-22	
GP said was chalazion? and may require opthalmic review for ?lancing if not resolving. Child not complaining of pain no discharge reported. Mother concerned not improving at all. Can you advise course of action please.	
Specialist's notes	
The 3 lumps are a little unusual for chalazia. I would try a warm compress and lid massage first. If no better, best to get it seen by an ophthalmologist.	

Fig. 13.4. Information exchanged for the patient.

Benefits and drawbacks of paediatric tele-ophthalmology

Childhood blindness is a major social and economic problem. In 1992, it was estimated that there were approximately 1.5 million blind children in the world.[12] The prevalence of blindness in children is estimated to range from 0.2 to 0.3 per 1000

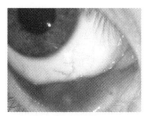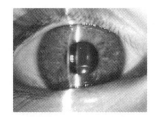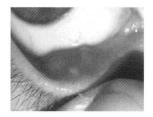

Fig. 13.5. Images obtained from a portable digital slit lamp built at the Lions Eye Institute. Lumps on the inner palpebral conjunctiva (right eye), optical section of the crystalline lens and eversion of the lower lid (right eye). Patient's permission to use the photographs was obtained.

children in industrialized countries and 1.0 to 1.5 per 1000 children in developing countries.[13] It has been predicted that, without extra interventions, the global number of blind individuals will increase from 44 million in 2000 to 76 million in 2020.[14] It therefore seems likely that there will be an enormous demand for telemedicine in paediatric ophthalmology. With the help of telemedicine, specialist care can be brought to the patient's doorstep.

The main drawback of paediatric tele-ophthalmology is the lack of digital non-invasive imaging devices. Easy-to-operate, low-cost and non-invasive ophthalmic imaging devices would increase the use of telemedicine for paediatric eye care. Nurses and allied medical professionals could use such devices for screening childhood eye conditions. Early detection of eye diseases is important for appropriate treatment and prevention of blindness.

Conclusion

In the future, tele-ophthalmology is likely to be used widely to identify and manage the causes of childhood blindness and visual impairment. It will help to identify the preventable and treatable causes of childhood blindness in rural, remote and underserved regions of the world. Apart from blindness, telemedicine tests will also be useful in detecting amblyopia – a common condition in children.

More research is needed to evaluate the use of real-time and store-and-forward techniques in diagnosing childhood eye disorders. Information is needed about appropriate technical standards, clinical effectiveness and cost-effectiveness.

Perhaps the most important principle in treating children with ocular problems is the recognition that children are not just little adults. They have unique concerns, problems and needs. When implementing a tele-ophthalmology service for a paediatric population, the service providers should familiarize themselves with the unique health and ocular problems of childhood. These have an important effect on the examiner's technique and rapport with the child and their family. More portable and non-invasive imaging devices will assist in obtaining good quality images and video pictures.

Further information

Lions Eye Institute in Perth, Western Australia. http://www.lei.org.au/ (last checked 5 August 2004).

Jules Stein Eye Institute, LA, California, US. http://www.jsei.org/ (last checked 5 August 2004).

Department of Ophthalmology, Hospital for Sick Children and University of Toronto, Toronto, Ontario: http://www.sickkids.on.ca/ (last checked 5 August 2004).

Moorfields Eye Hospital, London: http://www.ucl.ac.uk/ioo/index.html (last checked 5 August 2004).

References

1   Simons BD, Flynn JT. Retinopathy of prematurity and associated factors. *International Ophthalmology Clinics* 1999; **39**: 29–48

2   Schwartz SD, Harrison SA, Ferrone PJ, Trese MT. Telemedical evaluation and management of retinopathy of prematurity using a fiberoptic digital fundus camera. *Ophthalmology* 2000; **107**: 25–28.

3   Yen KG, Hess D, Burke B, *et al.* The optimum time to employ telephotoscreening to detect retinopathy of prematurity. *Transactions of the American Ophthalmological Society* 2000; **98**: 145-50; discussion 150–151.

4   Cheung JC, Dick PT, Kraft SP, *et al.* Strabismus examination by telemedicine. *Ophthalmology* 2000; **107**: 1999–2005.

5   Dawson E, Kennedy C, Bentley C, *et al.* The role of telemedicine in the assessment of strabismus. *Journal of Telemedicine and Telecare* 2002; **8**: 52–55.

6   Helveston EM, Orge FH, Naranjo R, Hernandez L. Telemedicine: strabismus e-consultation. *Journal of AAPOS* 2001; **5**: 291–296.

7   Saari JM, Kerola MT, Broas M, Saari KM. Hand-held digital video-camera for eye examination and follow-up. *Journal of Telemedicine and Telecare* 2002; **8**: 237–240.

8   Yogesan K, Cuypers M, Barry CJ, *et al.* Tele-ophthalmology screening for retinal and anterior segment diseases. *Journal of Telemedicine and Telecare* 2000; **5** (suppl. 1): 96–98.

9   Constable IJ, Yogesan K, Eikelboom R, *et al.* Fred Hollows Lecture: digital screening for eye disease. *Clinical and Experimental Ophthalmology* 2000; **28**: 129–132.

10   Yogesan K, Constable IJ, Barry CJ, *et al.* Evaluation of a portable fundus camera for use in the teleophthalmologic diagnosis of glaucoma. *Journal of Glaucoma* 1999; **8**: 297–301.

11   Yogesan K, Constable IJ, Barry CJ, *et al.* Telemedicine screening of diabetic retinopathy using a hand-held fundus camera. *Telemedicine Journal* 2000; **6**: 219–223.

12   World Health Organization. *Prevention of Childhood Blindness*. Geneva: World Health Organization, 1992.

13   Foster A, Gilbert C. Epidemiology of childhood blindness. *Eye* 1992: **6** (Pt 2): 173–176.

14   Frick KD, Foster A. The magnitude and cost of global blindness: an increasing problem that can be alleviated. *American Journal of Ophthalmology* 2003; **135**: 471–476.

▶14

Teleradiology

Liam Caffery

Introduction

Teleradiology is an umbrella term for the transfer of medical images over a communication network. Teleradiology can be used to improve patient care by providing radiology or other specialist medical opinions to areas that are unable to support a full-time medical specialist. In Australia, dedicated children's hospitals with a full range of paediatric subspecialties are located only in capital cities. Paediatric radiologists at these hospitals have all been asked to perform second reads on studies reported by general radiologists. The Children's Hospital at Westmead (in Sydney) was an early exponent of paediatric teleradiology in Australia and successfully completed teleradiology trials with a number of regional hospitals in New South Wales as well as hospitals in the Sydney area. The Children's Hospital aims to expand this service to other regional hospitals and to link teleradiology to radiologists at home for on-call purposes.[1]

Teleradiology in paediatrics is implemented to:

▶ reduce the costs of providing radiological services

▶ provide access to images for tertiary medical opinion

▶ reduce radiation doses to patients by obviating repeat examinations.

Paediatric teleradiology is a proven technique, and studies in the US have shown that the diagnostic accuracy of paediatric imaging is improved when a specialist paediatric radiologist reviews images over a teleradiology link.[2]

In teleradiology, the financial savings arise from increased productivity of specialist medical services, reduced or eliminated transport costs and reduced repeat examinations. Bergmo calculated that teleradiology in Norway was cheaper than providing a visiting radiologist service when the workload exceeded 1500 patients per year; it had the added advantage of having examinations reported sooner.[3] A pilot study on the paediatric teleradiology service between Nepean Hospital in Penrith and the Royal Alexandra Hospital for Children in central Sydney concluded that teleradiology saved 20 patient transfers per year at a cost of $7000–$10,000 per transfer.[4]

The Royal Children's Hospital, Brisbane, the Royal Children's Hospital, Melbourne, the Women's and Children's Hospital, Adelaide and the Princess Margaret Hospital for Children, Perth all have or use teleradiology. The purpose of this teleradiology is not to provide a routine radiology reporting service but, in collaboration with other paediatric subspecialties, to manage referred cases in which tertiary medical opinion is needed.

In paediatrics, reduced repeat examinations are important not just economically but for radiation protection of the patient. Due to the cumulative effect of radiation, adverse effects are larger in children than the general population.

Implementing teleradiology

A teleradiology system in its simplest form consists of two computers connected by a network that can transmit and receive images. Teleradiology can be implemented in numerous ways. The main decision in implementation is whether or not the system will be used to provide primary diagnosis or to review already interpreted radiology images. This decision will dictate the image quality needed. Primary diagnosis is defined by the American College of Radiologists (ACR) as the interpretation of images for which a written report is prepared.[5]

Primary diagnosis images in teleradiology, according to the guidelines set out by the ACR and the Royal Australian and New Zealand College of Radiologists (RANZCR), should use the DICOM standard (see below). DICOM image files are larger than those in other image formats, such as JPEG, so that the networks over which images are transferred need higher bandwidth and the display software and monitor at the receiving end need higher specifications than in a system used primarily for review. All of these higher specifications obviously mean higher image quality but also a higher cost.

Teleradiology of review images is dictated only by clinical acceptance of image quality. Lower-cost teleradiology systems can meet these needs because of their ability to use image formats such as JPEG and the higher compression ratios of these image files. This results in lower bandwidth requirements for the communication network and the ability to use standard personal computer monitors as review stations.

The digital image

Medical images must be in a digital format before they can be transmitted by a teleradiology system. A digital image is made up of a number of rows and columns called an image matrix. Each element of the image matrix is a pixel ('picture element'). Each pixel represents a single homogenous shade of grey.

In medical imaging, images are classified as small or large in matrix size. A small matrix, eg 512×512 pixels, results from computed tomography (CT), magnetic resonance imaging (MRI), ultrasound, nuclear medicine and digital fluoroscopy. A large matrix, eg 2048×2048 pixels, results from applications in computed radiography (CR). CR is a means of acquiring plain X-ray images in a digital format.

Image quality is improved by reducing the pixel size, ie reducing the pixel size improves spatial resolution (Fig. 14.1). Spatial resolution is measured in line pairs per millimetre (lp/mm) (Fig. 14.2). An image is said to have a spatial resolution of 2.5 lp/mm if one can visually distinguish distinct black and white lines on a test pattern where the bars are spaced to accommodate 2.5 line pairs per millimetre.

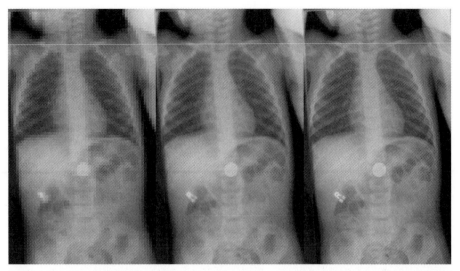

Fig. 14.1. Image quality is improved by increasing the image matrix and effectively reducing pixel size.

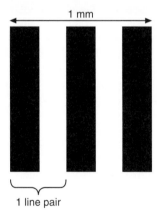

Fig. 14.2. Test pattern used to test a spatial resolution of 2.5 lp/mm.

Image quality is also determined by contrast resolution. Contrast resolution is the number of shades of grey that each pixel can represent. If a pixel can be one of 256 (2^8) shades of grey then the image is said to be an 8-bit image or to have a bit depth of 8. Similarly a 12-bit image can have 4096 different shades of grey. The human eye is capable of distinguishing about 256 shades of grey. Good quality images will be composed of 10- or 12-bit pixels (Fig. 14.3).

The overall size of an image file is proportional to the number of pixels in the image matrix and the number of bits needed to represent each pixel (Fig. 14.4).

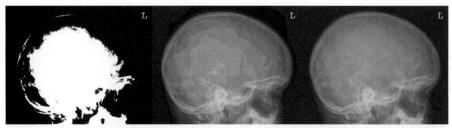

Fig. 14.3. Images with bit depths of 1, 4 and 8 bits show how increasing the bit depth improves image quality.

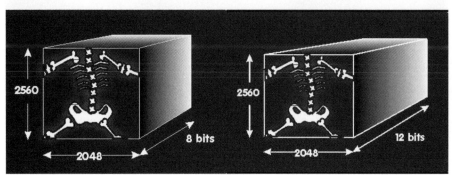

Fig. 14.4. An 8-bit CR image that has a matrix size of 2048×2560 would occupy 5.2 MBytes (2048×2560×8-bit = 41 943 040 bits or 5.2 MBytes; 8 bits = 1 Byte), whereas a 12-bit CR image that has a matrix size of 2048×2560 would occupy 7.9 MBytes (2048×2560×12-bit = 62 914 560 bits or 7.9 MBytes).

Image compression

Compression techniques can be used to reduce the size of an image file. Reducing the file size not only reduces the storage capacity needed for an image file but also decreases file transfer time across a network. Image compression is classified as lossless or lossy. Using lossless compression means that the decompressed image has exactly the same pixel values as the original image, whereas lossy compression aims to produce a decompressed image that is visually indistinguishable from the original image although the pixel values may vary somewhat from those in the original image.

Compression is usually expressed as a ratio. A compression ratio of 3:1 means that the image is compressed to one-third of its original size. Lossy compression techniques yield higher compression ratios than lossless compression techniques.

Run length encoding

Run length encoding (RLE) is a lossless compression technique that replaces a run of repeated pixel values in an image with two values – one representing the pixel value and the second the length of the run (Fig. 14.5). This technique can be useful where

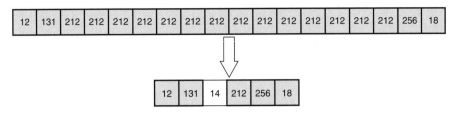

Fig. 14.5. Graphical representation of run length encoding (RLE).

there are large areas of the same pixel value, eg the blackness on the periphery of a chest X-ray.

JPEG

JPEG is a standardized image compression technique named after the committee that developed it – the Joint Photographic Experts Group. The technique is designed to exploit the fact that the eye perceives changes in colour less accurately than changes in brightness. JPEG compression involves dividing an image into 8×8 blocks of pixels and then applying a discrete cosine transform (DCT) to the blocks. The DCT is a mathematical formula that transforms the pixel values into sine waves of varying amplitude and frequency. Some of the higher frequency data are discarded, which results in reduced image size. During JPEG compression, a quality factor is applied; this determines how much information is thrown away, ie a low quality factor results in small images, but they may be of relatively poor quality compared with the original. Because the image is initially broken into 8×8 pixel blocks, higher compression ratios can lead to blocking artefacts.

Different DCT algorithms give rise to the different members of the JPEG family. JPEG2000 is the most recent revision of the JPEG family. It is more relevant to medical imaging because it supports compression of images up to 16-bit depth.

Wavelet compression

Wavelet compression is similar to JPEG compression, as it breaks down an image mathematically using a discrete wavelet transform (DWT). One of the main advantages of wavelet compression is that because the image is not divided into 8×8 pixel blocks before a DWT is applied, it can produce highly compressed images without a blocking artefact.

Effect of compression on medical images

Numerous studies have shown that lossy compression techniques can be used without degrading the diagnostic value of a medical image. Erickson stressed, however, that a single compression technique cannot be applied to every medical image and that some images are more 'compression-tolerant' than others.[6] In particular, digitized plain X-rays can be acceptably compressed up to 40:1, while compression ratios of 20:1 are more acceptable for CT, MRI and ultrasound images. These findings are consistent with other studies on compressed image quality.

DICOM

The acronym DICOM stands for Digital Imaging and Communication in Medicine. It is a standard for image storage and transfer that was originally developed by the ACR and the National Electrical Manufacturers Association (NEMA). The standard has evolved over the years and the current version is DICOM 3.0.

The aim of DICOM is to provide a standardized way of transferring medical images and associated data, eg patient demographics and study information, between different medical imaging devices regardless of manufacturer. It works at an application software level and assumes that a network connection exists between the relevant medical imaging devices.

A DICOM image has two parts. The first is the DICOM header that contains text-based information, such as patient demographics, study and image information. The second is the pixel data of the image, often in JPEG format. The DICOM header logically groups elements relating to an object. The object may be a patient, a visit, a study or an image. DICOM defines which elements are required for each object. The patient object contains elements such as the medical record number, name, date of birth, age and sex, whereas the image object contains elements such as image number, acquisition time, matrix size and bit depth.

DICOM supports different image compression techniques. This is referred to as the transfer syntax. Both the sending and receiving device must support the same compression technique for a transfer of images to occur. DICOM looks at what tasks need to be accomplished in a medical imaging network and assigns a service class to govern that task. The DICOM storage service class governs the storage of images in an image archive, the DICOM query-retrieve service class governs viewing images stored in an image archive and the DICOM print service class governs printing images on a networked printer.

A service object pair (SOP) is a combination of a DICOM object and a service class, eg store a CT image. The presentation context of a DICOM transaction is a combination of the SOP and transfer syntax, eg store a CT image using JPEG lossless compression. DICOM works by exchanging messages (Fig. 14.6).

Before two DICOM devices can exchange information, they must establish an association. This process involves both devices agreeing on a presentation context. Once the association has been established, the data are transferred from one device to another and the association is then terminated. DICOM defines a greyscale standard display function to facilitate display monitors of workstations displaying images in a visually consistent manner.

Vendors of medical imaging devices and teleradiology systems provide a DICOM conformance statement specifying which service classes and transfer syntaxes their device supports. However, DICOM does not guarantee connectivity between two

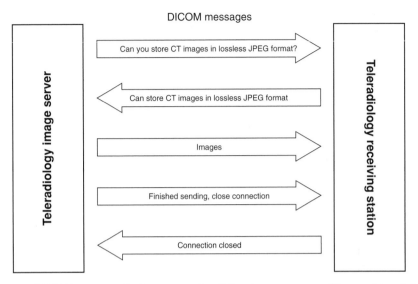

Fig. 14.6. DICOM image transfer between a teleradiology image server and the receiving station. CT=computed tomography.

devices. For primary diagnosis, DICOM is the method of choice for implementation of teleradiology.

Components of teleradiology systems

A teleradiology system is made up of a number of components (Fig. 14.7). These include:

▶ acquisition modalities

▶ image server

▶ communication network

▶ receiving station

▶ review station.

Acquisition modalities

Modalities such as CT, MRI, ultrasound, nuclear medicine and digital fluoroscopy all produce digital images. If these modalities are DICOM-compliant, they can transfer images using the DICOM standard into a teleradiology image server. The use of DICOM is strongly recommended for primary diagnosis teleradiology systems. The use of DICOM, however, may also provide the most economical way of transferring images from modality to the image server in review teleradiology systems.

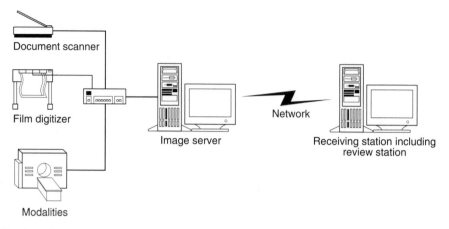

Fig. 14.7. Components of a teleradiology system.

CR is a means of acquiring traditionally analogue plain radiography, eg chest X-ray films, in a digital format. It uses conventional X-ray equipment, but instead of a film/screen cassette, a re-usable phosphor based imaging plate is used inside the cassette. The latent image is produced in the same way as in film/screen radiography. The plate is read by a CR digitizer to produce a digital X-ray. CR is mostly a DICOM-compliant modality and can transfer images to a teleradiology system using the DICOM standard.

CR requires significant capital investment, so it is often the case that the digital modalities will transfer DICOM images to a teleradiology system and printed plain X-rays will be digitized by a film digitizer for sending to the teleradiology system.

Film digitizers

If X-rays are produced on plain film, some means of digitizing the image is required. A wide range of film digitizers are available. They are used to scan a sheet of film to produce a digital image that can be transferred via a teleradiology system (Fig. 14.8). A high-specification film digitizer is capable of producing a DICOM image with the necessary bit depth and image matrix for primary diagnosis. At low workloads, this type of digitizer represents a more economical way of producing digital plain X-rays than CR. A low-cost film digitizer may produce a DICOM image without enough bit depth or matrix size for primary diagnosis or it may produce an image file, eg a bitmap, TIFF or JPEG image.

These images should only be used for review purposes, as they do not have the inherent file structure that allows window width and level adjustments or the ability to perform accurate measurements. The patient demographic information may also be separated from the image file.

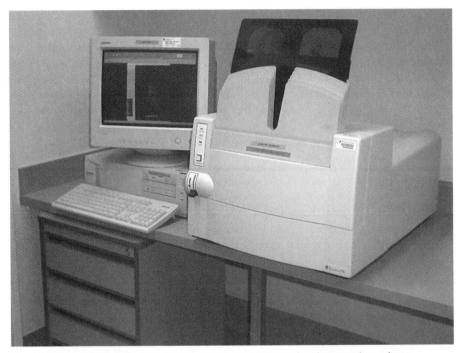

Fig. 14.8. Film digitizer with a coupled personal computer running the scanning software.

Document scanners

Documents scanners can be coupled to a teleradiology system for the purpose of scanning paper documents such as request forms or radiologist reports for transfer via teleradiology. As with film digitizers, the resultant image may be a DICOM image or some other image file format.

Image server

A teleradiology image server is also known as a transmit server or compression server. The role of the image server is to:

▶ store images from modalities, film digitizers and document scanners

▶ compress the images, if required

▶ establish a network connection with a receiving teleradiology application

▶ transfer the images to the receiving station.

Teleradiology software on the image server allows the user to configure one or more receiving destinations and different compression techniques and ratios. The image server can be a DICOM-compliant device that establishes a DICOM association with the receiving application or more simply a device for transmitting image files, eg JPEG images.

The sequence of image transfer where the image server transmits images to receiving application is called the 'push' method. A 'pull' method of image transfer occurs when images are transferred in response to a request from the receiving application. This is the method used by web-based teleradiology systems in which a web client requests images stored on the image server based on certain criteria, eg patient name and date.

Communication network

A number of options are available for the network used to connect the transmitting and receiving stations of teleradiology systems. The method of choice will be dictated by cost, speed and security of transmission required for appropriate delivery of service. Network transmission speed or bandwidth is measured in bits per second (bit/s). Bandwidths are commonly expressed as kilobits per second (kbit/s) or megabits per second (Mbit/s)

1 Mbit/s = 1000 kbit/s = 1 000 000 bit/s

The time taken to transfer an image from an image server to the receiving station depends on the image file size and the network bandwidth. Larger files obviously take longer to transmit; using a high bandwidth network will make image transfer time shorter. Roughly speaking:

Transfer time = image size divided by bandwidth

An 8-bit CR image that has a matrix size of 2048× 2560 would occupy 41 943 040 bits. To transfer this image uncompressed via a 10 Mbit/s network would take approximately 4 seconds, whereas the same image sent across a 100 Mbit/s network would take approximately 0.4 second. Note that these timings assume that the network is perfectly efficient. In practice, the transfer time is longer than the above calculations suggest because of the overhead needed by the network protocols to establish a connection between devices, check for errors in the data received, retransmit any data lost due to collisions, reconstruct any packets of data as required and acknowledge receipt of messages.

Receiving station

The role of a teleradiology receiving station is to:

▶ store images that have been transmitted from the image server

▶ allow review stations to display images so that they can be viewed by the user.

A receiving station may be a distinct server or it may be coupled with the display device. A web client is an example of a coupled device in which the images are cached on the client computer's hard disk for viewing inside a web browser. Alternatively, the receiving station may store the images in an archive to serve multiple display stations.

Review station

A review station is used to view the images sent via a teleradiology service. It is a combination of software that allows viewing and manipulation of images as well as a monitor on which to view them. Again the role of either primary diagnosis or review will dictate the sophistication of the review station software and the quality of the monitor and associated video card.

Recommendations from professional bodies

What standards apply to the practice of teleradiology? The ACR Technical Standard for Teleradiology provides the reference specification for teleradiology equipment to be used for primary diagnosis.[5] The RANZCR has adopted the ACR standard as its policy on teleradiology.[7]

The ACR has stressed that the specifications are not 'set in stone', because teleradiology continues to evolve and there may also be circumstances where the clinical need for teleradiology may take precedence over the availability of the ideal equipment. There are no recommendations for images that are not intended for primary diagnosis. A successful teleradiology system, however, needs to provide images of sufficient quality to satisfy clinical need.

Image acquisition

One aim of the use of standards in teleradiology is to ensure that there is no loss of quality between the acquisition of an image and its display. The ACR recommends the use of DICOM-compliant modalities for image acquisition and preserving the matrix size and bit depth of the image when the image is transferred to the teleradiology system and when it is displayed at the receiving application.

For CT, MRI, ultrasound, nuclear medicine and digital fluoroscopy, the image should be at least 512×512 pixels with an 8-bit pixel depth. For digital X-rays, such as CR, the image should have a minimum of 10-bit pixel depth. If the teleradiology systems will use digitized sheet film, then CT, MRI, ultrasound, nuclear medicine and digital fluoroscopy need to maintain the matrix size of the original matrix and have an 8-bit pixel depth.

These specifications apply to each individual image. That is, it is inappropriate to digitize a sheet of film on which has been printed say 20 images, eg 20 CT slices. Digitized plain X-rays should have a matrix size that will allow spatial resolution of 2.5 lp/mm and have 10-bit pixel depth.

Image display

The ACR makes further recommendations for the display of images at the receiving teleradiology application. These recommendations are again for images intended for primary diagnosis. They include:

▶ greyscale monitor with a luminance of 175 cd/m^2 (candelas per square metre)

▶ ability to adjust the window width and level of the image

▶ ability to magnify and pan the image

▶ ability to flip and rotate the image

▶ ability to perform linear, angle and pixel value measurements

▶ ability to display mandatory patient information on the screen with the images.

The ACR also recommends that the display station be housed in a room in which reflection from surrounding lighting does not degrade the image display. The display station should have a monitor capable of a displaying a minimum of 8-bit greyscale image in a 1000×1000 pixel matrix. Images not intended for primary diagnosis need not meet the above recommendations and in this situation it would be acceptable to use a standard personal computer monitor as the display station.

Image compression

The ACR and the US Food and Drug Administration (FDA) allow the use of both lossless and lossy image compression in teleradiology applications. Neither body makes recommendations about the technique or the degree of image compression, allowing the radiologist to be the ultimate judge as to whether or not the image is clinically acceptable. The FDA insists, however, that compressed images be annotated as such when they are displayed.[8]

For review images, higher rates of compression can be applied and these are not governed by the recommendations for primary diagnosis images.

Security

Local privacy legislation will dictate the level of security needed to maintain patient confidentiality in a teleradiology network. If mandated by legislation, encryption techniques such as secure socket layer (SSL) or pretty good privacy (PGP) may be needed on a public network such as the Internet. Alternatively it may be necessary to employ a private network for teleradiology. A software security technique such as password protection needs to be used on the teleradiology software.

Image archive

Local legislation will dictate how long an image needs to be archived. It is generally considered that an image only needs to be stored at the transmitting or receiving site – not both; however, local legislation may override this assumption. If the teleradiology system employs a film digitizer, then the hard copy film may or may not meet the legislative image archive requirements.

Methods of implementation

Teleradiology can be implemented in various different ways.

Dedicated teleradiology systems

Commercial teleradiology systems are available from numerous vendors. These systems are available as 'off-the-shelf' solutions and vary in their quality and sophistication. The choice of system is dictated by the following criteria:

▶ whether or not the system is to be used for primary diagnosis or review

▶ whether or not the image matrix size and bit depth meet the recommendations of the relevant professional bodies

▶ network bandwidth that allows acceptable transmission speed

▶ network options that meet local legislative requirements for the security of patient data

▶ encryption techniques that meet local legislative requirements for security of patient data

▶ DICOM compliance

▶ connectivity of film digitizers that produce an image suitable for need

▶ connectivity of document scanners to meet local needs

▶ image compression technique acceptable for clinical need

▶ software that annotates images with details of the compression technique when required

▶ software that allows image manipulation functions recommended by professional bodies

▶ storage capacity to meet image retention legislation

▶ internal redundancy and backup devices to maintain an image archive

▶ display monitors suitable for need

▶ software security

▶ reliability and redundancy appropriate for the clinical need.

Use of existing infrastructure

There is an increasing trend for radiology departments to introduce picture archiving and communication systems (PACS). Radiology departments that are PACS-based are fully digital, with DICOM-compliant modalities sending images to a central image archive and the images viewed by radiologists and other clinicians on review stations (Fig. 14.9).

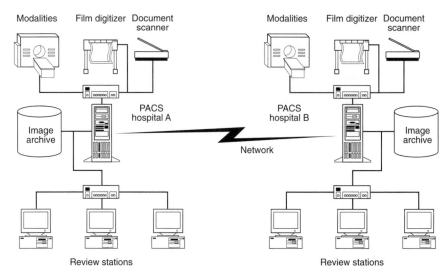

Fig. 14.9. Teleradiology implementation using existing PACS infrastructure.

The existing PACS infrastructure of these departments can be used to support teleradiology, with external images archived and reviewed on the same equipment as local images. The use of existing PACS infrastructure to support teleradiology has obvious advantages in reducing the capital cost of implementing teleradiology, but it also has advantages in workflow, because a clinician does not require training and access to separate PACS and teleradiology applications.

A PACS infrastructure can be used to support teleradiology in a number of ways:

▶ Data warehousing: images from geographically separate sites can be archived centrally allowing access to all images from all sites.

▶ PACS to PACS image transfer: a remote PACS can be set up to mimic a modality that archives images to a PACS. The external PACS transfers images over a wide area network (WAN).

▶ Remote modality: a modality can archive images over a WAN in the same way a local modality can. For example, a CT scanner at Hospital A some 50 km or more from Hospital B can still archive images to Hospital B's PACS.

▶ Remote review station: images on PACS can be viewed on a review station geographically distant from the PACS as long as there is a WAN connection between the review station and the PACS.

Case study: teleradiology in Queensland

In 2000, the Queensland State Health Department began installing PACS in its major hospitals. The first installations were at the four tertiary referral hospitals in Brisbane, the state capital: the Royal Brisbane and Women's Hospital, the Royal Children's

Hospital, the Prince Charles Hospital and the Princess Alexandra Hospital. An additional PACS system was installed at the Townsville Hospital located 1500 km north of Brisbane (Fig. 14.10). All of these hospitals are connected via the Health Department's WAN.

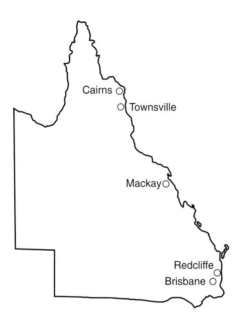

Fig. 14.10. Locations of hospitals participating in teleradiology.

Transferring images between these sites is necessary because of the large number of patients that are transferred for specialty services only available at one of the hospitals. Teleradiology was implemented as an extension to the existing PACS and network infrastructure. Queensland Health developed a web-based teleradiology management system that would transfer images from one PACS to another and would also convert a radiologist's report into a DICOM image and transfer this along with the radiology images.[9] The image and report transfer take place in a single operation.

Neurosurgical services for Redcliffe Hospital are provided by staff at the Royal Brisbane Hospital, located 35 km away. For this reason, the CT scanner at Redcliffe is connected via the Queensland Health WAN to the PACS at the Royal Brisbane Hospital. Another example of a remote modality connection to a PACS occurs at the Cairns Base Hospital, where, for the same reason, their CT scanner is connected to the PACS at the Townsville Hospital. The two sites are 290 km apart. A neurosurgeon can review images from the remote sites and advise on treatment, or request that the patient be transferred for neurosurgical intervention.

The Princess Alexandra Hospital (PAH) provides after-hours radiology reporting for Mackay Hospital. Emergency images are transferred from Mackay Hospital to the

PACS at the PAH, where the on-call radiologist reports them. A report is then faxed back to the referring doctor once the images have been reviewed.

Web-based teleradiology

A web-based teleradiology system simply means viewing images using a web browser such as Internet Explorer or Netscape. The image server in this model of teleradiology is also a web server and allows clients to connect and view images in the same way they can view other web pages on the web (Fig. 14.11). Web-based teleradiology may be implemented as a full DICOM-based system, or the DICOM images from modalities may be converted to JPEG or other format for display. The latter requires much less bandwidth than a DICOM-based system.

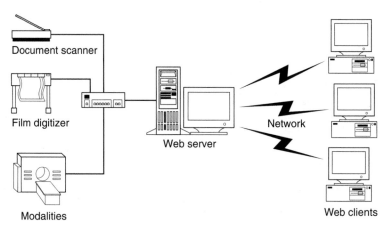

Fig. 14.11. Web-based teleradiology system.

Web-based teleradiology systems use a 'pull'-based image transfer model, in which images are transferred to the client web browser on the basis of criteria such as patient name and date, as entered by the client. Web-based teleradiology has the advantage that no special teleradiology software needs be installed on the client computer. The viewing functions (eg window width, level adjustments, magnification) come from an applet or plug-in that is loaded by the client web browser at run time.

Extenuating circumstances

A patient's treatment in an impoverished country or a war zone where no dedicated teleradiology infrastructure exists may be advantaged by review of radiology. Informal teleradiology has been used in these circumstances by sending an image as an email attachment.[10,11] The email attachment may come from a digital modality, but more often than not it is produced by photographing an X-ray film on a light box with a digital camera.

Conclusion

Paediatric subspecialists tend to work in tertiary hospitals. Because of this, teleradiology is a useful tool not only in providing paediatric radiology review but also in assisting other paediatric specialities provide tertiary medical opinions for patients in remote or rural areas. This has advantages in improving patient care and improving the economics of providing that care. Teleradiology also reduces repeat radiology examinations when a child's treatment is transferred to another facility – an important consideration in reducing the radiation dose to the patient. In addition, teleradiology may assist in the wellbeing of the child by allowing examinations to be performed close to the child's home before transfer.

References

1　Children's Hospital at Westmead. *Outreach Service. A Hospital Without Walls.* http://www.chw.edu.au/about/outreach.htm (last checked 2 August 2004).
2　Franken EA, Berbaum KS. Subspecialty radiology consultation by interactive telemedicine. *Journal of Telemedicine and Telecare* 1996; **2**: 35–41.
3　Bergmo TS. An economic analysis of teleradiology versus a visiting radiologist service. *Journal of Telemedicine and Telecare* 1996; **2**: 136–142.
4　Crowe BL, Hailey DM, de Silva M. Teleradiology at a children's hospital: a pilot study. *Journal of Telemedicine and Telecare* 1996; **2**: 210–216.
5　American College of Radiologists. ACR Technical Standard for Teleradiology. In: *ACR Practice Guidelines and Technical Standards,* 2002: 645–653. http://www.acr.org/departments/stand_accred/standards/pdf/teleradiology.pdf (last checked 2 August 2004).
6　Erickson BJ. *Irreversible Compression of Medical Images.* Society for Computer Applications in Radiology. http://www.scarnet.org/pdf/SCAR%20White%20Paper.pdf (last checked 2 August 2004).
7　Royal Australian and New Zealand College of Radiologists. Position on Teleradiology. In: *Policies – Diagnostic Imaging.* http://www.ranzcr.edu.au/open/policies/diagnostic_imaging/pol6.htm (last checked 2 August 2004).
8　U.S. Department Of Health and Human Services. Food and Drug Administration. *Guidance for the Submission of Premarket Notifications for Medical Image Devices.* http://www.fda.gov/cdrh/ode/guidance/416.pdf (last checked 2 August 2004).
9　Caffery L, Manthey K. Implementation of a Web-based teleradiology management system. *Journal of Telemedicine and Telecare* 2004; **10** (suppl. 1): 22–25.
10　Corr P, Couper I, Beningfield SJ, Mars M. A simple telemedicine system using a digital camera. *Journal of Telemedicine and Telecare* 2000; **6**: 233–236.
11　Swinfen P, Swinfen R, Youngberry K, Wootton R. A review of the first year's experience with an automatic message-routing system for low-cost telemedicine. *Journal of Telemedicine and Telecare* 2003; **9** (suppl. 2): 63–65.

▶15

Tele-otology for Children with Chronic Ear Disease

Robert H Eikelboom and Marcus D Atlas

Introduction

Otolaryngology is a medical specialty concerned with diseases of the ear, nose and throat (ENT). Otology is one subspecialty that deals with disease of the ear and hearing. Otolaryngology relies heavily on various imaging modalities: an otoscope for examining the ear canal and tympanic membrane (ear drum), an optical fibre examination scope for examining the nose, larynx and pharynx, and various X-ray and magnetic resonance scanners for viewing pathologies such as cancers and tumours in the skull base and neck.

There have been very few telemedicine applications in the ENT field, probably for a number of reasons:

▶ There is no culture of recording images for analysis or record keeping, as there is in other fields such as ophthalmology or radiology.

▶ Medical specialists may consider that real-time teleconsultations do not fit in efficiently with their medical practice.

▶ Many consultations, particularly those associated with the ear and balance, require one or more physical tests such as tuning fork tests, audiometry, tympanometry and vestibular tests.

▶ There are a number of other obstacles, including legal liability, cross-border medical licensure, a lack of government fee rebates for service and a lack of validated protocols.

There is, however, a demonstrable need to improve access to specialist ENT services for people in rural and remote areas, particularly as these are often in areas of greater need. As ear-related conditions are by far the most common paediatric otolaryngology problem in remote areas, it is a very suitable field for telemedicine. This chapter describes the magnitude of the problem, current management practices and their shortcomings, the potential role of tele-otology, and the important elements when planning a tele-otology system.[1]

The burden of ear disease in children

There is a high level of middle ear disease in children. The most common type of middle ear disease is otitis media. In its chronic and most serious form, it is called chronic suppurative otitis media (CSOM), a condition that can affect children soon after birth and commonly continues on through to adulthood.[2,3] The World Health Organization reports that 51 000 children worldwide under the age of 5 years die annually as a result of complications arising from otitis media.[4]

In 1990, 24.5 million cases of otitis media were reported in the US (increasing from 9.9 million in 1975), with children below the age of four years being the most vulnerable.[5,6] CSOM is most common in developing countries and indigenous peoples. Otorrhoea (ear discharge) has been found in up to 6% of children and youths in developing countries.[7] It is 15 times more prevalent in North American Indians and the Inuit (Eskimo) group than in the general population.[8,9] In Australian aboriginal children, a prevalence of 60% has been reported,[10-13] with those in rural and remote areas having higher prevalence than those in urban areas.[14]

We have used tele-otology in the assessment of Australian Aboriginal children. These children have an average of 32 months with otitis media between the ages of 2 months and 20 years, compared with an average of 3 months for non-Aboriginal children in the same age range. Furthermore, 41% of school-aged Aboriginal children have a hearing loss of 25 dB in at least one ear compared with about 4% in the general population of the same age group.[11, 15]

In most cases, chronic otitis media leads to perforation of the tympanic membrane, chronic otorrhoea and hearing loss. The aetiology of CSOM is not fully understood. In the Aboriginal population, however, environmental and cultural factors, crowding leading to frequent contact with other children, lack of breast feeding, lack of water, lack of hygiene and poor nutrition are all implicated.[8,16] In the wider population, the factors implicated seem to be upper respiratory tract infection, climate and prematurity.[17]

The major effects of hearing loss in children are on learning, speech and language development,[18] which can lead to further social and community problems. Untreated CSOM has many potential complications, which may include facial nerve paralysis and intracranial infections.

Management of ear disease

Management of chronic otitis media requires a thorough assessment of the condition, medical interventions using antibiotics, various surgical interventions and audiological interventions including the use of hearing amplification.[19] The primary tool for assessment is a visual examination of the ear canal and tympanic membrane by otoscopy, but assessment also includes tympanometry and pure tone audiometry. Unless intensive management is maintained and surgery is undertaken to close the perforation, many ears will resume discharging.

There is, however, poor access to specialist medical services for people in rural and remote areas. In 2001, the medical specialist-to-population ratio for remote areas was 1:8 compared with 1:1 for city and regional areas.[20] The Australian Bureau of Statistics classifies 82% of the total land area of Australia as remote or very remote. Only 2.8% of Australia's population lives in these areas. However, 47% (or 107,000) of these are indigenous people, which represents 26% of the total indigenous population of Australia.[21,22]

Otolaryngologists conduct regular clinics in some of the major regional centres, with occasional visits to remote areas. The number of patients attended to by the specialist during these visits can vary widely because of unexpected situations arising in the communities, such as funerals or other significant community events.[23] Long distances to travel to many small communities add to the difficulties of providing adequate ENT services. The task of primary care falls on general practitioners or other healthcare workers.

The potential of telemedicine

Views of the external ear through an otoscope are important in the diagnosis of external and middle ear disease, such as otitis media. A telemedicine system with appropriate equipment and software able to capture still or moving images can provide an efficient, inexpensive source of diagnostic information to healthcare workers, general practitioners, audiologists and patients. The important role of healthcare workers in this work has been recognized by others:

> 'A comprehensive primary health care approach (exemplified by Aboriginal controlled health services) is likely to both maximise community acceptance and ownership, and improve knowledge of the community among health workers. These are critical factors in achieving compliance with effective therapy.'[23]

The specific benefits are:

▶ Tele-otoscopy can be placed in the hands of local primary healthcare workers. These people usually provide the day-to-day health needs for remote communities. The people in these communities have a strong cultural and social relationship with the local primary healthcare workers.

▶ The provision of specialist services using tele-otoscopy will expand the reach of medical treatment enormously. At present, ear and hearing specialists must travel to remote communities, but these sessions are limited by the human resources available and the distances involved. Tele-otology is potentially available if a trained healthcare worker is present at the remote site.

▶ Tele-otoscopy will assist in a more efficient use of ENT resources. At present, healthcare staff work with general practitioners to manage many ear conditions, especially otitis media with effusion and perforation of the eardrum. Some of these patients, however, have cholesteatoma or other dangerous middle ear infections that can only be diagnosed by an ear examination with an otoscope, usually only by a specialist. Tele-otoscopy allows early detection of dangerous cases, thus increasing efficiency and safety.

▶ There are problems with surgery, including changes in ear conditions between the dates of consultation and operation (sometimes a number of months or even years). The provision of thorough postoperative care may also be disrupted because of irregular surgical visits and irregular attendance by patients because of distance and communication problems. Tele-otoscopy allows accurate preoperative assessment and reduces surgical cancellation, as well as enhancing the provision of regular postoperative care by health workers at or close to the homes of the patients.

The costs of providing healthcare to remote communities are high. Major costs include surgeons, audiologists, travel for health workers and patients, clinic facilities, surgical facilities, and accommodation. Tele-otoscopy potentially allows much more efficient use of resources targeted at known ear disease, the provision of better surgery and extensive patient follow-up.

Use of telemedicine in ENT work

There seems to be relatively little use of telemedicine in the ENT field. A few have reviewed the area,[24,25] and there have been some reports of pilot studies, although little evidence that a sustainable programme has been established.[26–28] Whitten *et al* established a videoconferencing service for children in underprivileged inner city areas and found that about 30% of the consultations were ENT-related.[29,30]

Three centres are currently active in reporting their work in the field of ENT telemedicine. Melcer and colleagues operate in a military setting and have reported that more than 90% of their consultations are ENT-related.[31,32] This may be partly due to the presence of an enthusiastic ENT specialist in the team. About 4% of the consultations were for those aged 1–17 years. Melcer *et al* use real-time videoconferencing for their consultations and an endoscope for imaging. They report positive attitudes of medical personnel towards telemedicine. As an index of success, they use the number of diagnoses that were changed by the specialists after the referring provider had made an initial diagnosis. Overall, 45% of diagnoses were changed, which suggests that telemedicine could reduce the number of unnecessary medical evacuations.

The second active telemedicine programme is in Alaska.[33] Patricoski *et al* use a multipurpose telemedicine cart, which includes a video-otoscope and user-friendly software to store and transmit still images. They compared assessments made in person with an examination microscope to two follow-up assessments from still images of tympanostomy tubes (grommets or ventilation tubes) at 6 months and 12 months after surgery. The follow-up of patients after tympanostomy surgery is important, but this is difficult to manage after they return to their remote communities or when the surgeon cannot be present. The results showed that still images could be used with confidence for following up these tympanostomy patients. The Alaskan study also questioned the assessors about their confidence in making the correct diagnosis. This was recorded as 'confident' or 'very confident' for 73% of cases at the first assessment and for 82% of cases at the second assessment. There was also a significant correlation between this confidence and the quality of the image.

The third active ENT telemedicine programme is being undertaken by our own group in Perth. The premise is that an ear specialist should be able to make a diagnosis and provide management advice by using a series of still images of the tympanic membrane taken by a trained healthcare worker together with a detailed clinical history and an audiogram. This programme has concentrated on the development and validation of a store-and-forward telemedicine system for the assessment of middle ear disease, particularly otitis media with effusion and chronic otitis media. At an early stage, the limits of compression of digitized images of the tympanic membrane were determined, video-otoscopes were tested for suitability to telemedicine, particularly considering safety and quality, and an ENT telemedicine training course for healthcare workers was developed.[34-36] A validation study was also undertaken to evaluate the assessments, diagnoses and management advice given by otolaryngologists. This showed that no patients with ear disease were missed by assessment by telemedicine, but the advice offered did vary. Furthermore, the quality of the images recorded was related to the age of the patient, with lower-quality images being captured from the very young. This is similar to the experience of Patricoski and colleagues in Alaska.[33] It is important, because successful treatment of chronic ear disease and avoiding hearing loss and the ensuing social disadvantages is related to early intervention and management of the disease from a very young age.

Essential elements of tele-otology

As a clinical diagnosis always consists of three elements – history, examination and tests – a telemedicine diagnosis must be made from images, a detailed clinical history and the results of tests.

Video-otoscope

A set of good-quality images is essential for the assessment of the external ear canal and tympanic membrane. The important factors to consider when selecting a video-otoscope are:

▶ image quality

▶ safety

▶ method of focusing

▶ colour balance

▶ depth of field

▶ the balance of the device with the attached cables when it is held in one hand

▶ versatility for other telemedicine applications.

A large range of devices are available. An adaptation of the standard video-otoscope is battery-powered, which makes it portable (Fig. 15.1). It is relatively inexpensive but suffers from poor image quality, especially when the batteries are not fully charged. Devices based on the Hopkins Rod optical system produce high – quality images, but the narrow and long shape of the scopes make them potentially dangerous instruments, especially when used in uncooperative patients.

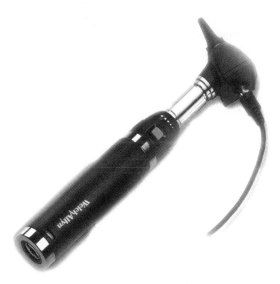

Fig. 15.1. The WelchAllyn battery-powered video-otoscope.

A number of dedicated video-otoscopes are available (Figs 15.2–15.4). They produce high-quality images by using an external light source to deliver light via a fibre-optic cable and employ good-quality lenses and cameras. The optical systems are designed to hold a standard speculum. This eases safety concerns, but they should still be used with caution.

Whichever instrument is used, the primary aim of a video-otoscope is to capture good-quality images in a safe manner. Safety includes ensuring that the patient is not injured with the otoscope, taking steps to prevent cross-infection between patients and between the ears of a patient, and ensuring that the patient feels at ease and is seated comfortably. The operator should be seated so that both the patient's ear and the computer monitor can be seen (Fig. 15.5). Discharging ears should be cleaned and wax obscuring the view of the tympanic membrane should be removed before starting. A typical image has the tympanic membrane filling no more than 80% of the image area, with some of the adjacent ear canal skin also visible. Video-otoscopes can be used for real-time videoconferencing or in a store-and-forward telemedicine system.

Image digitizing

For store-and-forward systems, an image digitizer (also called a frame grabber) is needed to convert the analogue video signal from the camera on the video-otoscope into a digital file suitable for displaying and recording the images. The quality and cost

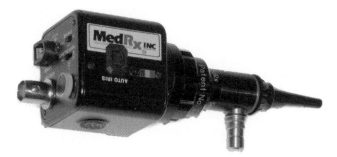

Fig. 15.2. The MedR$_x$ video-otoscope

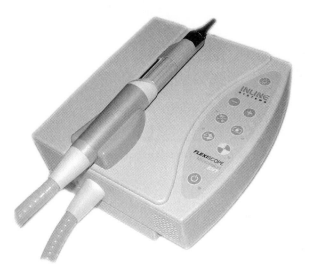

Fig. 15.3. The InLine video-otoscope

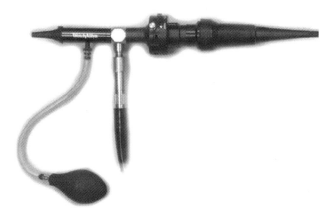

Fig. 15.4. The AMD video-otoscope

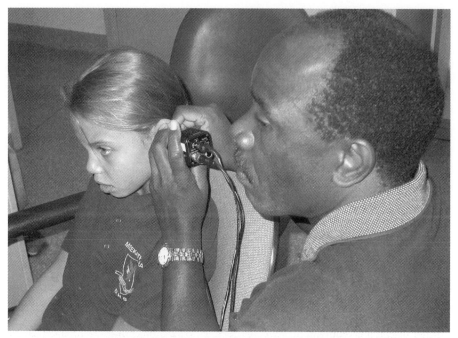

Fig. 15.5. Safe practices must be observed when using a video-otoscope; this includes ensuring that the operator can easily observe both the patient and image on the monitor.

of the digitizers vary and are reflected in their speed and accuracy of digitizing of colour and intensity. The various components of a store-and-forward system are shown schematically in Fig. 15.6.

Software

The primary requirements for the software are that it is easy to use and captures and transmits all the images and data with the minimum of operator intervention. The

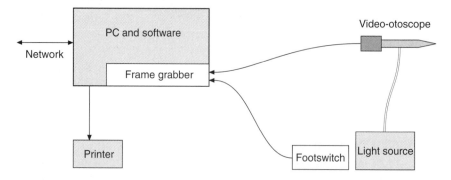

Fig. 15.6. The components of a tele-otology system at the remote site.

imaging functions should allow the operator to concentrate on safe practice and producing good-quality images. A foot switch to control the digitizing of a series of images can facilitate this. There should be provision for entry and storage of the patient details, a clinical history and other data, such as audiometry and tympanometry results. Compression of the digitized images is advisable to avoid having to transmit and store very large amounts of data.[34] The transmission of the images and data to a server, assessment of images and data, and the reporting functions should be integrated into the software.

Training

The focus of training should be the safe use of the video-otoscope to collect excellent quality images. The training should cover the set up and care of the equipment and the use of the software. Other aspects could be background information on ear anatomy, hearing and hearing loss, diseases of the middle ear, and management of middle ear disease.

Future developments

There have been a number of studies that have validated aspects of tele-otology. Further research is required, however, to determine the effects that tele-otology has on chronic ear disease in remote communities. Most interventions to date have not proved as successful in remote communities as they have been in urban settings. It remains to be seen whether or not the improved access to ear specialists that telemedicine provides also assists in improving the delivery of these interventions. Special attention should also be paid to improving the protocols for young children.

The introduction of tele-otology is associated with a substantial set-up cost: each telemedicine station may cost US$15 000. An economics analysis is needed to show the short-term and long-term benefits. In economic terms, the goal of tele-otology should be to decrease the high cost to society of deafness, missed education and social problems.

The question of cost-effectiveness is also relevant to the sustainability of tele-otology. The cost of setting up tele-otology will have to be met by community, regional or state health authorities. Models will have to be developed to suit the structure of health funding in the country concerned. Nationalized health systems with salaried specialists will have particular priorities, such as efficiency and triaging of patients. Health systems in developing countries face other obstacles, including the patients' capacity to pay. For the foreseeable future, implementation of telemedicine may continue to be reliant on aid from overseas government and non-government organizations.

In countries where the health system is a mixture of publicly funded and private healthcare, the public system is usually responsible for the care of those in rural and remote areas. Although the promise of telemedicine has been recognized by public health authorities,[37–39] shifts in funding policies will be needed. The role of the private sector in the health system is interesting. In Australia, teleradiology and telecardiology operate successfully from major regional or metropolitan primary care centres, and other telemedicine applications such as tele-otology may be able to use the same model. The centralizing of medical skills may benefit patients through shorter waiting times, less travel and lower fees.

Conclusion

There is a demonstrable need to improve the ear healthcare of children. Telemedicine technology is capable of providing a part of the solution, and healthcare staff for the most part are willing to be involved in tele-otology. The issues that remain to be resolved before there can be a widespread implementation of tele-otology are a more complete validation of the protocols, short-term and long-term economic analyses and development of appropriate funding models.

Further information

Lions Ear and Hearing tele-otology project. http://www.lehi.com.au/research/telemedicine.asp (last checked 6 August 2004).

Alaska Federal Health Care Access Network telehealth project. http://www.afhcan.org (last checked 6 August 2004).

Audiology Forum: video-otoscopy. http://www.rcsullivan.com/www/ears.htm (last checked 6 August 2004).

American Academy of Pediatrics examination of middle ear disease. http://www.aap.org/otitismedia/www/vc/ear/index.cfm (last checked 6 August 2004).

References

1   Eikelboom RH, Atlas MD, Mbao MN, Gallop M. Tele-otology: planning, design, development and implementation. *Journal of Telemedicine and Telecare* 2002; **8** (suppl. 3): 14–17.

2   Boswell J, Nienhuys T, Rickards F, Mathews J. Onset of otitis media in Australian Aboriginal infants in a prospective study from birth. *Australian Journal of Otolaryngology* 1993; **1**: 232–237.

3   Boswell J. Presentation of early otitis media in 'Top End' Aboriginal infants. *Australian and New Zealand Journal of Public Health* 1997; **21**: 100–102.

4   World Bank. *World Development Report 1993: Investing in Health*. Oxford: Oxford University Press, 1993: 215–222.

5   Stool SE. *Otitis Media with Effusion in Young Children*. Rockville, Maryland: US Department of Health and Human Services, 1994.

6   Teele DW, Klein JO, Rosner BA. Epidemiology of otitis media in children. *Annals of Otology, Rhinology and Laryngology. Supplement* 1980; **89**: 5–6.

7   Berman S. Otitis media in developing countries. *Pediatrics* 1995; **96**: 126–131.

8   Manning P, Avery M, Ross A. Purulent otitis media: differences between populations in different environments. *Pediatrics* 1974; **53**: 135–136.

9   Ward B, McPherson B, Thomason JE. Hearing screening in Australian Aboriginal university students. *Public Health* 1994; **108**: 43–48.

10 Sunderman J, Dyer H. Chronic ear disease in Australian Aborigines. *Medical Journal of Australia* 1984; **140**: 708–711.

11   Watson DS, Clapin M. Ear health of aboriginal primary school children in the Eastern Goldfields Region of Western Australia. *Australian Journal of Public Health* 1992; **16**: 26–30.

12   Kelly HA, Weeks SA. Ear disease in three aboriginal communities in Western Australia. *Medical Journal of Australia* 1991; **154**: 240–245.

13   Casselbrant ML, Brostoff LM, Cantekin EI, *et al.* Otitis media with effusion in preschool children. *Laryngoscope* 1985; **95**: 428–436.

14   Kamien M. Ear disease and hearing in aboriginal and white children in two schools in rural New South Wales. *Medical Journal of Australia* 1975; **1**: 33–37.

15   McPherson B. Hearing loss in Australian Aborigines: a critical evaluation. *Australian Journal of Audiology* 1990; **12**: 67–78.

16   Coates HL, Morris PS, Leach AJ, Couzos S. Otitis media in Aboriginal children: tackling a major health problem. *Medical Journal of Australia* 2002; **177**: 177–178.

17   Pestalozza G, Romagnoli M, Tessitore E. Incidence and risk factors of acute otitis media with effusion in children of different age groups. *Advances in Oto-Rhino-Laryngology* 1988; **40**: 47–56.

18   McCafferty GJ, Lewis AN, Coman WB, Mills C. A nine-year study of ear disease in Australian aboriginal children. *Journal of Laryngology and Otology* 1985; **99**: 117–125.

19   Morris P. Management of otitis media in a high risk population. *Australian Family Physician* 1998; **27**: 1021–1029.

20   *Medical Labour Force 2001*. Canberra: Australian Institute of Health and Welfare, 2001. http://www.aihw.gov.au/publications/hwl/mlf01/mlf01-c00.pdf (last checked 9 June 2004).

21   Australian Bureau of Statistics. ASGC Remoteness Classification: Purpose and Use. In: *Census Paper no. 03/01*. Canberra: Commonwealth of Australia, 2003: 7, 10.

22   Australian Bureau of Statistics. *CDATA01 – Your Census at Work*. Canberra: Commonwealth of Australia, 2002.

23   Couzos S, Metcalf S, Murrary R. *Systematic Review of Existing Evidence and Primary Care Guidelines on the Management of Otitis Media in Aboriginal and Torres Strait Islander Populations*. Canberra: Commonwealth Department of Health and Aged Care, 2001.

24   Burgess LP, Holtel MR, Syms MJ, *et al.* Overview of telemedicine applications for otolaryngology. *Laryngoscope* 1999; **109**: 1433–1437.

25   Holtel MR, Burgess LP. Telemedicine in otolaryngology. *Otolaryngologic Clinics of North America* 2002; **35**: 1263–1281.

26   Crump WJ, Driscoll B. An application of telemedicine technology for otorhinolaryngology diagnosis. *Laryngoscope* 1996; **106**: 595–598.

27   Crump WJ, Levy BJ, Billica RD. A field trial of the NASA Telemedicine Instrument Pack in a family practice. *Aviation, Space, and Environmental Medicine* 1996; **67**: 1080–1085.

28   Blakeslee DB, Grist WJ, Stachura ME, Blakeslee BS. Practice of otolaryngology via telemedicine. *Laryngoscope* 1998; **108**: 1–7.

29   Whitten P, Cook DJ, Shaw P, *et al.* Telekid Care: bringing health care into schools. *Telemedicine Journal* 1998; **4**: 335–343.

30   Whitten PS, Cook DJ. School-based telemedicine: using technology to bring health care to inner-city children. *Journal of Telemedicine and Telecare* 1999; **5** (suppl. 1): 23–25.

31   Melcer T, Crann B, Hunsaker D, *et al.* A retrospective evaluation of the development of a telemedicine network in a military setting. *Military Medicine* 2002; **167**: 510–515.

32   Melcer T, Hunsaker D, Crann B, *et al.* A prospective evaluation of ENT telemedicine in remote military populations seeking specialty care. *Telemedicine Journal and e-Health* 2002; **8**: 301–311.

33   Patricoski C, Kokesh J, Ferguson AS, *et al.* A comparison of in-person examination and video otoscope imaging for tympanostomy tube follow-up. *Telemedicine Journal and e-Health* 2003; **9**: 331–344.

34   Eikelboom R, Mbao M, Atlas M, *et al.* Compression of video-otoscope images for tele-otology: a pilot study. *Proceedings of the Annual EMBS International Conference* 2001: 3517–3520.

35   Mbao MN, Eikelboom RH, Atlas MD, Gallop MA. Evaluation of video-otoscopes suitable for tele-otology. *Telemedicine Journal and e-Health* 2003; **9**: 325–330.

36   Eikelboom RH, Weber S, Atlas MD, *et al.* A tele-otology course for primary care providers. *Journal of Telemedicine and Telecare* 2003; **9** (suppl. 2): 19–22.

37   Western Australia Department of Health. *The Country Health Services Review. Vision, Goals, Directions for Developing WA Country Health Services*. Perth: Department of Health, 2003: 41, 47.

38   Planning and workforce group: Western Australia Department of Health. *Innovative Models of Care*. Perth: Western Australia Department of Health, 2003: 17–19.

39   Health Reform Commission. *A Healthy Future for Western Australians*. Perth: Western Australia Department of Health, 2004: 43–44.

▶16

Telemedicine and Children with Special Healthcare Needs

James P Marcin, Marina Reznik and Philip O Ozuah

Introduction

Although many people in industrialized countries live in rural communities, they are faced with significant inequities in access to healthcare compared with those living in urban and suburban communities.[1] For example, in the US, 20% of the population live in designated rural communities, yet only 9% of physicians work in these areas. These disparities are part of the reason that mortality for children and adults in the US is higher in rural communities than in suburban and urban communities. Furthermore, patient-specific measures of quality of care and health outcomes are worse in rural hospitals, with rural patients receiving poorer healthcare and having poorer outcomes for a variety of medical and surgical services.[2-7]

Rural health services are difficult to maintain because of low patient volumes, limited numbers of healthcare providers and unfavourable economies of scale. Compounding these problems is the fact that patients who live in rural communities often bypass local healthcare providers by travelling to urban settings to receive care.[8,9] This occurs for several reasons. In some cases, the specialty care or advanced technology that is needed to diagnose or treat a particular condition is not available in rural settings. Rural patients may also have perceptions that local healthcare is poor, directly affecting the sustainability of local providers and healthcare institutions.[10] Furthermore, the perception that 'bigger is better' may incorrectly influence rural residents, who presume that a large urban hospital will retain better-qualified physicians and offer the newest in medical technology advances.[8,11]

Children who live in rural and medically underserved regions experience even greater disparities than adults and are at particular risk because there are relatively fewer paediatric specialty and subspecialty services available.[12] Moreover, the closest services that are available are typically more distant from their rural residence than for adults.[13] This is particularly true for children with special healthcare needs (CSHCN) who live in rural communities, for whom obtaining specialty or subspecialty care is especially challenging. Special needs children include those with asthma, congenital heart disease, hearing impairments, epilepsy, diabetes mellitus, cerebral palsy or leukaemia. In rural communities, obtaining appropriate care may be difficult for several reasons.[14] First, these children require more frequent routine and urgent medical assessments than children without special needs. Second, these children often have medical conditions and needs that are unique, uncommon and require specialist or specialty team knowledge and collaboration. Third, it is more difficult to transport CSHCN because they often require medical devices, such as wheelchairs, oxygen, suction, monitoring devices (eg pulse oximetry) and sometimes mechanical ventilators. Telemedicine has the potential to solve these problems by providing a link between families of CSHCN and specialty care providers, thus allowing the delivery of comprehensive services to children with complex medical illnesses. By importing primary and specialty paediatric expertise through telemedicine, rural clinics and hospitals can increase their capacity to treat patients locally without having to invest in expensive specialty clinics or transport all patients to a referral centre.

Background

There are several reports about the use of telemedicine for adults and children with special healthcare needs in other countries as well as in the US. Rialle *et al* describe the concept of 'smart' home systems that provide health services for people with special needs who wish to remain independent and living in their own home.[15] A smart system is a monitoring and medical surveillance system for the home. It features sensors connected by a communication system such as the Internet. The sensors are connected wirelessly in the home to a base station that performs signal analysis and detects critical situations such as falls, sudden palsy, stroke or hypothermia. Alarms are set off if the patient's activity deviates from the norm. The home base station communicates with a remote medical control station in charge of making an appropriate response.

The bioengineering and telemedicine group in Madrid, Spain have developed a multimodal system that allows remote monitoring of ECG signals as well as a direct link to health services via telemedicine for people with special needs. In the pilot study, participants were satisfied with the system and found it to be helpful and efficient in providing support for their independent living.[16] In the US, in Tampa, Florida, the use of videoconferencing to bridge the transition to home for families caring for a relative with a prolonged state of reduced consciousness due to a brain injury was found to be successful by reducing the number of perceived family needs compared with a control group.[17]

Telemedicine has been used increasingly by several institutions as a means of providing paediatric specialty support for rural facilities to improve the care of children with special needs.[18-21] The Georgia Telehealth Project provides consultations between subspecialists at the Medical College of Georgia's Department of Pediatrics and nurse facilitators at a rural clinic affiliated with Georgia's Children's Medical Services.[19] The subspecialty groups most frequently consulted include allergy and immunology, respiratory medicine, neurology and genetics. In this project, telemedicine was found to be an acceptable means of delivering certain paediatric subspecialty services to children with special healthcare needs who lived in rural areas distant from tertiary centres.

Farmer *et al* reported the findings from a 1997–98 survey of healthcare providers from seven US states who were developing interdisciplinary telehealth programmes for CSHCN living in rural areas.[20] The health problems that were being addressed by the responders included neurodevelopmental disorders, paediatric primary care issues, emotional/behavioural concerns and chronic illnesses such as asthma, cancer, diabetes and cystic fibrosis. The authors concluded that telehealth systems have the potential to increase access to specialized services and to enhance community-based services for rural and underserved children.

Two remote telemedicine clinics were established and linked to a tertiary care centre in Texas with the goal of improving access for special healthcare needs children.[21] These clinics were evaluated to determine whether or not the tertiary interdisciplinary team could effectively plan interventions for CSHCN and to assess user satisfaction with telemedicine. The authors found that the interdisciplinary team, the patients and their families were highly satisfied with healthcare delivery via telemedicine. In this chapter, we describe our experience at the University of California Davis Children's Hospital (UCDCH) with caring for CSHCN.

Caring for children with special healthcare needs: one hospital's experience

In 1999, staff at the UCDCH established a telemedicine programme to a rural and medically underserved community with the objective of providing paediatric subspecialty telemedicine consultations to CSHCN.[18] This project was started to improve access to specialty care for CSHCN and as a step towards the US goal of providing a 'medical home' for every child with special healthcare needs.[22] (A medical home provides access to comprehensive, high-quality healthcare and a primary care provider who offers integrated healthcare services and who will develop a sustained partnership with patients, practising in the context of family and community.) In addition, the use of telemedicine to provide specialty consultations for CSHCN with their primary care provider in their own community can facilitate care that is more accessible, family-centred and coordinated, thereby reinforcing other efforts to provide a medical home.[23]

Before implementing the telemedicine programme, a prospective medical needs survey of CSHCN and their parents or guardian was conducted to assess the role they perceived for telemedicine in the care of their children. We also assessed the success of the telemedicine programme and reported the parent or guardians' perceptions of the appropriateness and quality of telemedicine consultations for their children after the telemedicine programme was initiated.

A telemedicine clinic for CSHCN was established in Oroville, California, a community located 150 km north of the UCDCH in Sacramento. The city of Oroville and its surrounding communities have been designated as health professional shortage areas by the US government. The population of Oroville is 13 000, and the population of the greater Oroville area is 45 000. The telemedicine connection linked two adjacent local primary care offices (one office with two general paediatricians and one physician assistant, and another office with one general paediatrician and one physician assistant) caring for local CSHCN to an established UCDCH paediatric subspecialty clinic office.

The telemedicine programme started in 1999. A part-time telemedicine site coordinator was hired in Oroville to assist in the telemedicine activities such as scheduling and coordinating appointments. The telemedicine connection uses three ISDN lines (384 kbit/s) that provide videoconferencing with a peripheral general patient examination camera (Fig. 16.1). At each telemedicine consultation, the patient, the patient's parents or guardians, the referring healthcare provider (physician or physician assistant) and the UCDCH subspecialist participate. At the end of the encounter, either a handwritten or dictated consultation note from the subspecialist is faxed to the Oroville site for inclusion in both the Oroville and UCDCH medical records.

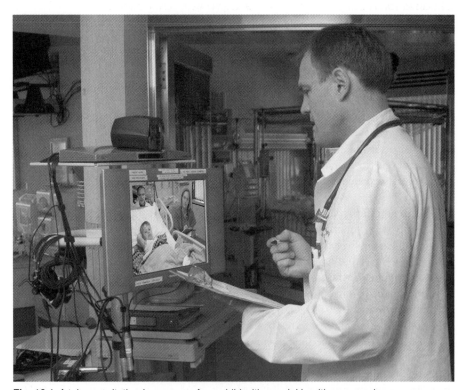

Fig. 16.1. A teleconsultation in progress for a child with special healthcare needs.

Pre-telemedicine survey

Forty-two parents or guardians of CSHCN were randomly selected from the Oroville community and participated in a telephone survey. It was clear from the survey that making medical appointments was a significant burden for the parents or guardians.

Eighty-three percent of them stated that travel time to the specialist's office at the UCDCH exceeded one hour. Forty percent of all parents or guardians and 96% of working parents or guardians typically missed work to attend their children's appointments. Fifty-two percent of the parents or guardians considered themselves as primarily responsible for coordinating care among the different medical services for their children. Most of the parents or guardians reported that they relied on emergency department services or home regulation of drugs, or both, for their children in the absence of direct access to their subspecialist provider.

Perceived advantages and disadvantages of receiving subspecialty care using telemedicine varied substantially. Positive comments about telemedicine included: 'Could see two doctors at one time', 'Saves time and gas', 'Wouldn't have to miss work', 'We could see the same doctors we always see and not have to re-explain things to new doctors' and 'If there is a doctor who knows more and is far away, I would do it to get the best care'. Perceived disadvantages of telemedicine included the following comments: 'If it is an emergency, I would rather be face-to-face with the doctor', 'Potential failure of the electronic system,' 'If I'm not talking face-to-face, [the doctor] is not going to tell me the truth' and 'I prefer face-to-face meetings…I want to talk with [the doctor] with nothing in between us'. Twenty-one caregivers (50%) indicated that they would be 'very likely' to use telemedicine in the future when available, 15 (36%) indicated that they would be 'likely' to use telemedicine in the future and four (9%) stated it would be 'unlikely' for them to use telemedicine when offered in the future.

Telemedicine programme

During a three-year period of telemedicine (April 1999–April 2002), 55 CSHCN received a total of 130 teleconsultations from paediatric subspecialists. The proportion of patients who failed to arrive for their scheduled telemedicine appointment (17%) was very similar to what is experienced by the UCDCH paediatrics subspecialty clinic, which has a mean failure to show rate of 15%. The frequency of teleconsultations increased steadily after the programme's inception. The median number of visits per individual was two (range 1–12). The variety of illnesses that affected these patients warranted different paediatric subspecialty consultations, including paediatric endocrinology–obesity, psychiatry, gastro-enterology, haematology–oncology, nephrology and infectious disease.

The median consultation time was 30 minutes (range 15–70). Some sort of technical difficulties were experienced in 38 consultations (29%). In 22 encounters (17%), either the subspecialist or the Oroville healthcare provider complained of pixelation or blockiness of the videoconference image. Difficulties with audio occurred in 10 encounters (8%) and in one encounter a simultaneous telephone connection was required for audio. More than one attempt was needed to establish the telemedicine connection in six encounters (5%). All of the encounters during which technical difficulties were experienced eventually completed the telemedicine consultation during the scheduled visit.

Satisfaction with telemedicine

Satisfaction surveys were administered to both the parents or guardians and the Oroville providers.[24] The questions used five-point Likert scales (1 = excellent, 5 = very poor). One hundred and thirty parent or guardian surveys (from 55 individual parents or guardians) and 81 provider surveys were collected. Overall, satisfaction was very high, with all of the parents or guardians rating satisfaction of telemedicine care as either 'excellent' or 'very good.' All but one of the responders stated that they wished to continue to receive their consultations using telemedicine. Ninety percent of overall telemedicine satisfaction scores were 'very good' or 'excellent'. All but two of the provider respondents rated their satisfaction with telemedicine as 'excellent' or 'very good'. The lowest satisfaction score from the providers was their perception that telemedicine allowed an adequate examination by the UCDCH physician.

Conclusions

The data collected from our pre-telemedicine survey suggest that most parents or guardians of CSHCN living in a rural, medically underserved community would be either likely or very likely to receive their children's subspecialty care using telemedicine. Furthermore, data from our CSHCN telemedicine clinic show that paediatric subspecialty telemedicine consultations to a rural, underserved community are feasible and considered highly satisfactory by both the parents or guardians and the rural healthcare providers. Ninety-eight percent of the parents or guardians stated that they wished to continue to receive their consultations using telemedicine rather than having to travel to the UCDCH subspecialty clinic for routine face-to-face appointments.

There are several potential advantages in the use of telemedicine as a means of providing subspecialty consultations to CSHCN living in rural, underserved communities. First, by increasing local access to subspecialty healthcare expertise, telemedicine may provide a means of supporting a medical home in communities that otherwise have limited access to comprehensive care. Telemedicine may promote increased care coordination between the primary care physicians and subspecialists and allows primary care providers to coordinate and directly participate in the team management of CSHCN. Telemedicine may also provide an educational benefit to the rural primary care providers, reduce provider isolation and potentially increase their knowledge in a medical subspecialty. Telemedicine decreases the travel and work loss burdens for the parents or guardians of CSHCN and potentially lessens the chances for medical errors because of poor communication between the subspecialist and primary care provider. Finally, telemedicine allows patients to remain in the care of their primary care physicians, assists community providers to retain patients and may improve patients' and parents' or guardians' perception of their primary care providers.

The data from our pre-telemedicine survey are consistent with previous studies that investigated the perceived advantages and disadvantages of telemedicine.[25] The issues of missed work, costs and time for transportation, and the time needed to schedule a face-to-face appointment, act as barriers. In a survey conducted by Allen and Hayes on patient satisfaction with telemedicine in a rural clinic, faster and easier access to a subspecialist was noted as the primary advantage of telemedicine.[26] That study reported that patients 'would rather see specialists on the TV system than wait for a few days to see him or her in person'.

Karp *et al* reported similar overall parent or guardian satisfaction when using telemedicine to provide subspecialty consultations to CSHCN.[19] Their experience was analogous to ours insofar as most of the consultations were conducted by only a few subspecialty groups. In Karp's report, allergy–immunology and respiratory medicine accounted for 64% of the consultations, and, in our work, 89% of the consultations were performed by endocrinology–obesity and child psychiatry. These results are consistent with previous telemedicine research that has shown that some healthcare providers are more likely to adopt telemedicine, while others are slow to adopt or never adopt it.[27,28] In our experience, some clinicians prefer to have personal contact with their patients and have varying degrees of comfort with new technologies, which may partly explain why some subspecialists were more or less likely to adopt telemedicine. Other reasons for the unequal use of telemedicine among subspecialists include the varying need for different subspecialists in Oroville, the families' willingness to participate in telemedicine, the referring physicians' preference to refer patients using telemedicine, the subspecialists' comfort with using telemedicine and the frequency with which patients need to be seen for their condition.

There are several limitations to the generalizability of our telemedicine programme. First, certain subspecialties at the UCDCH have been relatively more successful at incorporating telemedicine into their work. This variation between subspecialty areas may have been caused by the reluctance of parents or guardians or subspecialty providers, or both, to use and maintain telemedicine because of factors related to their specific subspecialties. Furthermore, while the referring physicians from Oroville were general paediatricians, one might expect that the perceptions of the need for telemedicine (or subspecialty consultation) would be different between referring paediatricians or other primary care physicians, or both. We believe that the success of a telemedicine programme depends on financial and personnel resources, patients' and parents' or guardians' attitudes, the referring and consulting healthcare providers' commitment to telemedicine and the specific medical condition being considered for telemedicine consultation.

In conclusion, telemedicine has the potential to increase access to subspecialty providers for children with special healthcare needs who live in rural and underserved communities. The use of telemedicine as a means of providing specialty care services to underserved populations is a viable solution to inequities in the availability of care. Moreover, telemedicine can assist in the development of partnerships between primary and specialty healthcare providers by improving continuity of care and providing comprehensive and integrated services for children with special needs.

References

1   Thompson T. *HHS Issues on Community Health in Rural, Urban Areas.* Washington DC: CDC/NCHS Press Office, 2001.

2   Keeler EB, Rubenstein LV, Kahn KL, *et al.* Hospital characteristics and quality of care. *Journal of the American Medical Association* 1992; **268**: 1709–1714.

3   Stoddard JJ, St Peter RF, Newacheck PW. Health insurance status and ambulatory care for children. *New England Journal of Medicine* 1994; **330**: 1421–1425.

4   Zhang P, Tao G, Irwin KL. Utilization of preventive medical services in the United States: a comparison between rural and urban populations. *Journal of Rural Health* 2000; **16**: 349–356.

5   Rutledge R, Fakhry SM, Baker CC, *et al.* A population-based study of the association of medical manpower with county trauma death rates in the United States. *Annals of Surgery* 1994; **219**: 547–567.

6   Baker SP, Whitfield RA, O'Neill B. Geographic variations in mortality from motor vehicle crashes. *New England Journal of Medicine* 1987; **316**: 1384–1387.

7   Rogers FB, Shackford SR, Osler TM, *et al.* Rural trauma: the challenge for the next decade. *Journal of Trauma* 1999; **47**: 802–821.

8   Rieber GM, Benzie D, McMahon S. Why patients bypass rural health care centers. *Minnesota Medicine* 1996; **79**: 46–50.

9   Aucar JA, Doarn CR, Sargsyan A, *et al.* Use of the Internet for long-term clinical follow-up. *Telemedicine Journal* 1998; **4**: 371–374.

10 Rissam HS, Kishore S, Bhatia ML, Trehan N. Trans-telephonic electro-cardiographic monitoring (TTEM) – first Indian experience. *Studies in Health Technology and Informatics* 1998; **50**: 361–363.

11 Geyman JP, Norris TE, Hart LG. *Textbook of Rural Medicine.* New York: McGraw-Hill, 2001.

12 *Annual Report of the American Board of Pediatrics to the Association of Medical School Pediatric Department Chairs.* American Board of Pediatrics, 2001.

13 Eberhardt MS, Ingram DD, Makuc DM, *et al. Urban and Rural Health Chartbook. Health, United States, 2001.* Hyattsville, MD: National Center for Health Statistics, 2001.

14 Saywell RM Jr, Zollinger TW, Schafer ME, *et al.* Children with special health care needs program: urban/rural comparisons. *Journal of Rural Health* 1993; **9**: 314–325.

15 Rialle V, Duchene F, Noury N, *et al.* Health 'Smart' home: information technology for patients at home. *Telemedicine Journal and e-Health* 2002; **8**: 395–409.

16 Rodriguez-Ascaso A, Villalar JL, Arredondo MT, *et al.* An assistive home care environment for people with special needs. *Journal of Telemedicine and Telecare* 2002; **8** (suppl. 2): 72–74.

17 Hauber RP, Jones ML. Telerehabilitation support for families at home caring for individuals in prolonged states of reduced consciousness. *Journal of Head Trauma Rehabilitation* 2002; **17**: 535–541.

18 Marcin JP, Ellis J, Mawis R, *et al.* Using telemedicine to provide pediatric subspecialty care to children with special health care needs in an underserved rural community. *Pediatrics* 2004; **113**: 1–6.

19 Karp WB, Grigsby RK, McSwiggan-Hardin M, *et al.* Use of telemedicine for children with special health care needs. *Pediatrics* 2000; **105**: 843–847.

20 Farmer JE, Muhlenbruck L. Telehealth for children with special health care needs: promoting comprehensive systems of care. *Clinical Pediatrics* 2001; **40**: 93–98.

21 Robinson SS, Seale DE, Tiernan KM, Berg B. Use of telemedicine to follow special needs children. *Telemedicine Journal and e-Health* 2003; **9**: 57–61.

22 United States. Department of Health and Human Services. *Healthy People 2010: Understanding and Improving Health.* Washington, DC: US Department of Health and Human Services, 2000.

23 Ziring PR, Brazdziunas D, Cooley WC, *et al.* American Academy of Pediatrics. Committee on Children With Disabilities. Care coordination: integrating health and related systems of care for children with special health care needs. *Pediatrics* 1999; **104**: 978–9781.

24 Nesbitt TS, Hilty DM, Kuenneth CA, Siefkin A. Development of a telemedicine program: a review of 1,000 videoconferencing consultations. *Western Journal of Medicine* 2000; **173**: 169–174.

25 Hassol A, Gaumer G, Grigsby J, *et al.* Rural telemedicine: a national snapshot. *Telemedicine Journal* 1996; **2**: 43–48.

26 Allen A, Hayes J. Patient satisfaction with telemedicine in a rural clinic. *American Journal of Public Health* 1994; **84**: 1693.

27 Poulsen PB. *Health Technology Assessment and Diffusion of Health Technology.* Odense, Denmark: Odense University Press, 1999.

28 Cain M, Mittman R. *Diffusion of Innovation in Health Care.* Oakland, CA: Foundation and Institute for the Future, 2002.

▶17

Telemedicine for Children Presenting to Rural Emergency Departments or Intensive Care Units

James P Marcin, Marina Reznik and Philip O Ozuah

Introduction

Past studies have suggested shortcomings in the provision of high-quality care to acutely ill and injured children presenting to rural hospitals.[1-6] At times, rural emergency departments (EDs) are inadequately equipped for paediatric emergencies and underserved with respect to paediatric specialty services.[1,2] Furthermore, personnel working in rural EDs, including physicians, nurses, pharmacists and support staff, may be less experienced in paediatric emergencies. The relative lack of equipment, infrastructure and personnel well versed in delivering specialty care to children may result in delayed or incorrect diagnoses, suboptimal therapies and imperfect medical management.[7-14] As a consequence, acutely ill or injured children may receive lower quality of care than children presenting to non-rural hospitals that specialize in paediatric medicine.[5,6,15-17]

Telemedicine has been shown by several centres to be a feasible means of addressing quality of care issues in adults and children who present to rural and urban EDs that require specialty consultations.[18-21] For example, Brennan *et al* conducted a controlled trial of telemedicine in two EDs where patients were randomized to receive care from a physician via telemedicine or face-to-face. There were no significant differences between the two groups when outcomes were compared, including the need for additional care, the frequency of return ED visits and the overall patient satisfaction.[20] The authors of this trial concluded that for some non-emergency diagnoses, the use of telemedicine in the ED is feasible and results in patient satisfaction similar to that from face-to-face consultations.

Stamford *et al* also described their experience in providing rural EDs with telemedicine consultations for adult patients.[22] In their descriptive analysis, telemedicine consultations resulted in diagnostic and therapeutic changes in 18% and 52%, respectively. Similarly, in a different descriptive report, trauma surgeons from an urban tertiary hospital performed consultations using telemedicine on patients being treated in the rural EDs.[23]

Emergency department telemedicine

The University of California Davis Children's Hospital (UCDCH) established telemedicine links to four rural EDs in northern California starting in 2003. The goal was to provide the rural EDs with paediatric critical care expertise shortly after a child presents with either acute illness or injury. When such a child presents to one of these EDs, an appropriate consultant is called and a telemedicine consultation is initiated 24 hours per day, seven days per week. All consultants have telemedicine access available at one of eight telemedicine stations at the UCDCH or at their homes, or both.

Each of the EDs has a purpose-built, telemedicine unit mounted on a wall with a flat-screen monitor that can be pulled over an acute care ED trolley (Figs 17.1 and 17.2). Connections use either a T1 line or three ISDN lines. Children who have received telemedicine consultations for acute illness or injury in the rural ED telemedicine network have been the more ill or severely injured, including children with diagnoses such as acute epiglottitis, diabetic ketoacidosis with coma, traumatic brain injury or coma. However, there have been cases of consultations being conducted on mildly and moderately ill children with management and disposition questions (eg should this patient be discharged home or hospitalized?). Findings to date suggest that the use of telemedicine under these circumstances can improve the access to specialty physicians, improve the quality of care and maintain patient/parent satisfaction.

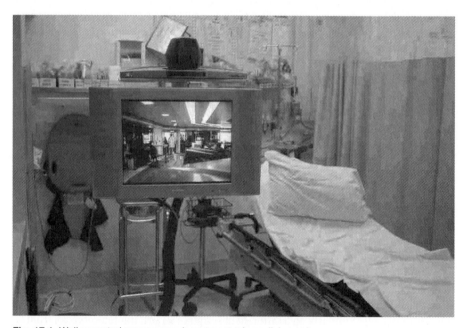

Fig. 17.1. Wall-mounted emergency department telemedicine unit.

Rural intensive care units

Intensive care units (ICUs) are typically regionalized to improve efficiency and patient outcomes.[8,12,24–27] Paediatric ICUs are even more regionalized than adult ICUs because children require critical care services much less frequently than adults.

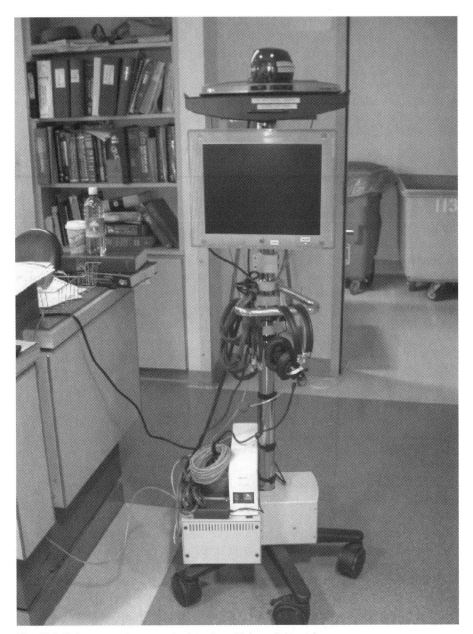

Fig. 17.2. Pole-mounted emergency department telemedicine unit.

Therefore, when a child with an acute illness or injury requires admission to a paediatric ICU from a rural hospital, the transferring facility must initiate treatment, stabilize the patient and arrange transport to a paediatric referral centre. This is often the case even if the transferring rural facility is an adult referral centre with adult ICU capabilities.

Under special circumstances, however, transporting an acutely ill or injured child from a rural facility with adult ICU capabilities to a paediatric ICU referral centre may not be necessary or possible. For example, children are often admitted to an ICU for monitoring or because of the need for special nursing care. These children may be only 'moderately ill', eg a child with asthma requiring continuous salbutamol or a child with known diabetes and moderate diabetic ketoacidosis. In these cases, long-distance patient transport may be considered unnecessary or an overutilization of resources.

At the other extreme, a child presenting to a rural hospital may require emergency stabilization or an emergency intervention or procedure, or may be too critically ill to tolerate transport to a paediatric referral centre. In these cases, transporting an acutely ill or injured child before stabilization or before urgently needed interventions or procedures may contribute to morbidity or mortality. For example, given a child presenting with a traumatic subdural haematoma and shock, it may be more appropriate for the rural hospital to have the shock reversed and the haematoma evacuated before subjecting the patient to a long, potentially dangerous journey. Although such a patient would probably require ICU admission after resuscitation and surgery, they may no longer need transport to a paediatric centre, yet they may require some ongoing support from a paediatric referral centre. In such cases, where a paediatric patient may either be 'not so critically ill' or where interfacility transport might contribute to a patient's morbidity or even mortality, telemedicine is a means of providing paediatric critical care support to a rural centre.

Although there is a growing literature on telemedicine in general,[28] there is limited information on the use of telemedicine in intensive care units for adults, and even less for children.[29-34] Berg et al reported remote critical care consultations between the Naval Hospital in Guam and the Tripler Army Medical Center in Hawaii.[29] During a 10-week study period, a total of 87 teleconsultations were conducted on 25 patients from the Naval Hospital's ICU. The results of this study showed that a broad range of critical care patients could be managed effectively through daily remote critical care consultation. Below, we discuss a healthcare model, clinical outcomes and financial analyses as they pertain to our experience at the UCDCH, where telemedicine has been used to support the care of particular children admitted to a rural, adult ICU.

In rural Northern California, the Mercy Medical Center in Redding (MMCR) is a centrally located hospital that serves as a regional adult specialty referral centre and as a paediatric referral centre for some paediatric specialty services. The closest paediatric ICU to the MMCR is in Sacramento, about 260 km to the south, which requires long-distance patient transport and the displacement of families from their community. In the alternative healthcare model, children (eg those not so critically ill or those too critically ill to transport) are cared for in the adult ICU at the MMCR with paediatric critical care support from the paediatric ICU at the UCDCH. This telemedicine programme and some health outcomes analyses have been reported recently.[35,36]

Intensive care unit telemedicine

Telemedicine consultations to a UCDCH paediatric critical care physician are conducted for select children admitted to the adult ICU at the MMCR at the discretion of the MMCR attending physician (a neonatologist, general paediatrician, adult intensivist or adult trauma surgeon) depending on the patient's age, diagnoses and medical condition (Fig. 17.3). The paediatric critical care physician from the UCDCH is paged when a consultation is requested, and a telemedicine consultation is initiated, typically within 15 minutes of being contacted.

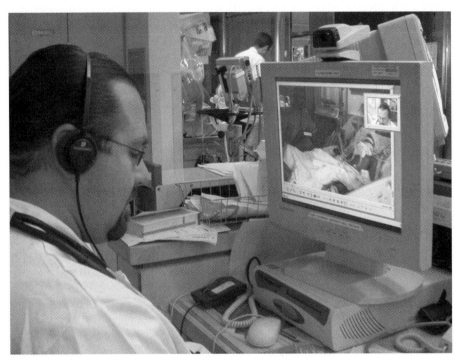

Fig. 17.3. Telemedicine consultation between two intensive care units.

Each consultation consists of a full history (with referring physician, nurse and parent or guardian), physical examination, and review of pertinent radiographs, medical records and laboratory results. With each consultation, a written note is completed and faxed to the MMCR to be included in the patient's medical record. Follow-up consultations are conducted at the discretion of the consulting critical care physician (sometimes multiple consultations per day) or can be requested by the referring physician or bedside nurse. At any time after the initial or follow-up consultation, the patient can be transported to the UCDCH paediatric ICU at the discretion of the referring or consulting physicians.

We have recently reported a comparison of the outcomes of three cohorts of patients cared for at the MMCR adult ICU.[35] The first cohort was those patients who were cared for in the MMCR ICU who received telemedicine consultations during a two-year study period (April 2000–April 2002). The second cohort was those patients cared for in the MMCR ICU during the period in which telemedicine was available; this included both telemedicine patients – the first cohort – and those who were managed in the MMCR concurrently without telemedicine, as not all paediatric patients cared for in the ICU received consultations. The third cohort was those patients cared for in the Redding ICU during a time when a sole paediatric intensivist worked in the Redding ICU, ie it was a historical control population.

The analyses adjusted for severity of illness using the paediatric risk of mortality, version III (PRISM III).[37,38] A PRISM III score is calculated from demographical, physiological and laboratory data collected in the first 12 hours after admission, with a higher score representing a more ill patient. The PRISM III score predicts mortality and length of stay (LOS). Observed mortality and length of stay can then be compared with those predicted. Efficiency of care was also calculated for each of the patient cohorts. Efficiency of care is the ratio of the number of patient care days when mechanical ventilation and/or vasoactive infusions were used to the total number of patient care days.

Telemedicine patients

In the ICU telemedicine study period, 70 telemedicine consultations were conducted on 47 patients (Table 17.1). The median number of consultations per patient was 1 (range 1–7). The patients that received telemedicine consultations had a mean PRISM III score of 9.6, and the average efficiency of care was 54%. Common diagnoses included pneumonia/bronchiolitis (19%) and trauma (19%). During the study period, 180 total infants and children were admitted to the rural adult ICU, including the 47 patients who received consultations (Table 17.1). The mean PRISM III score for the entire group was 7.7, and the efficiency of care was 28%. The mean PRISM III score and efficiency of care for the patients excluding those who received telemedicine consultations were 7.0 and 21%, respectively. Common diagnoses included trauma (32%) and pneumonia/bronchiolitis (13%).

Pre-telemedicine controls

From October 1997 to September 1998, while a lone paediatric intensivist attended the adult ICU, there were 116 admissions (Table 17.1). Nineteen patients (16%) were transferred from another facility. The mean PRISM III score was 7.5, and the efficiency of care was 30%. The common primary admission diagnoses were pneumonia/bronchiolitis (27%) and trauma (20%). The satisfaction survey showed the importance of the paediatric patient remaining in the local community. Parents or guardians and nurses all stated that it was important or very important to them that the child be cared for locally (4.3 and 4.4 on the five-point Likert scale, respectively). This was less important to the MMCR physicians (3.9 on the five-point scale, $p < 0.01$).

Table 17.1. Demographic, diagnostic and outcome data for three cohorts of paediatric patients admitted to the MMCR adult ICU

Variable	Patients receiving telemedicine consultations (%)	All ICU patients in rural hospital during telemedicine period (%)	Pre-telemedicine controls with paediatric ICU attending (%)
Number of patients	47 (70 consultations)	180	116
Dates	April 2000– April 2002	April 2000– April 2002	October 1997– September 1998
Baseline demographic and clinical features			
Age in months, mean (median)±SD	63.9 (32.4) ±62.1	99.0 (112.9) ±68.1	65.8 (44.5) ±61.4
Emergency admissions	46 (98%)	165 (92%)	110 (95%)
Transfers from other facility	7 (15%)	12 (7%)	19 (16%)
PRISM III, mean (median) ±SD	9.6 (8.0) ±8.4	7.7 (5.5) ±6.2	7.5 (5.0) ±7.3
Paediatric ICU efficiency	54%	28%	30%
Admission diagnoses			
Postoperative	9 (19%)	54 (28%)	24 (21%)
Trauma	9 (19%)	57 (32%)	23 (20%)
Pneumonia/bronchiolitis	9 (19%)	23 (13%)	31 (27%)
Asthma	3 (6%)	10 (6%)	7 (6%)
Clinical and PRISM III outcomes			
Observed mortality	1 (2%)	3 (2%)	3 (3%)
Predicted deaths	4.2 (9%)	8.4 (5%)	8.2 (7%)
Observed or predicted deaths (95% CI)	0.24 (0.01–0.81)	0.36 (0.09–0.76)	0.37 (0.09–0.76)

ICU financial data

The average daily costs at the UCDCH Paediatric ICU were estimated using the average daily costs over a two-year period. The average daily costs at the MMCR ICU were estimated using actual patient charges and published inpatient cost to charge ratios. Transport costs were also estimated from actual transport charges and known cost to charge ratios.[39] The total revenue for the 25-month period for the paediatric patients in the Mercy Redding ICU is also shown in Table 17.2. This represents hospital revenue that would otherwise not be realized had a telemedicine programme not been in place. For those patients who received telemedicine consultations, the revenue generated during the 25-month period was $388 000 – ie a revenue of $186 000 annually. For half of the paediatric patients who remained in the ICU, the 25-month revenue was $580 000, or $279 000 annually.

Conclusions

In developing our telemedicine programme, there were many technical challenges, particularly in providing a 24 hours a day, seven days a week service. This included

Table 17.2. Healthcare costs saved and revenue generated due to telemedicine for patients admitted to MMCR ICU

Patient group	n	Patient-days	Difference in ICU costs ($)	Transport costs avoided ($)	Total savings (annual savings) ($)	Total revenue to rural hospital (annual revenue) ($)
Patients receiving telemedicine consultations	47	147	141 000	217 000	358 000 (172 000)	388 000 (186 000)
Half of paediatric ICU patients in rural hospital during telemedicine period	90	220	211 000	415 000	626 000 (300 000)	580 000 (279 000)

complex on-call systems for the technical personnel at both sites and the physicians from the UCDCH paediatric ICU. Expensive T1 lines were used to ensure speed and reliability. We do not use sophisticated peripheral telemedicine devices, such as stethoscopes and oto-ophthalmoscopes. The high-resolution detachable examination camera was abandoned, as it was easier to ask the physician or nurse in the rural ICU to describe the pupillary responses than attempt to use the camera. X-ray films were placed on a viewing box and examined with the general videoconferencing camera. Rather than using direct data transmission from monitors and ventilators, the remotely controlled video camera was used to obtain close up pictures of the displays. We feel that the biggest benefits of telemedicine compared with traditional telephone consultations are that with telemedicine, a more comprehensive medical review is conducted and there is direct visualization of the patient and medical equipment.

The UCDCH ICU telemedicine programme shows that teleconsultations for a rural adult ICU can successfully provide supportive care for critically ill children. Mortality and length of stay were comparable with severity-adjusted benchmark data from 33 national paediatric ICUs, as well as historical controls. Both rural providers and parents or guardians were very satisfied with telemedicine in terms of quality of care and the ability to keep patients in the local community. In addition, by avoiding transport costs and the higher costs of a referral hospital, overall patient costs and charges were less with telemedicine and the revenue from patient charges was ultimately retained in the rural hospital. Finally, because of this programme, some lengthy, risky and expensive patient (and family) transports were avoided.

References

1   Athey J, Dean JM, Ball J, et al. Ability of hospitals to care for pediatric emergency patients. Pediatric Emergency Care 2001; 17: 170–174.
2   McGillivray D, Nijssen-Jordan C, Kramer MS, et al. Critical pediatric equipment availability in Canadian hospital emergency departments. Annals of Emergency Medicine 2001; 37: 371–376.
3   Esposito TJ, Sanddal ND, Dean JM, et al. Analysis of preventable pediatric trauma deaths and inappropriate trauma care in Montana. Journal of Trauma 1999; 47: 243–253.

4   Moody-Williams JD, Krug S, O'Connor R, et al. Practice guidelines and performance measures in emergency medical services for children. Annals of Emergency Medicine 2002; 39: 404–412.

5   Durch J, Lohr KN, eds. Emergency Medical Services for Children. Washington, DC: National Academy Press; 1993.

6   Durch JS, Lohr KN. From the Institute of Medicine. Journal of the American Medical Association 1993; 270: 929.

7   Keeler EB, Rubenstein LV, Kahn KL, et al. Hospital characteristics and quality of care. Journal of the American Medical Association 1992; 268: 1709–1714.

8   Pollack MM, Alexander SR, Clarke N, et al. Improved outcomes from tertiary center pediatric intensive care: a statewide comparison of tertiary and nontertiary care facilities. Critical Care Medicine 1991; 19: 150–159.

9   Pollack MM, Getson PR. Pediatric critical care cost containment: combined actuarial and clinical program. Critical Care Medicine 1991; 19: 12–20.

10 Kronick JB, Frewen TC, Kissoon N, et al. Influence of referring physicians on interventions by a pediatric and neonatal critical care transport team. Pediatric Emergency Care 1996; 12: 73–77.

11 Tilford JM, Roberson PK, Lensing S, Fiser DH. Improvement in pediatric critical care outcomes. Critical Care Medicine 2000; 28: 601–603.

12 Tilford JM, Simpson PM, Green JW, et al. Volume–outcome relationships in pediatric intensive care units. Pediatrics 2000; 106: 289–294.

13 Phibbs CS, Bronstein JM, Buxton E, Phibbs RH. The effects of patient volume and level of care at the hospital of birth on neonatal mortality. Journal of the American Medical Association 1996; 276: 1054–1059.

14 Hampers LC, Trainor JL, Listernick R, et al. Setting-based practice variation in the management of simple febrile seizure. Academic Emergency Medicine 2000; 7: 21–27.

15 Seidel JS, Henderson DP, Ward P, et al. Pediatric prehospital care in urban and rural areas. Pediatrics 1991; 88: 681–690.

16 Seidel JS, Hornbein M, Yoshiyama K, et al. Emergency medical services and the pediatric patient: are the needs being met? Pediatrics 1984; 73: 769–772.

17 Gausche M, Seidel JS, Henderson DP, et al. Pediatric deaths and emergency medical services (EMS) in urban and rural areas. Pediatric Emergency Care 1989; 5: 158–162.

18 Lambrecht CJ. Emergency physicians' roles in a clinical telemedicine network. Annals of Emergency Medicine 1997; 30: 670–674.

19 Lambrecht CJ. Telemedicine in trauma care: description of 100 trauma teleconsults. Telemedicine Journal 1997; 3: 265–268.

20 Brennan JA, Kealy JA, Gerardi LH, et al. Telemedicine in the emergency department: a randomized controlled trial. Journal of Telemedicine and Telecare 1999; 5: 18–22.

21 Brennan JA, Kealy JA, Gerardi LH, et al. A randomized controlled trial of telemedicine in an emergency department. Journal of Telemedicine and Telecare 1998; 4 (suppl. 1): 18–20.

22 Stamford P, Bickford T, Hsiao H, Mattern W. The significance of telemedicine in a rural emergency department. IEEE Engineering in Medicine and Biology Magazine 1999; 18: 45–52.

23 Rogers FB, Ricci M, Caputo M, et al. The use of telemedicine for real-time video consultation between trauma center and community hospital in a rural setting improves early trauma care: preliminary results. Journal of Trauma 2001; 51: 1037–1041.

24 American Academy of Pediatrics. Committee on Pediatric Emergency Medicine. American College of Critical Care Medicine. Society of Critical Care Medicine Consensus report for regionalization of services for critically ill or injured children. Pediatrics 2000; 105: 152–155.

25 Yeh TS. Regionalization of pediatric critical care. Critical Care Clinics 1992;8:23–35.

26 Pearson G, Shann F, Barry P, et al. Should paediatric intensive care be centralised? Trent versus Victoria. Lancet 1997; 349: 1213–1217.

27 Pollack MM, Katz RW, Ruttimann UE, Getson PR. Improving the outcome and efficiency of intensive care: the impact of an intensivist. Critical Care Medicine 1988; 16: 11–17.

28 Wootton R, Yellowlees P, McLaren P (eds). Telepsychiatry and e-Mental Health. London: Royal Society of Medicine Press, 2003.

29 Berg BW, Vincent DS, Hudson DA. Remote critical care consultation: telehealth projection of clinical specialty expertise. Journal of Telemedicine and Telecare 2003; 9 (suppl. 2): 9–11.

30 Rosenfeld BA, Dorman T, Breslow MJ, et al. Intensive care unit telemedicine: alternate paradigm for providing continuous intensivist care. Critical Care Medicine 2000; 28: 3925–3931.

31 Breslow MJ, Rosenfeld BA, Doerfler M, et al. Effect of a multiple-site intensive care unit telemedicine program on clinical and economic outcomes: an alternative paradigm for intensivist staffing. Critical Care Medicine 2004; 32: 31–38.

32   Becker C. Remote control. Specialists are running intensive-care units from remote sites via computers, and at least one health system with the e-ICU is reaping financial rewards – and saving lives. *Modern Healthcare* 2002; **32**: 40–42, 44, 46.

33   Wetzel RC. The virtual pediatric intensive care unit. Practice in the new millennium. *Pediatric Clinics of North America* 2001; **48**: 795–814.

34   Rosenfeld B. A remote possibility. *Cost and Quality* 2000;**6**:38–39.

35   Marcin JP, Nesbitt TS, Kallas HJ, *et al*. Use of telemedicine to provide pediatric critical care inpatient consultations to underserved rural Northern California. *Journal of Pediatrics* 2004; **144**: 375–380.

36   Marcin JP, Schepps DE, Page KA, *et al*. The use of telemedicine to provide pediatric critical care consultations to pediatric trauma patients admitted to a remote trauma intensive care unit: a preliminary report. *Pediatric Critical Care Medicine* 2004; **5**: 251–256.

37   California Children's Services Manual of Procedures. *Pediatric Intensive Care Unit Standards*. Chapter 3.32. Sacramento: Department of Health Services, State of California; January 1999. http://www.dhs.ca.gov/pcfh/cms/onlinearchive/pdf/ccs/numberedletters/1998/manualofprocedures/picu.pdf (last checked 7 August 2004).

38   Pollack MM, Patel KM, Ruttimann UE. PRISM III: an updated Pediatric Risk of Mortality score. *Critical Care Medicine* 1996; **24**: 743–752.

39   Office of Statewide Health Planning and Development (OSHPD). *Hospital Annual Financial Data*. Sacramento, CA: California Department of Health Services; 2000. See http://www.oshpd.cahwnet.gov/HQAD/HIRC/hospital/financial/annual/Pivot/ (last checked 7 August 2004).

▶18

Telemedicine and Underserved Communities in Developing Nations

Marina Reznik, James P Marcin and Philip O Ozuah

Introduction

The World Health Organization (WHO) has emphasized 'the importance of reducing social and economic inequities in improving the health of the whole population' to ensure high-quality healthcare for all.[1] This is particularly relevant to many developing countries and medically underserved populations who face growing health disparities and whose children are disproportionately affected by these inequalities. There were 57 million deaths in the world in 2002, of which 10.5 million were among children aged less than 5 years. More than 98% of these child deaths were in developing countries.[2]

Advances in information and communications technology have provided new ways of healthcare delivery.[3] The WHO has recognized the role of 'health telematics' in improving access to medical and healthcare, health education, global health promotion, training of health personnel and the management of emergency situations.[4] Telemedicine has become increasingly popular in both industrialized and developing countries.[3] Telemedicine has important effects on many aspects of health systems in the developing nations.[5] It has the potential to improve healthcare by removing time and distance barriers, providing medical education and medical care, and optimizing the use of limited health services.[6] Many authors have suggested the potential advantages of telemedicine for delivering healthcare in the developing world.[7–9] However, few reports describe actual clinical experience of using telemedicine in developing countries.[10–13]

Reports of the use of telemedicine for children in developing countries are even more scarce. Lee *et al* used low-bandwidth telemedicine to evaluate surgical patients from Kenya before the visit of a surgical team from the US.[14] Fifty-one patients, including seven paediatric patients were pre-screened. Sixty-five percent of patients were thought to be unsuitable for surgery because of advanced disease or the absence of the necessary local medical resources. Overall, 60 patients, including 9 (15%) paediatric patients, underwent surgery. Paediatric cases included various laparoscopic, oncologic and soft tissue reconstructions. The authors concluded that low-bandwidth, Internet-based telemedicine was a cost-effective technique that could be used efficiently and effectively for pre-screening of surgical patients in developing countries.

Person *et al* described two cases involving girls aged five and six years who accidentally suffered broken legs and how they were helped with the use of telemedicine.[15] This report illustrated a simple store-and-forward telemedicine technique that provided consultation, referral and education in the developing world of the Pacific Rim. The Swinfen Charitable Trust has reported similar favourable experience with the use of email to support hospital doctors in a number of developing countries.[16] About one-third of the cases handled by the trust are paediatric (see Chapter 19).

Medical Missions for Children

The Medical Missions for Children (MMC) is a US not-for-profit organization supported entirely by charitable donations. Its goal is to improve healthcare for children in medically underserved communities by using telemedicine as a 'virtual information bridge'. The virtual bridge is the MMC Global Telemedicine and Teaching Network, which is a network of 25 American hospitals that mentor participating hospitals in underserved countries.[17] The MMC provides videoconferencing equipment for the participating hospitals in the developing world, as well as satellite time for the communication. Videoconferencing equipment (donated by Polycom) includes ViewStation EX, ViewStation FX and VS 4000 equipment, which communicates at bandwidths from 128 kbit/s to 2 Mbit/s. Physicians from the mentoring hospitals volunteer their time and expertise to participate via videoconference in remote examinations of patients, consultations about diagnosis and treatment, and education about new procedures, drugs and medical equipment.

The MMC was founded in March 1999 as a way of screening ill children from developing countries before having doctors travel to treat them.[18] Five years later, the MMC serves children in hospitals in 17 countries in Latin America, eastern Europe, South Africa, Nigeria and India. Two or three patient consultations or diagnostic sessions are held by videoconference each month. Five to ten children participate in each session. Thus, on average, each hospital will treat 25 patients a month or 300 patients annually with telemedical support.

Most of the MMC network time, about 80%, is used for educational videoconferences, lectures and symposiums to provide healthcare professionals in the developing countries with new information on diagnosis, techniques and treatment of paediatric diseases. This exchange of information allows physicians to share knowledge and ideas that can be applied to future patients, thus improving the overall level of care. The mentoring hospitals conduct an average of 50 educational videoconferences per month or a total of approximately 600 educational videoconferences per year. Since its inception, the programme has provided direct and indirect medical consultations and services to approximately 1500 children per month or a total of 18 000 children annually.

Case report

Yordano is an 11-year-old boy from rural Panama whose life was changed with the help of the MMC. Yordano was born with a cranial deformity that resulted in absence of one eye, difficulty in swallowing and mental retardation.[19] Yordano comes from a family of six. His father is a painter and his mother is a seamstress. He has an 18-year-old brother, a 5-year-old brother and a healthy twin brother. Yordano was the first child to use the MMC telemedicine network in November 2000. He was examined by the physicians at St Joseph's Children's Hospital in New Jersey, and it was decided that he could be helped. A computer model of his head was created with the help of interactive telemedicine to collect measurements. The model skull was reshaped with computer imaging to correct the problems. Then, using a computer, physicians designed titanium implants to correct his problem. A physical model was made to confirm that all the parts fitted properly. Yordano's doctors in Panama were involved with the preparation. However, it was decided that the surgery should be performed at St Joseph's Children's Hospital. In November 2001, Yordano and his mother arrived in the US. Yordano had two operations to reconstruct his skull and jaw. The first, conducted in November 2001, changed the shape of Yordano's skull to create an eye socket for a prosthetic eye. Yordano returned to the US in July 2003 for the second operation to receive a new titanium jaw (Figs 18.1–18.3). After the surgery was completed, an educational session was held by the surgeons from the US who used the MMC telemedicine network to review the procedure with 50 physicians from Panama.

MMC and the Children's Hospital at Montefiore

The Children's Hospital at Montefiore in the Bronx, New York, is a mentoring hospital for the University College Hospital in Ibadan, Nigeria. Although this programme is

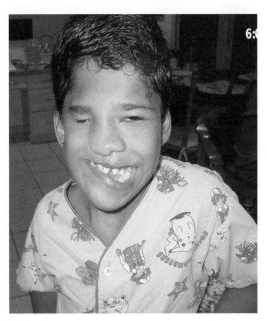

Fig. 18.1. Yordano before surgery.

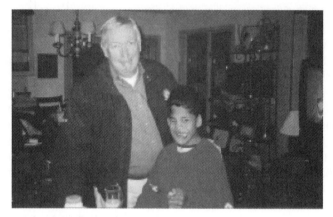

Fig. 18.2. Yordano arriving for surgery.

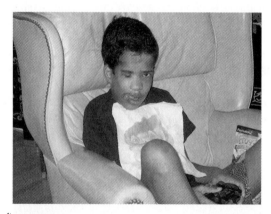

Fig. 18.3. Yordano after surgery.

relatively new, we expect it to provide health education and better access to medical care for children in Nigeria. Telemedicine is used to facilitate encounters between the faculty at the International Center for Child Health at the Children's Hospital at Montefiore (CHAM) and Nigerian medical professionals. The work includes a forum for medical information exchange in the form of training sessions, seminar series, symposiums and consultations via videoconferencing.

Working in partnership with the MMC, the CHAM is sponsoring the College of Medicine/University College Hospital in Ibadan. The MMC has provided the telemedicine equipment for the hospital in Nigeria. A curriculum for the hospital's educational needs and interests is being developed by medical staff in collaboration with CHAM faculty members. An existing agreement between the MMC and the World Bank allows the CHAM to connect with the Medical Missions site (via three ISDN lines using PictureTel TeamStation equipment) and access the World Bank satellite to reach the College of Medicine/University College Hospital via Ibadan's satellite dish. The World Bank pays for the cost of the satellite use during these encounters.

Our Nigerian partner has responsibility only for providing space for the telemedicine equipment and administrative support to ensure the high quality, efficiency and long-term sustainability of the programme. They also provide an appropriate mechanism for assessing and discussing the medical and educational needs and interests in Nigeria to ensure that the programme contributes to the enhancement of paediatric healthcare.

Conclusion

Although some authors have described the potential advantages and benefits of telemedicine as a useful technique for delivering healthcare in the developing world,[7-9] much work remains to be done. The WHO, in its Health-for-all policy for the 21st century, emphasized 'the importance of reducing social and economic inequities in improving the health of the whole population' to ensure high-quality healthcare for all.[1] There are obvious potential advantages of using telemedicine for delivering healthcare in the developing world, but few reports that describe actual clinical experience; there are even fewer reports about the use of telemedicine for children in developing countries. The MMC, a non-profit organization, has a telemedicine network between mentoring hospitals in the US and hospitals located in developing nations. Since its inception, the programme has provided direct and indirect medical consultations and services to approximately 18 000 children annually.

References

1   World Health Organization. *Health-for-all Policy for the Twenty-first Century.* (document WHA51.7). Fifty-first world health assembly. Geneva: World Health Organization, 1998.
2   World Health Organization. *The World Health Report 2003: Shaping the Future.* Geneva: World Health Organization, 2003.
3   Wootton R, Craig J, eds. *Introduction to Telemedicine.* London: Royal Society of Medicine Press, 1999.
4   World Health Organization. *Health-for-all Policy for the Twenty-first Century: 'Health Telematics'.* (document EB101/INF.DOC./9). Geneva: WHO, 1998.
5   Edworthy SM. Telemedicine in developing countries. *British Medical Journal* 2001; **323**: 524–525.
6   Zhao Y, Nakajima I, Juzoji H. On-site investigation of the early phase of Bhutan Health Telematics Project. *Journal of Medical Systems* 2002; **26**: 67–77.
7   Einterz EM. Telemedicine in Africa: potential, problems, priorities. *Canadian Medical Association Journal* 2001; **165**: 780–781.
8   Fraser HS, McGrath SJ. Information technology and telemedicine in sub-Saharan Africa. *British Medical Journal* 2000; **321**: 465–466
9   Groves T. SatelLife: getting relevant information to the developing world. *British Medical Journal* 1996; **313**: 1606–1609
10 Wootton R. The possible use of telemedicine in developing countries. *Journal of Telemedicine and Telecare* 1997;**3**:23–26.
11 Wootton R. Telemedicine and developing countries – successful implementation will require a shared approach. *Journal of Telemedicine and Telecare* 2001; **7** (suppl. 1): 1–6.
12 Vassallo DJ, Swinfen P, Swinfen R, Wootton R. Experience with a low-cost telemedicine system in three developing countries. *Journal of Telemedicine and Telecare* 2001; **7** (suppl. 1): 56–58.

13   Patterson V, Hoque F, Vassallo D, *et al*. Store-and-forward teleneurology in developing countries. *Journal of Telemedicine and Telecare* 2001; **7** (suppl. 1): 52–53.

14   Lee S, Broderick TJ, Haynes J, *et al*. The role of low-bandwidth telemedicine in surgical prescreening. *Journal of Pediatric Surgery* 2003; **38**: 1281–1283.

15   Person DA, Hedson JS, Gunawardane KJ. Telemedicine success in the United States Associated Pacific Islands (USAPI): two illustrative cases. *Telemedicine Journal and e-Health* 2003; **9**: 95–101.

16   Graham LE, Zimmerman M, Vassallo DJ, *et al*. Telemedicine – the way ahead for medicine in the developing world. *Tropical Doctor* 2003; **33**: 36–38.

17   Medical Missions for Children: Global Telemedicine and Teaching Network. http://www.mmissions.org/ (last checked 8 June 2004).

18   Davis AW. Providing medical assistance to the underserved. *Conferencing Buyer* 2003: **1**: 4–5. http://www.mmissions.org/cb.pdf (last checked 7 August 2004).

19   Medical Missions for Children. *Yordano's Story*. http://www.mmissions.org/yordano.htm (last checked 7 August 2004).

▶19

Store-and-forward Telemedicine

Karen Youngberry, Roger Swinfen, Pat Swinfen and Richard Wootton

Introduction

There are two fundamentally different methods of performing telemedicine. In a real-time interaction, the parties are connected by some communications medium – perhaps the humble telephone or perhaps a high-speed video link – and can interact with one another in real time. In a store-and-forward interaction, on the other hand, the reply may not be received until some considerable time after the transmission of the query. A common example of store-and-forward interaction is the use of email, where the recipient reads the message and replies at leisure. Another common example is the use of text messaging to mobile phones or the recording of telephone voice messages.

Store-and-forward telemedicine systems for diagnosis or management usually involve the transmission of textual information supplemented by digital images or video. Not many store-and-forward systems are designed purely for paediatric work and most usually advise on both adult and paediatric patients. For example, there is a long history of telepathology using Internet communication of various forms.[1,2] Communication via store-and-forward telemedicine can be between doctors and specialists, between patients and healthcare professionals, or between specialists. It can involve medical personnel from anywhere in the world. The systems can also double as both a diagnostic and educational tool.

The limited availability of specialist services in developing countries has led to the development of many store-and-forward telemedicine systems to provide this advice, often on a charitable basis, ie the specialists participate as volunteers. For store-and-forward systems in or between industrialized countries, however, telemedicine is more likely to be performed on a commercial basis, with the cost of a consultation usually falling on the patient.[3]

Telemedicine in the developing world

Telemedicine is by definition unrestricted by national boundaries and has been used in both the industrialized and developing world. For reasons of geography and lack of resources, it may be particularly important in the developing world. In the past, telemedicine has been used mostly for educational purposes, as information shortage is common in these countries.[4] Only relatively recently has telemedicine been used to help improve access to clinical healthcare.[5]

The developing world can benefit from store-and-forward telemedicine through e-consultations with doctors in the industrialized world, provision of healthcare to rural areas of the country and provision of a means for further education and training of medical personnel.[6] These systems allow healthcare workers from countries facing similar medical and lifestyle hardships to communicate and support each other professionally.[7] The humanitarian component of these projects also enhances the links between the industrialized and developing worlds.[8]

Store-and-forward systems are generally more appropriate than real-time telemedicine for developing countries – not only because of the cost of real-time techniques, but also because different time zones between countries often impede real-time communication.[7]

Clinical and educational telemedicine

Long before the Internet became a viable tool for providing clinical advice, it was being used as a means for disseminating information and education. Many of the store-and-forward systems that use the Internet for clinical purposes also provide education. However, systems designed purely for educational purposes rarely provide clinical advice.

Many reviews of the quality of medical information on the Internet have been conducted, and they indicate that there is little control over, or regulation of, the vast range of information available.[8] It is difficult for health professionals, especially in the developing world, to determine what is authentic, high-quality medical advice. Store-and-forward systems can assist by providing patient-specific clinical advice and, through this, general medical knowledge.[9] In addition, the Internet can act as a vehicle for asking questions from a purely educational standpoint, with specialists directing users to relevant information. An extra benefit is that specialists in the industrialized world can update their knowledge of rarely seen diseases and conditions, thus giving them the opportunity to learn as well as teach.[10]

The Internet also represents a portal to allow medical students and patients and their families to access medical information. Some store-and-forward systems operate an educational system in parallel with their clinical system. For patients, this has been found to be a feasible and effective means of providing medical education, especially for those in rural or remote areas.[11] It has also been used to provide medical students undertaking overseas placements the opportunity of gaining extra educational information as well as clinical advice and reassurance.

Email versus web-based systems

One of the important decisions to make when establishing a store-and-forward telemedicine system is whether to use email or web-based interfaces for communication. A number of services have been established around the world using these different modalities. Although access to the Internet is relatively reliable and easily available in the industrialized world, this is not always the case in developing countries (especially in rural areas). Thus the geographical areas in which a store-and-forward system will be employed may determine the type of system to be used. As described below, email tends to be preferred for telemedicine systems in the developing world, while the industrialized world tends to opt for web-based systems.

Web-based systems

Web-based interfaces usually involve a browser window accessed via the Internet and specifically designed for the service being provided. Through this web page, referring doctors can input patient case information, specialists can review and advise on cases, and referring doctors can receive their replies. Some services combine this with an email notification system to advise participants about the status of their cases. This sort of work involves a background database, and a storage and retrieval system to collate the information.

Some examples of web-based store-and-forward systems in which significant paediatric work has been carried out include the following:

▶ A recent study of at-home monitoring of paediatric patients with asthma (in an industrialized country) showed that this is becoming a viable technique as Internet access becomes more common in patient's homes.[11] In this study, patients kept a diary of their symptoms and peak flow readings, and uploaded these together with a digital video recording of inhaler use to their case manager at regular intervals for comment and follow-up. The system was reported as being just as effective as face-to-face monitoring, but was more flexible, as patients and their case managers did not need to be available at the same time.[11]

▶ MedTech Outreach is an organization that provides a low-cost teleconsulting system for doctors in Vietnam who can access free specialist advice from Sydney, Australia. The specialists provide their advice on a voluntary basis. A secure website was developed as a single point of contact, so that participants could upload and review case information. All the case data were kept in a central repository that could be accessed later for case review, evaluation and educational purposes. The use of standard browser software provided a scalable system with few technical limitations.[9] MedTech provided Internet connections to the hospitals involved, as web access was not previously available. Developers of web-based systems involving the developing world may need to create the necessary infrastructure.

▶ As most store-and-forward services are established on a research or charity basis, patients do not usually have to pay money to participate. In the US, however, there is a commercial web-based store-and-forward telemedicine system in which doctors (on behalf of their patients) can seek advice from consultants from the industrialized world.[3] The system uses an interface that patients can log onto in order to give permission for their doctors to discuss their case with a specialist. Like other systems, a web-based system was chosen due to the growing availability of the Internet in patients' homes and in doctors' surgeries.[11] There is a cost associated with consultations (generally not covered by insurance), which falls on the patient.[3] Although it has been a successful example of store-and-forward telemedicine, it is not an approach that would be suitable for most poorer patients in the developing world.

Email-based systems

Reliable Internet access is a problem in the developing world and can often be costly. This inhibits the ability of services that use high-bandwidth and real-time interaction. Although satellite communications are available, they remain particularly expensive. Email-based systems are often used instead. Doctors can send requests by email for medical advice, their messages containing deidentified history (to allay privacy concerns) and digital images as appropriate. These systems may or may not contain the background database integral to most web-based systems.

In the following examples of email-based store-and-forward systems, significant paediatric work has been carried out:

▶ Lee *et al* established a surgical prescreening store-and-forward system to supplement an existing surgical outreach programme between the US and Kenya.[12] Some weeks before the scheduled trip to Kenya, the case histories of potential patients were sent by email to the surgeons for assessment. Those whom the surgeons deemed appropriate for surgery were included on the theatre list and notified to attend. This prevented patients travelling to the hospital unnecessarily and saved consultant time during the outreach clinic. The system was found to be inexpensive and effective.[12]

▶ As with web-based systems, the other use for email store-and-forward systems is to allow patients direct communication with specialists. Borowitz and Wyatt established a system to allow parents (as well as physicians and other healthcare professionals) to obtain free email advice about paediatric gastroenterology cases. Due to the expansion of Internet access, the email system was converted to a web-based system after about 12 months of operation. This research discovered that the average time spent dealing with an email case was comparable to that of a telephone consultation, but more flexible.[13]

▶ Email can be used to provide advice from specialists in the industrialized world and can also be used by specialists in a developing country to provide advice to their colleagues in rural areas. Deodhar described a store-and-forward telemedicine system in a neonatal intensive care unit in a major hospital in India, which provided advice to a primary care neonatal unit in a rural hospital. This use of email for correspondence was simple and effective, and allowed additional information relating to patient care to be obtained from a centre of expertise. Email was the mode of choice because of technical and logistical problems relating to the reliability of telephone lines and power supplies. The study showed that it was a simple and inexpensive method of improving the quality of neonatal care in the rural areas of India.[14]

Satellife (http://www.healthnet.org) is an organization that established an email communication network for healthcare workers around the world, called Healthnet. When it was first set up, it used a low-earth-orbit satellite to provide email connections to areas throughout Africa. It also provides access to health information resources to a wide range of health professionals and medical students across the developing world in an attempt to overcome 'information poverty'. The operation continues to this day, but most of the data traffic is now carried by standard telephone lines, as access to these has improved.[4]

Establishing a store-and-forward system

The equipment commonly used in store-and-forward systems is a digital camera and a computer with email or web access. These are reasonably common items that can be acquired at relatively low cost. They may already be available as part of the infrastructure of the healthcare system. The only additional cost then is the price of the Internet connection. In comparison, other forms of telemedicine involving real-time transmission such as satellite, ISDN or broadband connections are much more expensive. Equipment requirements here include videoconference systems, cabling, call charges and peripheral equipment such as document cameras.

Although many store-and-forward systems report being successful overall, they often meet similar problems during their development. The common problems include protocols for digital photography, medicolegal issues, appropriateness of the advice and system evaluation.

Protocols for digital photography

Digital cameras have become common over the last few years. Most digital cameras are relatively easy to use, even for the novice photographer. Images that are to be used for clinical purposes, however, require some more advanced skills. Issues of focus, colour and field depth are important in clinical photographs, and taking pictures of X-ray films needs particular care. Doctors therefore need training in the use of their digital cameras and how to control and monitor the images they produce. One method of doing this is to provide a basic digital photography guide either on paper or on the web.[15,16] Establishing a system for sending test images so that new participants can receive feedback and advice about the quality of their images before sending in their first referral is also helpful.

Medicolegal issues

Medicolegal questions that are commonly raised in connection with store-and-forward services include licensure and indemnity, medical negligence, responsibility for patient care, security, and confidentiality. Issues such as licensure and indemnity, medical negligence, and responsibility for patient care can be resolved in a number of ways, depending on the countries involved. In Australia – although this remains to be tested in a court of law – specialists are covered by their Medical Defence Organisation for 'good Samaritan' work. Individual store-and-forward systems have resolved these issues in different ways. For example, doctors in the developing country may provide indemnities under the law of the country of the specialists for each submitted case or they may rely on a disclaimer placed at the end of all email messages.[9,17] These issues can be resolved and should not form an excuse to avoid developing a telemedicine service.[18]

Security and confidentiality concerns can also be resolved. Borowitz and Wyatt found that about 90% of patients freely communicated personal and sensitive information directly to their physicians via email without concerns.[13] If all patient information is deidentified, this avoids the risk of breaches of confidentiality should someone else gain access to the system. Internet banking and payment systems are becoming commonplace, and if these can be functional and secure, there is no reason why a store-and-forward medical system cannot be the same.[18]

Appropriateness of advice

One issue that is more relevant for store-and-forward systems operating in the developing world, rather than the industrialized world, is that of the appropriateness of the advice given. Doctors in developing countries generally have far fewer resources then their counterparts in industrialized countries. Access to drugs, laboratory services and certain testing procedures varies, as does the availability of specialist surgeons. Doctors from industrialized areas need to take into consideration the availability of their suggested treatment when providing advice. The MedTech organization found that identifying existing relationships between the doctors in each country not only increased the willingness of the specialists to participate, but also meant that they generally had a better knowledge of the environment in which their colleagues practised.[9] Obviously this is not always possible, but providing participant specialists with an understanding of where the referral is coming from will certainly help them give the most appropriate advice.

System evaluation

One of the challenges associated with store-and-forward telemedicine systems is that of effective evaluation. A system that does not track, in some way, the communication processes will have great difficulty in evaluating the service being provided. This is the advantage of using a system with a background database to collect information automatically about the system traffic. Statistical information for the evaluation can then be obtained easily. Most web-based systems and some email systems[19] have the necessary architecture. Some web systems even have a built in survey tool that is completed for each case submitted.[9] This information is stored in the database ready for analysis as required. Evaluation at a system level therefore is relatively straightforward. It is a fundamental weakness of almost all telemedicine work in the developing world so far, however, that there are no outcomes data, ie evaluation at a patient level.

Limitations

Store-and-forward telemedicine systems have certain limitations, such as obtaining the appropriate information from referring doctors about each case so that the specialists have enough information to provide advice. The information required for each case referral can be specified, eg the medical history, test results and images (both X-ray and clinical), but this does not guarantee that it will be forthcoming. A template with subheadings could ensure that all relevant information is collected, but this means either using web interaction or providing special software to the referrer – neither are likely to be satisfactory approaches in practice.

Another potentially important issue is the availability of resources in the referrer's location. Specialists obviously wish to provide appropriate advice, ie to not recommend diagnostic tests or treatments that are simply unobtainable. In practice, this does not seem to be a problem, and specialists are sympathetic to the clinical environment of the referrers (see above). Many systems use volunteer specialists to provide advice, and therefore the specialist's willingness to participate becomes an issue.[20] Do the advice providers gain from participating in the service? A real practical problem for administrators of these systems is ensuring a minimum turnaround time, as it is rarely possible to enforce a time limit on those providing the responses.

Problems with Internet access can inhibit the use of web-based systems in some countries. There may also be difficulties with the electricity supply for running equipment, such as computers and modems. An appropriate communication method should be chosen that will be easily available, will be reliable and will not exceed the finances available to the participants.

Language barriers may also be a concern. Most systems currently being used depend on communication in English. It seems that most referring doctors who have been involved with telemedicine to date speak good English and that it is an effective form of communication. Written communication allows time for translation and avoids problems of speech and accents, so that miscommunications can be avoided.[7]

Example: the Swinfen Charitable Trust

The Swinfen Charitable Trust (SCT) was established in 1997 by Lord and Lady Swinfen in the UK. The aim of the trust is to assist the poor, sick and disabled people of the developing world. One of the ways this has been achieved is by providing a low-cost telemedicine service to hospitals in the developing world. In return, these hospitals agree to treat patients for free if they cannot afford to pay for their own medical care. Hospitals in developing countries can apply to the trust to become part of the service. If they do not already have access to a digital camera and email, the trust can provide what is necessary. All of the staff and specialists who work for the SCT do so on a volunteer basis. Specialists come from all over the industrialized world.

As of May 2004, the SCT had a network of 24 hospitals from 12 countries that were accessing specialist advice. A panel of over 100 specialists from 6 countries provides this advice. The system uses an automatic message-handling system to coordinate and track the referrals and responses being sent to the service.

Store-and-forward system

From 1999, when the SCT first started, until 2002, the email messages were handled manually. During 2002, an automatic message-handling program was developed to solve some of the problems associated with manual operations, reduce the labour for the operators and create a system that could be expanded in the future.[21,22]

Email was chosen over a web-based interface because of difficulties with web access in some of the more remote areas of the developing countries that were participating in the service. The system operators, who live 10 time zones apart, can track and allocate cases from anywhere in the world. As any email program can be used to send email messages to the system, there are no software compatibility issues to deal with.

How does the system work? Everyone involved uses a single email address. When an email message is sent in by a referring doctor, it is manually allocated to a specialist by one of the system operators on the basis of specialty and availability. The system then gives the case a unique identification number. From this point on, the AutoRouter takes over handling of the case by forwarding traffic back and forth between specialist and referring doctor on the basis of the identification number of the case. Information on each case, such as the referring doctor, specialist, date and times of messages, allocations and replies, is collected automatically. Some referrals (cases) require responses from multiple specialists or a specialist may be unable to respond, so there may be multiple messages from different doctors before a case is resolved.

Usage for paediatrics

Although the SCT deals with referrals from all areas of medicine, paediatric work accounts for a large proportion of cases. To quantify this, we extracted details of all paediatric cases from July 2002 to January 2004 (20 months). Patients younger than 18 years were considered to be paediatric cases in accordance with the World Health Organization guidelines.

During the 20-month study period, 237 cases were sent to the SCT. The total number of paediatric cases was 99 (42%): 93 of which were about specific patients and 6 of which were requesting general educational material about paediatric patients. Overall, 51% of cases concerned male patients, 46% concerned female patients and in 3% of cases the sex of the patient was not provided in the email history.

The cases were sent from 18 different hospitals in 10 developing countries (Fig. 19.1). They covered 22 different specialty and subspecialty areas. These included orthopaedics (30%), surgery (12%), dermatology (12%) and neurology (6%). In total, 33 specialists responded to the cases, some cases requiring multiple specialists' responses due to the complexity of the case. The specialists came from five different countries: 69% from Australia, 21% from the UK and the remainder from Austria, New Zealand and Canada.

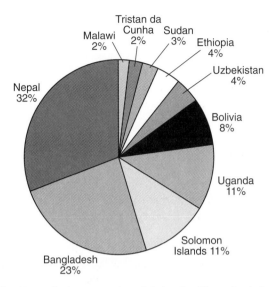

Fig. 19.1. Origin of the 99 paediatric cases referred during the 20 month study period.

The median time delay between the arrival of an email message and the time when the referring doctor received a reply from a specialist was less than two days (interquartile range 0.9–5).

Discussion

During its five years of service, the Swinfen Charitable Trust has proved itself to be a sustainable and efficient means of providing low cost telemedicine to the developing world. It shows that simple and cheap telemedicine methods can provide good quality medical advice.[4]

Case study

The following is an example of a paediatric case sent via email to the Swinfen Charitable Trust (Fig. 19.2):

I would be grateful for advice on the (L) thumb of the following patient.

11-year old boy who has a intrinsic paralysis of his left hand due to ulna nerve damage secondary to leprosy. He is scheduled for an intrinsic replacement.

Incidentally, he has congenital abnormalities of both hands:

Accessory hypoplastic thumb on right, which I have removed.

Left thumb shows abnormal proximal phalangeal head with ulna deviation of distal phalanges. He opposes with a pulp to side grip. The X-ray suggests a clinodactyly without a delta phalanx.

My plan was to do a corrective osteotomy of the proximal phalanges and bone grafting, with circlage wiring or an external fixator for stabilization.

I would be grateful for advice on approach, stabilization etc.

Kind regards

Mark

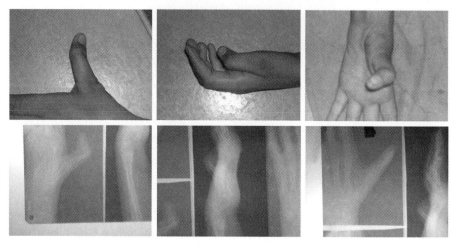

Fig. 19.2. Pictures of paediatric case sent to the Swinfen Charitable Trust.

The response was as follows.

Dear Mark

Your question about the boy's thumb has been passed to me for comment.

My first thought is that if the boy can only oppose by a clip action, there is probably significant muscle weakness or paralysis in the thenar group. You mention that he has an intrinsic paralysis for which you are going to do an intrinsic replacement.

Correcting the deformity of the interphalangeal joint of his left thumb will not improve his opposition. It will merely lengthen the thumb in line with the proximal phalanx and may indeed reduce function by causing an obstruction in the palm to flexion of the fingers.

I would suggest great caution and wait until you can assess the benefit he receives from the intrinsic replacement before embarking on surgery to the thumb.

If you do decide to correct the thumb deformity, I would do a wedge osteotomy close to the neck of the proximal phalanx of the thumb. If you have a 'mini' fixator, I would stabilize the osteotomy with this using the distal phalanx for the distal wires. As to the approach, I suggest that as you will be excising a wedge from the proximal phalanx and closing it, the approach should be where you plan to place the base of the wedge. From the pictures, it would appear that this would be on the ulnar side of the thumb.

I think it is unlikely that with this technique a graft would be needed, and certainly I see no place for a cerclage wire.

With very best wishes

Stephen

The referral letter received the following response.

Dear Stephen

Thanks for your prompt reply on the thumb. ... He has an isolated ulna nerve palsy and an intact median nerve with normal function of his thumb. In the light of this, I proceeded with a closing wedge osteotomy and took your advice with an external fixator. I'll let you know how it turned out. Did a Four tail Zancoli-Lasso procedure for his intrinsic loss.

Regards

Mark

Conclusion

Store-and-forward telemedicine is a viable technique both in and between industrialized and developing countries. It is an efficient means of providing low-cost telemedicine that can be used for both educational and clinical purposes. Systems can be web-based or email-based, and the equipment requirements for each are modest compared with other forms of telemedicine. There are potential problems and limitations with store-and-forward services, but these can be overcome with proper planning and design. Existing store-and-forward systems have shown this mode of telemedicine to be effective and useful and also to be sustainable – for both adult and paediatric medicine.

Further information

Satellife: The Global Health Information Network. http://www.healthnet.org (last checked 8 August 2004).
Telemedicine in Cambodia. http://www.camnet.com.kh/cambodiaschools/villageleap/telemedicine.htm (last checked 8 August 2004).
Swinfen Charitable Trust. http://www.uq.edu.au/swinfen (last checked 8 August 2004).

References

1   Kayser K. Interdisciplinary telecommunication and expert teleconsultation in diagnostic pathology: present status and future prospects. *Journal of Telemedicine and Telecare* 2002; **8**: 325–330.

2   Brauchli K, Christen H, Haroske G, *et al.* Telemicroscopy by the Internet revisited. *Journal of Pathology* 2002; **196**: 238–243.

3   Kedar I, Ternullo JL, Weinrib CE, *et al.* Internet based consultations to transfer knowledge for patients requiring specialised care: retrospective case review. *British Medical Journal* 2003; **326**: 696–699.

4   Groves T. SatelLife: getting relevant information to the developing world. *British Medical Journal* 1996; **313**: 1606–1609.

5   Wootton R. Telemedicine and developing countries – successful implementation will require a shared approach. *Journal of Telemedicine and Telecare* 2001; **7** (suppl. 1): 1–6.

6   Wright D. The International Telecommunication Union's Report on Telemedicine and Developing Countries. *Journal of Telemedicine and Telecare* 1998; **4** (suppl. 1): 75–79.

7   Zbar RI, Otake LR, Miller MJ, *et al.* Web-based medicine as a means to establish centers of surgical excellence in the developing world. *Plastic and Reconstructive Surgery* 2001; **108**: 460–465.

8   Letendre P. Web-based educational resources: an overview. *Vox Sanguinis* 2002; **83** (suppl. 1): 227–230.

9   Hersh D, Hersch F, Mikuletic L, Neilson S. A web-based approach to low-cost telemedicine. *Journal of Telemedicine and Telecare* 2003; **9** (suppl. 2): 24–26.

10   Mukundan S Jr, Vydareny K, Vassallo DJ, *et al.* Trial telemedicine system for supporting medical students on elective in the developing world. *Academic Radiology* 2003; **10**: 794–797.

11   Chan DS, Callahan CW, Sheets SJ, *et al.* An Internet-based store-and-forward video home telehealth system for improving asthma outcomes in children. *American Journal of Heath-System Pharmacy* 2003; **60**: 1976–1981.

12   Lee S, Broderick TJ, Haynes J, *et al.* The role of low-bandwidth telemedicine in surgical prescreening. *Journal of Pediatric Surgery* 2003; **38**: 1281–1283.

13   Borowitz SM, Wyatt JC. The origin, content, and workload of e-mail consultations. *Journal of the American Medical Association* 1998; **280**: 1321–1324.

14   Deodhar J. Telemedicine by email – experience in neonatal care at a primary care facility in rural India. *Journal of Telemedicine and Telecare* 2002; **8** (suppl. 2): 20–21

15   Wootton R, ed. *The Swinfen Charitable Trust Digital Camera Guide.* Canterbury: Swinfen Charitable Trust, 2004.

16   Nayler JR. Clinical photography: a guide for the clinician. *Journal of Postgraduate Medicine.* 2003; **49**: 256–262.

17   Helveston EM, Orge FH, Naranjo R, Hernandez L. Telemedicine: strabismus e-consultation. *Journal of the American Association for Pediatric Ophthalmology and Strabismus* 2001; **5**: 291–296.

18   Wallace S, Sibson L, Stanberry B, *et al.* The legal and risk management conundrum of telemedicine. *Journal of Telemedicine and Telecare* 1999; **5** (suppl. 1): 8–9.

19   Swinfen P, Swinfen R, Youngberry K, Wootton R. A review of the first year's experience with an automatic message-routing system for low-cost telemedicine. *Journal of Telemedicine and Telecare* 2003; **9** (suppl. 2): 63–65.

20   Robie DK, Naulty CM, Parry RL, *et al.* Early experience using telemedicine for neonatal surgical consultations. *Journal of Pediatric Surgery* 1998; **33**: 1172–1177.

21   Wootton R. Design and implementation of an automatic message-routing system for low-cost telemedicine. *Journal of Telemedicine and Telecare* 2003; **9** (suppl. 1): 44–47.

22   Swinfen P, Swinfen R, Youngberry K, Wootton R. A review of the first year's experience with an automatic message-routing system for low-cost telemedicine. *Journal of Telemedicine and Telecare* 2003; **9** (suppl. 2): 63–65.

Section 2: Primary and Community Services

20. **Telemedicine and Child Health – Telepaediatrics from a Secondary Level**
Michael L Williams

21. **Telemedicine and Paediatric Palliative Care**
Mark Bensink and Helen Irving

22. **Telerehabilitation for Paediatrics**
Edward Lemaire

23. **Telemedicine for Schoolchildren in Kansas**
Pamela Whitten and Ryan Spaulding

24. **Telephone Help Lines for Parents**
Robert Ferguson

25. **A National Telephone and Online Counselling Service for Young Australians**
Wendy Reid and Debra Caswell

▶20

Telemedicine and Child Health – Telepaediatrics from a Secondary Level

Michael L Williams

Introduction

Children and adolescents who live in regional and rural areas need specialist medical services that are often not available in their area. This creates difficulty in access to specialist care for these patients because of transport availability, distance and cost. General specialists and primary care providers in regional and rural areas need professional support at a subspecialty or specialist level. Health consumers have increasing expectations of medical services, including – for rural patients – equity of access to the specialist services available in metropolitan areas.

Paediatric outreach clinics have been used to address these issues and, more recently, in some areas, telepaediatric clinics have been added.[1] This chapter describes telepaediatric consultation in a regional child and adolescent health service that offers a model of service in regional and rural settings.

Outreach in a regional paediatric service

Paediatric outreach services have been provided from metropolitan and regional centres where distances create difficulty for patients to attend the specialist's centre. The aim is to provide the specialist service with fewer barriers to access created by distance. This ease of access is especially important for parents with young and disabled children, single parents with other children, the indigenous population and those travelling long distances. Often one or two days off work may be needed for the trip to see the specialist, which in Queensland may require up to 20 hours by surface travel.

The delivery of outreach clinics has direct costs, including specialist's payment, travel and accommodation, as well as other effects. Travelling imposes risks of accident for the specialist. Time away from the family and practice, sometimes aggravated by unexpected delays because of weather, has adverse effects on the specialist's private, as well as professional, life. Remuneration may be considered inadequate for the time committed. If the doctor is the only specialist in a region, time away from the regional centre will reduce the availability of that specialist service, resulting in possible delays in the management and transfer of patients to another centre.

Outreach visits allow an opportunity for direct contact between the visiting specialist and local healthcare providers, including joint case management planning and other educational outcomes. This enhances the local capacity to provide care to patients. Time constraints, however, may result in the visiting specialist consulting alone, with little contact with the local carers.

Telehealth clinics have been established to provide the benefits of outreach visits while overcoming their costs and difficulties. As with outreach visits, the aim of the telehealth clinics is to allow access to specialist care equivalent to that provided in a metropolitan area, but with efficiency. The reasons for developing a telepaediatric service include:

- Avoiding the difficulties and costs for patients of travelling to a distant centre – either the regional centre or a tertiary centre.

- Meeting patient expectation for specialist opinion, without increasing costs to the health service for patient travel and accommodation.

- Consolidating the role of general paediatricians as case managers supported by the subspecialist, rather than having case management based in the metropolitan centre.

- Supporting primary care health workers in geographically isolated settings.

- Avoiding fragmented care, with consultations by subspecialist, regional paediatrician and general practitioner occurring in isolation.

- Allowing patients and their families a further specialist opinion.

- Providing inservice education for healthcare workers through discussion of their patients' management.

- Maximizing time and cost efficiency.

The Child and Adolescent Health Service in Mackay

The Child and Adolescent Health Service (CAHS) of the Mackay Health District serves a large region in central Queensland (see Fig. 3.1). Telepaediatric services began in 1998. The telepaediatric service now provided at Mackay illustrates how telepaediatrics can be incorporated into the service delivery of a general paediatric service, especially where the area served is large.

The CAHS based at the Mackay Base Hospital provides general paediatric (level 2) care for children and adolescents from birth to age 18 years. It covers a region that extends more than 300 km to the west and 200 km to the north and south. It supports six other hospitals. It has a full-time consultant paediatrician as director, with two visiting consultant paediatricians and three junior medical staff, including a trainee registrar. It has a special care nursery, with 2200 births a year in the region. The annual admission rate is around 1600 patients a year to a child and adolescent ward, with a busy outpatient department adjacent to the inpatient unit.

Outreach to outlying towns has been provided since the first paediatrician came to the region in 1980. This led to reduced cover in the regional centre and an increased workload for an understaffed service. Outreach by a limited number of tertiary hospital subspecialists to the regional centre commenced in 1987, with one or two visits a year. This was recognized as demanding for the subspecialist. The face-to-face contact of outreach visits helped to build improved communication and understanding between the regional specialist and the subspecialist and primary care providers.

The development of telepaediatric services

The opportunity to increase contact with the tertiary centre specialists through the medium of telehealth was welcomed. Most initial contact took place on an ad hoc basis, usually with 1–2 patients. A regular eating disorders clinic was established. The specialists had limited support, often having to use unfamiliar equipment by themselves. This proved to be inefficient and time consuming. The introduction of the central support officer[2] (see Chapter 3) and planned clinics reduced the workload for both the regional paediatrician and the subspecialist. It allowed expansion to a greater number of regular clinics, serving many more patients, while still conducting occasional ad hoc clinics. We now have about 53 subspecialty telehealth clinics and 15 outreach clinics per year from the tertiary centres, covering 19 subspecialty areas. In addition 2–3 ad hoc clinics per month, usually with 1–2 patients, occur between Mackay and the tertiary centre in Brisbane. During the two years from February 2002, there were 514 telepaediatric patient consultations between the Royal Children's Hospital in Brisbane and Mackay. There were also 33 patient consultations, mainly neurosurgical, between Townsville Hospital (400 km to the north) and Mackay.

In areas of low-volume paediatric caseload, such as haematology and rheumatology, or if a clinician is not available for outreach, we use telepaediatric clinics alone, usually every three months. Where there is a medium caseload volume, such as in oncology or endocrinology, we have established one or two outreach visits per year and telepaediatric clinics every three months in between. The high-caseload areas, such as scoliosis, cardiology and paediatric surgery, are covered by three or four outreach visits a year and telepaediatric consultation in between, mainly for cardiac cases.

Local telepaediatrics

A monthly paediatric outreach service is provided to three towns north of Mackay. More than 200 km to the west are six towns up to 100 km apart, with three hospitals. Previously, a three-monthly outreach clinic visit was made to two of the towns, but this was found to be overly demanding on the paediatrician's time. Frequent outreach visits to each of the six towns cannot be justified with a limited number of paediatricians. The success of the telepaediatric service between the tertiary unit and our regional centre encouraged us to offer a regular telepaediatric service to our rural primary care providers. We have established 36 bookings for general paediatric and primary care clinics each year, holding 27 clinics in the past year. The clinic is cancelled if there are no patients or a lack of personnel. In the two years from February 2002, we have had teleconsultations with 81 patients in their home towns, with their general practitioner or child health nurse, or both, presenting the case. The telehealth contact is reinforced by one outreach visit a year, with a priority of meeting with medical and other health staff.

Telephone contact between the paediatrician and either subspecialist or GP, usually without notice, remains a frequent means of discussion about case management. This is helped if the patient has been seen in a telepaediatric consultation. Often a patient initially discussed by telephone will be booked into the next telepaediatric clinic. A planned telephone conference with a speakerphone could approximate to a telehealth consultation, but it lacks the visual component that allows person-to-person interaction and the ability to show clinical signs and images. Email, often with digital photographs of skin lesions or X-rays, is also used for case consultation. Telehealth consultation provides the specialist, patient and family with a better means of evaluating health problems and discussing management.

An annual calendar of telepaediatric and outreach clinics is developed by the director of the CAHS in conjunction with the central telepaediatric coordinator in Brisbane, who liaises with the subspecialists and the general practitioners who will be involved. A dedicated telehealth room has been established in Mackay in the child and adolescent outpatient and office area, next to the director's office, and adjacent to the inpatient unit. The room-based videoconferencing equipment is easy to use, only needing to be switched on at the wall and a pre-programmed ISDN number to be dialled. We videoconference at 384 kbit/s to the tertiary unit, which allows best quality, with links to the smaller centres at 128 kbit/s because of restricted telecommunications. The site where the patient is present will dial the call and hence pay the line charges.

Our outpatient administrative officer books patients in to the subspecialty clinics only after referral by the paediatricians following their consultation with the patient. Before the telepaediatric clinic, a one-page form is completed and faxed to the telepaediatric coordinator, including patient details, parents' names, clinical details and the clinical questions that we wish addressed. The paediatric registrar, who may act as clinical coordinator for the clinic, usually does this, and during the clinic presents patients and make notes in the patient's record, supervised by the clinician. The telehealth unit is used by the CAHS staff three times per week for educational meetings, which helps to increase their familiarity with the equipment and medium (see Chapter 26).

Clinical vignettes illustrating telepaediatrics – the regional view

Initially in the telehealth consultation, the referring clinician presents the clinical summary, questions and concerns. There is usually discussion between the clinicians about these issues and then the parents and patient are brought into the room to meet and talk with the specialist. X-rays and other documents may be shown via the document camera, and patient signs shown. Occasionally, a videorecording may be shown to illustrate clinical signs such as fits or a gait disturbance. It is unusual to find that management decisions are limited by not being face to face.

Examples of clinics are described below:

Endocrine clinic (1.5 hours)

New cases:

▶ Hypothyroid infant.

▶ Infant with probable congenital adrenal hyperplasia.

▶ Thyrotoxicosis in two-year-old child.

▶ Delayed puberty in a 15-year-old girl with CHARGE association.

Review case:

▶ Fourteen-year-old girl with multiple endocrine neoplasia (MENS) and delayed puberty.

Most of the new cases had been discussed by telephone with the subspecialist soon after presentation, so the telehealth consultation allowed the subspecialist and parents to meet for more detailed case review. Close-up views of the thyrotoxic girl's goitre and exophthalmos, and the masculinized infant girl's genitalia, were presented to the specialist. The subspecialist follows up many cases seen at telepaediatric clinics at an annual outreach visit.

Ad hoc clinic – chronic renal failure

A telehealth consultation was arranged with the paediatric nephrologist for a six-year-old boy with chronic renal failure who had returned from the tertiary unit with peritoneal dialysis. There were a number of clinical concerns. His parents found management difficult, so dialysis was undertaken in hospital. There was a need to assess current clinical state and look at application for renal transplant. This was the first child our unit had managed with peritoneal dialysis.

The consultation involved nursing and medical staff from the regional hospital. The boy's father was included in the consultation after initial discussion of management issues with staff. We agreed to apply for renal transplant after defining a means of ensuring drug compliance. This decision was best made with inclusion of all parties, which was enabled by the telepaediatric consultation.

Ad hoc clinic – neonatal cardiac consultations

A telehealth echocardiogram with the paediatric cardiologist at the tertiary centre was arranged late on a Saturday afternoon for a baby with persisting oxygen requirement but no respiratory distress and a normal chest X-ray. The clinician was concerned to rule out a cardiac disorder, especially going into the night in an isolated setting. The echocardiogram showed no cardiac disorder but features consistent with persistent pulmonary hypertension of the newborn. The baby was able to remain in Mackay, with staff reassured about the diagnosis.

A nine-day-old baby presented with signs of cardiac failure. A telehealth echocardiogram with the tertiary centre paediatric cardiologist was arranged within two hours of presentation. A critical cardiac lesion was identified, management, including prostaglandin infusion, was agreed to, transfer arrangements were made and the receiving unit and the surgical team was notified.[3]

Telehealth may help to decide whether or not to transfer a child, and, if so, to which facility. Mackay sends neonatal cases north to the nearest tertiary neonatal unit but cardiac cases south to the paediatric cardiology unit. A telehealth echocardiogram on an infant with a possible cardiac disorder, performed at 384 kbit/s, provides a rapid and accurate diagnosis, and hence correct transfer planning (see Chapters 3 and 4). After presentation of the case, the parents meet the cardiologist, the echocardiogram is performed and the cardiologist discusses the findings with the parents and referring doctor. This allows the receiving unit to plan their management, including urgent surgery, accordingly. An interested and experienced ultrasonographer is required at the remote end to provide the required images for the cardiologist. Our ultrasonographer gains experience by working with the visiting paediatric sonographer and cardiologist on their outreach clinics to our centre. The local ultrasonographer also performs *in utero* telehealth echocardiogram studies with a tertiary specialist, thus saving pregnant women the inconvenience of travel.

Multi-site consultation

A five-year-old girl had a posterior fossa tumour resected and treated at the tertiary centre in Brisbane. She came from a town 260 km west of Mackay. The tumour had recurred to the point that it was deemed incurable while she was still in Brisbane. She was commenced on a palliative care programme and plans for her transfer back to her home town were made. Her father had already returned home for work. Before her transfer, a multi-site teleconsultation was arranged with a three-way link between the tertiary oncology team and mother in Brisbane; the regional paediatrician, nursing and medical staff in Mackay; and the doctor, nurse and father in the rural town. Discussion surrounded current and potential symptoms, such as malignant meningitis and seizures, and their management, with participation of all. Although it was planned for her to remain in her home town, there was a possibility of her needing to come to Mackay or needing support from the Mackay clinicians.

A multi-site teleconsultation brings all parties involved in a case together with a face-to-face interaction. In this case, the inclusion of all parties allowed a mutual understanding and agreement about the management of this girl with difficult and potentially changing symptoms; both parents, despite being in different centres, were able to be fully involved in the establishment of the management plan.

General paediatric consultation

A 4-year-old boy was presented by the general practitioner in the monthly telehealth clinic at a rural town 200 km away from the regional centre. The boy had longstanding faecal retention with soiling. Two attempts at taking bowel washout fluid orally had not resolved the symptom. The paediatrician was able to discuss with the general practitioner and parent the nature of the problem and the need for bowel washout delivered via nasogastric tube. The general practitioner and parent were comfortable about this proceeding at the rural hospital, so a management plan was developed.

This consultation was supportive to the mother, who was not able to travel easily to the regional centre, as it allowed her an explanation of her child's condition and best management in a timely manner. It validated the general practitioner's views and supported him in managing the case locally without further delay.

Emergency patients and inpatients

Apart from infants with a suspected cardiac disorder, we infrequently use teleconsultations in emergency or acute cases. Staff are busy with case management, often it is afterhours, and contact by the regional paediatrician with a subspecialist usually occurs via telephone, which is quicker and easier. X-rays and other images may be photographed and sent by email. A mobile unit connected to the communication network at the child's bedside with available tertiary consultants may increase the use of telehealth for acute cases.[4] Occasionally, after 1–2 days of inpatient care, a case is discussed via a telehealth consultation with a subspecialist and the parents.

Telepaediatric services – primary healthcare perspective

We have had a mixed response to the offer of regular telepaediatric clinics to rural centres. Some general practitioners have been keen and have regularly referred patients for telepaediatrics, while others, especially those with a busy private practice, have not taken up telepaediatric use. Child health nurses have been enthusiastic and have been more available. Nurses have presented patients for the telepaediatric clinic when the doctor was not available. Junior doctors working in an isolated setting have appreciated the opportunity of clinical support and discussion.

Rural practitioners, including nurses, have indicated that a telepaediatric consultation:

▶ is clinically helpful, supporting and validating local case management

▶ provides education without the doctor having to leave the town. The topics discussed are relevant to their practice – for example, teaching umbilical venous catheterization (UVC) to practitioners in an isolated town in which they recently had a neonate who would have benefited from UVC

▶ is appreciated by patients who do not have to travel to see a specialist

▶ helps build a local team approach, often with both general practitioner and child health nurse, allowing joint discussion and planning of case management.

The doctors' main concern was a lack of reimbursement for their time. A child health nurse, salaried by the health department, as the remote clinical coordinator and presenter, with the general practitioner when available, may be the most suitable means for conducting regional to rural telepaediatric clinics.

Telepaediatric services – regional perspective

A significant reduction has been seen in numbers of patients travelling to the tertiary centre, and hence a reduction in the costs to the health district for travel subsidies, since the introduction of our outreach and telepaediatric clinics (see Chapter 3). On the other hand, far more patients are receiving tertiary specialist consultation than would do so if the only contact was by referral to the tertiary centre or outreach alone. The telepaediatric consultation is well received by parents, providing review of management plans and an opportunity to ask the tertiary specialist questions. Occasionally, the limitations of the consultation, or a need for further investigations or management, create a need for the patient to travel to the tertiary unit. If so, the telepaediatric consultation has allowed the patient and specialist to meet and plan the visit with appropriate expectations.

The use of outreach, and especially telepaediatric, consultation has reinforced the general paediatrician as a case manager and provides educational stimulation. Managing a broad range of paediatric cases, facilitated by outreach and telepaediatric subspecialty support, is fulfilling for the paediatrician. A closer collaborative interaction between the general paediatrician and tertiary specialists develops, which builds regional paediatric expertise. Consistency in the tertiary specialists who serve the region helps this relationship and patient follow-up. The addition of telepaediatric clinics to outreach and other services enhances a holistic regional service.

Telepaediatric clinics allow training opportunities for medical staff and students – both in the clinical use of the medium and through the cases presented. We have encouraged our registrars to act in a central coordination role. They write up the case summaries to be sent by fax before the clinic, present the cases and clinical questions to the specialist, and summarize the discussion and management plan. In this way, they are training more actively as case managers in a range of paediatric areas, supervised by the general paediatricians. Medical students may sit in, sometimes taking a more active role.

Parents and their children have mostly adapted quickly to the medium of telehealth. Children often find it fun. We have used our telepaediatric unit to allow children who are spending a prolonged period away from home to see and talk with their school friends or family in their hometown, which is fun for all. We have also used it to meet parents and for handover of their babies when transferring back from the neonatal intensive care to our regional nursery.

Establishing telepaediatrics in a regional centre

The introduction of telepaediatrics to a regional child and adolescent health service requires additional consultant time, with a paediatrician acting as regional coordinator, leading and showing others its role. It is preferable for the consultant to be full-time in the health service to allow adequate time and availability. The consultant will:

▶ identify where the need and opportunities for telepaediatrics lie, using travel subsidy information if available, as well as contacts with rural practitioners

▶ plan a yearly clinic programme (tertiary and primary levels to regional centre) according to expected need, integrated with outreach and other services

▶ liaise with the central telepaediatric coordinator about technical matters and clinic arrangements, including ad hoc clinics

▶ supervise each subspecialty clinic's bookings, ensuring appropriate referrals from a consultant

▶ ensure that a consultant and/or registrar is sitting in with each consultation – to present, introduce the patient and parents, and discuss and make records of the case plan

▶ notify general practitioners and others of the service and the referral process.

A central coordinator, based in the tertiary unit, can make all telehealth clinic bookings for the regional centre.[2] The coordinator can assist with technical queries – if need be, arranging for a local technician to provide onsite input (see Chapter 3). We have found that this position is an essential element to the sustainability and success of our service.

An administrative officer can assist the regional coordinator by:

▶ making patient bookings for telehealth clinics with charts available, as part of the child and adolescent outpatient service

▶ ensuring that all health professionals involved in the cases are notified of a clinic, such as the physiotherapist and occupational therapist for a rheumatology clinic

▶ faxing telehealth summary sheets on each patient to the central coordinator for the subspecialist or obtaining these from the rural centre

▶ checking the quality of connection between the central and peripheral units

▶ ensuring that the telepaediatric room and equipment is ready for use

▶ collecting data in conjunction with the central coordinator for evaluation.

We advocate use of a room designated primarily for telehealth, if not a dedicated telepaediatric room, with room-based videoconferencing equipment linked to dedicated communication lines with up to 384 kbit/s capacity, a small desk, chairs for six or seven people and some toys. It is best that this be located in the paediatric outpatient area, supported by the administrative officer, with a waiting area and ready access by medical staff. Our equipment is a videoconferencing unit, television screen, camera, video document camera, video cassette recorder and a connection for an ultrasound machine (Fig. 20.1) (see also Chapter 3).

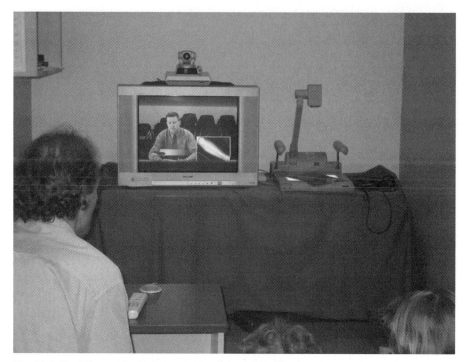

Fig. 20.1. The Mackay telehealth room during a consultation.

The siting of the telehealth service would usually be in the regional public hospital. The health department could support the service by:

- agreeing to a policy that patients need to see the local specialist and access outreach/telehealth clinics before a travel subsidy to the tertiary unit is provided, unless otherwise indicated by the local paediatrician

- ensuring that provision of telehealth clinics, in conjunction with outreach, is included in the job description for consultants and salaried rural doctors at all levels – tertiary, secondary and primary – especially the director of the regional service

- providing appropriate administrative and technical support

- paying for costs, especially line costs borne by the patient's remote site

- creating reimbursement for doctors for telehealth services that have shown clinical effectiveness (the Australian Medicare system has item numbers for telepsychiatry but no other telehealth consultation)

▶ supporting state-wide subspecialty services, which utilize telehealth and provide local ownership of the service delivery in each region, ensuring the best involvement of the regional specialist service. This mandates regional input into the planning, evaluation and remodelling of state-wide services.

The problems to avoid include:

▶ basing most activity on ad hoc consultation, which is less time-efficient

▶ not having user-friendly, ready-to-go equipment that can be connected with a single switch on and one dial (busy clinicians are often in a rush)

▶ either end not being on time, which is frustrating for the other party

▶ using a telehealth unit that is at a distance from the paediatric department.

Conclusion

Telepaediatrics enhances established paediatric services.[5] It creates a more effective and hence attractive role for the regional paediatrician. It builds and maintains better links with tertiary specialists and primary health workers. The benefits flow on through to primary health and hence the health of regional and rural communities.

As a means of outreach service delivery, telepaediatrics is preferred for the following reasons:

▶ It can be provided frequently and for urgent consultations.

▶ It addresses areas of low case volume in an efficient manner.

▶ It can be flexible, with cancellation of a clinic if not needed.

▶ It facilitates the inclusiveness of all parties involved with the patient, including the parents, if necessary by multi-site consultation.

▶ It provides a good means of follow-up, retaining the personal rapport previously established in face-to-face contact.

We have shown integration of a successful telepaediatric model into our mainstream regional health services for children and adolescents. We have achieved the aims without increased costs for the regional health service. There has been a substantial reduction in cost and loss of time for patients and their families.[6] For us, it is no longer a fringe activity but an integral part of routine service delivery.

References

1   Williams M, Smith A. Paediatric outreach services. *Journal of Paediatrics and Child Health* 2004; **40**: 501-503.
2   Smith AC, Isles A, McCrossin R, *et al*. The point-of-referral barrier – a factor in the success of telehealth. *Journal of Telemedicine and Telecare* 2001; **7** (suppl. 2): 75–78.

3   Smith AC, Williams M, Justo R. The multidisciplinary management of a paediatric cardiac emergency. *Journal of Telemedicine and Telecare* 2002; **8**: 112–114.

4   Marcin JP, Nesbitt TS, Kallas HJ, *et al*. Use of telemedicine to provide pediatric critical care inpatient consultations to underserved rural Northern California. *Journal of Pediatrics* 2004; **144**: 375–380.

5   Spooner SA, Gotlieb EM, for the Committee on Clinical Information Technology and the Committee on Medical Liability. Telemedicine: pediatric applications. *Pediatrics* 2004; **113**: e639–e643.

6   Smith AC, Youngberry K, Christie F, *et al*. The family costs of attending hospital outpatient appointments via videoconference and in person. *Journal of Telemedicine and Telecare* 2003; **9** (suppl. 2): 58–61.

▶21

Telemedicine and Paediatric Palliative Care

Mark Bensink and Helen Irving

Introduction

Paediatric palliative care is the active total care of children with life-limiting disease. It involves care of the child's body, mind and spirit, and evaluating and alleviating physical, psychological and social distress. Crucially, it includes consideration of the health and wellbeing of family members.[1] Most children and families who receive palliative care choose the option of returning to the familiarity and security of the home environment.[2,3] For these families, home care is a feasible option as long as adequate support is provided by health professionals with the appropriate expertise.[4-6] Ideally, this support is provided by an integrated, multidisciplinary team of healthcare professionals who work together to support the child and their family through the end-of-life experience.[7] As a systematic review of palliative care teams undertaken by Finlay *et al* identified, care provided by a multidisciplinary care team with specific palliative care training provides the best opportunity for improving outcomes in palliative home care.[8] A recent review of adult and paediatric services in Australia identified that over 12 000 patients were receiving palliative care in the community.[9] This translates to almost 7000 hours of care being provided each week across the nation. Geographical dislocation between the palliative care team, the patients and families they care for and the healthcare professionals who support them in the community is a major challenge for palliative home care. Telemedicine, which is 'the delivery of healthcare and the exchange of healthcare information across distances',[10] offers a promising and innovative solution.

Paediatric palliative home care

End-of-life care for children is a great challenge, with care often being very complex. Provision of palliative care in the home requires considerable commitment from the family, extended family and health professionals who support them in the community. Families are faced with personal and financial sacrifice, fatigue and burnout, and significant symptomatology.[11-15] Ongoing communication, support, care and flexibility are all critical.

Families isolated from specialist services and caring for dying children in the home have found that local community hospice and home care programmes are poorly designed to provide paediatric palliative care.[16] Palliative care services in general have developed mainly in urban areas, resulting in an inequity of services for rural populations.[17,18] Care of rural patients falls on primary care professionals in the community, who may feel overwhelmed or unsupported, or both.[19-23]

Despite these challenges, home care provides a number of advantages. Many parents see palliative care in the home as an extension of their normal parental role and generally are involved as direct caregivers and decision-makers.[2] They see home care as a positive experience, a means to spend more time with their child, allowing siblings to be involved and cared for, and providing the opportunity to grieve in their own time.[24] There is evidence that caring for a child at home facilitates better psychological adjustment for parents than hospitalization,[25] as well as improved adaptation for siblings.[26] From the perspective of the healthcare system, home palliative care has also been shown to be a less costly alternative to hospitalization.[14]

To ensure that families caring for dying children in the home receive the most appropriate support, they need the involvement of a specialist multidisciplinary paediatric palliative care team.

Telemedicine – applications in palliative care

To date, telemedicine has been applied almost exclusively to adult palliative care, primarily in three broad areas:

▶ extending specialist expertise and support to geographically isolated healthcare professionals

▶ providing education to geographically isolated healthcare professionals

▶ extending specialist expertise and support to geographically isolated patients and families in the home.

Different technologies have been used to provide these services. Ordinary telephones have been used to provide advice lines and afterhours support services for both families and community health professionals. Videophones that operate over the ordinary telephone network or the digital equivalent (ISDN network) have been used to provide virtual home visits. Larger ISDN videoconferencing systems have been used to provide support and training, and the Internet has been used to provide specialist palliative care support to isolated community health professionals.

By far the most successful clinical telemedicine programme in adult palliative care is the partnership between the Kansas University TeleMedicine Services Department and Kendallwood Hospice in the US.[27,28] This home-based telehospice service was first implemented as a pilot study in 1997, with videophones that use the ordinary telephone network connecting staff and patients in Missouri and Kansas (Fig. 21.1). The value of using videophones in the home to supplement traditional home visits by nursing staff and social workers was shown. Patients and staff also liked using the system, commenting that it was simple to use. Preliminary cost measurements in 2000 showed that visits using the videophone were much less expensive than visits made in person.[29] The telehospice service has continued as an integrated service modality. Between 2000 and 2002, services were provided to 277 patients, with over 1200 telemedicine visits.[30] Of these, approximately half were for physical assessment of the patient. Nurses were involved in 93% of calls and social workers in 12%. Most of the calls (68%) were scheduled check-ups, and only a very small number of calls were for emergencies (0.5%). Notably, the telehospice service contributed more to rural patients, where distance is a major challenge, than urban ones. An analysis of 15 randomly selected telemedicine visits showed that similar services were provided via telemedicine as were provided in person via traditional service delivery.

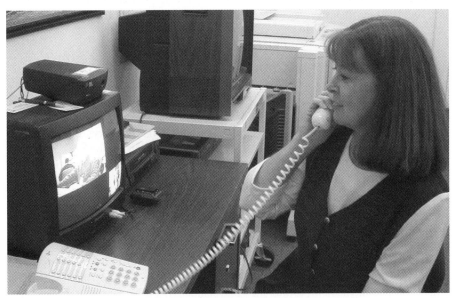

Fig. 21.1. Nurse using the telehospice unit to communicate with a palliative care patient in the home (courtesy of Dr D Cook, Kansas University Medical Center).

Given the success of telemedicine in adult palliative care, why then are there so few reports on the application of telemedicine to paediatric palliative care? There are a number of factors:

▶ Both telemedicine and palliative care are relatively new disciplines.

▶ Fewer children require palliative care, so paediatric palliative care services are not so well developed as adult palliative care services.

▶ Research into paediatric palliative care is a sensitive and challenging area.

Telemedicine, palliative care and paediatric palliative care

The vast majority of telemedicine has occurred in the last 20–30 years, making it a new area of medical research.[10] Likewise, palliative care as a specialist medical discipline is also relatively new: the UK formally recognized specialist palliative medicine in 1987, the American Academy of Hospice and Palliative Medicine was recognized as a specialty by the American Medical Association in 1996[31] and the Royal Australasian College of Physicians submitted an application to the Australian Medical Council in 2004 for recognition of palliative medicine as a full specialty.[32,33] In addition, the development of palliative services for children is not comparable to that of adult services. One reason is that fewer children than adults require palliative care.[34] Some have suggested that research in end-of-life care for children tends to be avoided, possibly for emotional reasons.[35] There is also more uncertainty about treatments for children – whether or not they are supportive, palliative, life-prolonging or curative.[36] All of these factors combine to make research in telepaediatric palliative care a new area, with few if any reports in the literature.

Telepaediatric home videophone project

The Paediatric Oncology Service at the Royal Children's Hospital provides a palliative care service for children in Queensland, areas of northern New South Wales and the southwest Pacific. Between January 2000 and June 2003, the service cared for 74 children and their families, of whom 68% came from rural and remote areas (Fig. 21.2).[37] Unfortunately, team members are unable to provide home visits for families outside the Brisbane metropolitan area because of the travel involved, which makes the telephone the main mechanism for communication. In order to investigate one possible solution to this problem, the Centre for Online Health has started an investigation using Internet-based videophones. The aim of the work is to determine whether or not Internet-based videophones can be used to improve the standard of paediatric palliative care in rural and remote areas, to investigate whether or not this form of telemedicine is a cost-effective model of service delivery and to discover whether or not telemedicine allows the same standard of palliative care to be delivered in rural and remote areas as that delivered in the metropolitan area.

Development of an Internet-based videophone

We have designed, built and tested a low-bandwidth Internet-based videophone for use in patients' homes. It is connected via the ordinary telephone network (Fig. 21.3). The videophone is based on readily available hardware, including a personal computer, web camera and modem (for more detailed information, see Bensink *et al*[38]). The main benefit of using a personal computer in the device is that the telecommunications can be controlled via software (eg modem characteristics), which provides improved reliability over current commercial units. A personal-computer-based device also allows more than simple videotelephony, so that applications such as the capture of high-resolution still images and short video sequences, web browsing and online chat are also possible.

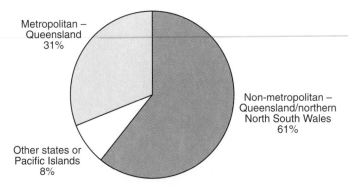

Fig. 21.2. Locations of Royal Children's Hospital Oncology Service palliative care patients in 2000–3.

Preliminary testing with the family of a paediatric palliative care patient has shown that the telepaediatric videophone is a feasible option for supporting paediatric palliative care in the home (Fig. 21.4).[38] Research is continuing to provide more information on telepaediatric palliative home care using the videophone and the impact on patients and families.

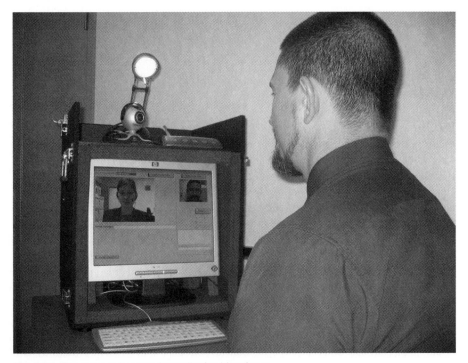

Fig. 21.3. The Internet-based telepaediatric videophone.

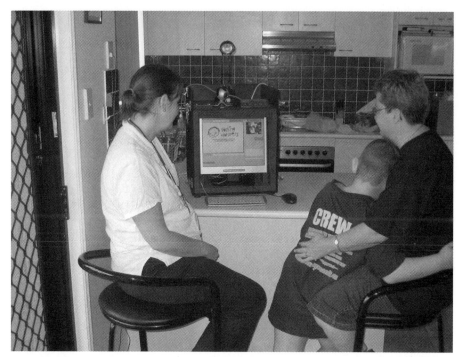

Fig. 21.4. Palliative home care patient with his mother and community nurse waiting for a videophone call.

Conclusion

Paediatric palliative care is fundamentally different from adult palliative care and requires special consideration. Given the choice, most families choose to return home for end-of-life care. Caring for a dying child in the home provides the opportunity for improved outcomes for the patient and their family, but presents its own unique set of challenges. To date, research into the application of telemedicine to palliative care has almost exclusively concerned adult patients. Although these applications have included telephone advice lines, the establishment of education and support networks using videoconferencing and the use of the Internet for specialist consultation, it is in the area of home care for adult palliative patients in rural and remote areas that telemedicine has been most successful. Given the limited specialist paediatric palliative care support available in rural and remote areas and the support needs of the patients, their families and the health professionals caring for them, telemedicine for home paediatric palliative care appears to hold great promise. Research is required to investigate what telemedicine can offer, what technologies are appropriate and what effect it has on the outcomes for paediatric palliative care patients, families and healthcare staff. Early research is encouraging.

References

1 World Health Organization. *Cancer Pain Relief and Palliative Care in Children*. Geneva: World Health Organization, 1998.

2 Hynson JL, Gillis J, Collins JJ, *et al*. The dying child: how is care different? *Medical Journal of Australia* 2003; **179** (suppl. 6): 20–22.

3 Goldman A. Home care of the dying child. *Journal of Palliative Care* 1996; **12**: 16–19.

4 Chambers EJ, Oakhill A, Cornish JM, Curnick S. Terminal care at home for children with cancer. *British Medical Journal* 1989; **298**: 937–940.

5 Goldman A, Beardsmore S, Hunt J. Palliative care for children with cancer – home, hospital, or hospice? *Archives of Disease in Childhood* 1990; **65**: 641–643.

6 Kopecky EA, Jacobson S, Joshi P, *et al*. Review of a home-based palliative care program for children with malignant and non-malignant diseases. *Journal of Palliative Care* 1997; **13**: 28–33.

7 American Academy of Pediatrics. Committee on Bioethics and Committee on Hospital Care. Palliative care for children. *Pediatrics* 2000; **106**: 351–357.

8 Finlay IG, Higginson IJ, Goodwin DM, *et al*. Palliative care in hospital, hospice, at home: results from a systematic review. *Annals of Oncology* 2002; **13** (suppl. 4): 257–264.

9 Commonwealth of Australia. *A Snapshot of Palliative Care in Australia: Summary of the National Palliative Care Plan Initiative a National Study into Palliative Care*. Canberra: Australian Government Department of Health and Ageing, 2003.

10 Wootton R, Craig J, eds. *Introduction to Telemedicine*. London: Royal Society of Medicine Press, 1999.

11 Stajduhar KI. Examining the perspectives of family members involved in the delivery of palliative care at home. *Journal of Palliative Care* 2003; **19**: 27–35.

12 Proot IM, Abu-Saad HH, Crebolder HF, *et al*. Vulnerability of family caregivers in terminal palliative care at home; balancing between burden and capacity. *Scandinavian Journal of Caring Science* 2003; **17**: 113–121.

13 Collins JJ. Palliative care and the child with cancer. *Hematology/Oncology Clinics of North America* 2002; **16**: 657–670.

14 Belasco JB, Danz P, Drill A, *et al*. Supportive care: palliative care in children, adolescents, and young adults – model of care, interventions, and cost of care: a retrospective review. *Journal of Palliative Care* 2000; **16**: 39–46.

15 Wolfe J, Grier HE, Klar N, *et al*. Symptoms and suffering at the end of life in children with cancer. *New England Journal of Medicine* 2000; **342**: 326–333.

16 Contro N, Larson J, Scofield S, *et al*. Family perspectives on the quality of pediatric palliative care. *Archives of Pediatric and Adolescent Medicine* 2002; **156**: 14–19.

17 Evans R, Stone D, Elwyn G. Organizing palliative care for rural populations: a systematic review of the evidence. *Family Practice* 2003; **20**: 304–310.

18 Fried O. Treatment and palliation of cancer in the remote setting. *Cancer Forum* 2002; **26**: 13–16.

19 Lloyd-Williams M, Wilkinson C, Lloyd-Williams F. General practitioners in North Wales: current experiences of palliative care. *European Journal of Cancer Care* 2000; **9**: 138–143.

20 Esteva Canto M, Llobera Canaves J, Miralles Xamena J, Bauza Amengual ML. Management of terminal cancer patients: attitudes and training needs of primary health care doctors and nurses. *Support Care Cancer* 2000; **8**: 464–471.

21 Shipman C, Addington-Hall J, Barclay S, *et al*. Educational opportunities in palliative care: what do general practitioners want? *Palliative Medicine* 2001; **15**: 191–196.

22 Trollor J. Clinical focus: rural general practitioners and palliative care. *Australian Journal of Rural Health* 1993; **1**: 23–29.

23 McRae S, Caty S, Nelder M, Picard L. Palliative care on Manitoulin Island. Views of family caregivers in remote communities. *Canadian Family Physician* 2000; **46**: 1301–1307.

24 Collins JJ, Stevens MM, Cousens P. Home care for the dying child. A parent's perception. *Australian Family Physician* 1998; **27**: 610–614.

25 Mulhern RK, Lauer ME, Hoffmann RG. Death of a child at home or in the hospital: subsequent psychological adjustment of the family. *Pediatrics* 1983; **71**: 743–747.

26 Lauer ME, Mulhern RK, Bohne JB, Camitta BM. Children's perceptions of their sibling's death at home or hospital: the precursors of differential adjustment. *Cancer Nursing* 1985: **8**: 21–27.

27 Doolittle GC. A POTS-based tele-hospice project in Missouri. *Telemedicine Today* 1997; **5**: 18–19.

28 Doolittle GC, Yaezel A, Otto F, Clemens C. Hospice care using home-based telemedicine systems. *Journal of Telemedicine and Telecare* 1998; **4** (suppl. 1): 58–59.

29   Doolittle GC. A cost measurement study for a home-based telehospice service. *Journal of Telemedicine and Telecare* 2000; **6** (suppl. 1): 193–195.

30   Whitten P, Doolittle G. *Telehospice: A Bistate Proposal to Improve End-of-life Care.* Wichita: Association of Kansas Hospices, 2002.

31   Holman GH, Forman WB. On the 10th anniversary of the organization of the American Academy of Hospice and Palliative Medicine (AAHPM): the first 10 years. *American Journal of Hospice and Palliative Care* 2001; **18**: 275–278.

32   Cairns W, Yates PM. Education and training in palliative care. *Medical Journal of Australia* 2003; **179** (suppl. 6): 26–28.

33   The Royal Australasian College of Physicians. *Adult Medicine Division and Australasian Chapter of Palliative Medicine Application to the Australian Medical Council for Specialty Recognition of Palliative Medicine,* 2004. http://www.amc.org.au/forms/Applicationfpm.pdf (last checked 10 August 2004).

34   Liben S. Pediatric palliative medicine: obstacles to overcome. *Journal of Palliative Care* 1996; **12**: 24–28.

35   Goldman A, ed. *Care of the Dying Child.* Oxford: Oxford University Press, 1994

36   Behrman RE, Kliegman RM, Jenson HB, eds. *Nelson Textbook of Pediatrics.* 17th edn. Philadelphia PA: Saunders, 2004.

37   Irving H, Pedersen L. Paediatric oncology palliative care in Queensland: the challenges, success and innovation of service provision. *Medical and Paediatric Oncology* 2003; **41**: 288.

38   Bensink ME, Armfield N, Russell T, *et al.* Paediatric palliative home care with Internet-based videophones: lessons learnt. *Journal of Telemedicine and Telecare* 2004; **10** (suppl. 1): 10–13.

▶ 22

Telerehabilitation for Paediatrics

Edward Lemaire

Introduction

Over the past decade, rehabilitation using telemedicine has become a viable alternative to conventional face-to-face practice. Elimination of distance barriers for physical rehabilitation services will enhance the lives of people with disabilities, help families deal with the consequences of disability and help people with disabilities reintegrate into society. Children have much to gain from improved access to rehabilitation services. As children grow, they require regular modifications to assistive devices, therapy programmes and psychosocial support structures. In many cases, the rehabilitation team must adapt treatment approaches after the child receives other medical interventions, such as orthopaedic surgery for cerebral palsy gait deviations, auditory surgery that affects communication therapy and drug changes for brain injury. The combination of growth and intervention factors leads to a long-term relationship between the family and rehabilitation staff. For this relationship to succeed, the healthcare system and consumer must make an effort to improve human interactions while maintaining quality.

Telerehabilitation can be used to offer the right service, at the right time, in the right place and at the right cost. The right service could involve a combination of health professionals on the rehabilitation team, such as those specializing in medicine, nursing, physical therapy, occupational therapy, speech and language pathology, prosthetics and orthotics, psychology, and social work.[1-10] The right place could be at an acute care hospital following surgery, at a clinic in the child's local community at school or at home. As scheduling is often difficult for families and health professionals, time flexibility is important. The right cost varies on the basis of the location and application. For example, a more expensive approach may be needed for initial assessments between healthcare institutions. A less expensive approach could be used for follow-up and ongoing therapy.

Challenges in physical rehabilitation

Physical rehabilitation presents certain challenges that are not associated with other telehealth applications. For example:

   assessment of pathological human motion

> assistive devices

> team assessments

> cross-discipline communication.

Assessment of pathological human motion

Rehabilitation patients are often required to walk, wheel or move during a consultation. Typical videoconferencing rooms are not large enough for these activities. Camera panning and large movements in the video field decrease image compression efficiency. This can result in higher bandwidth utilization, lower frame rates or image distortion. Lighting is more difficult to optimize over a large area, thereby decreasing image quality at certain points in the gait cycle. In some cases, one staff member at the local site must operate the video camera while another staff member supports or monitors the patient (ie increased personnel requirements). This increases human resource requirements. Motion analysis can also add time to the consultation, as front, side and panning video views could be required to understand the patient's movement problems.

Assistive devices

In many cases, rehabilitation specialists must assess a client's assistive device as part of a consultation (eg wheelchairs, prostheses, orthoses, walkers and canes). Assessment processes and evaluation information for assistive devices differ from typical telehealth encounters. Examples include structural evaluation, device fitting aspects, detecting rubbing or grinding sounds in joints, and methods for making adjustments at the remote site.

Team assessments

Of the people who require a telerehabilitation consultation, many have complex disabilities that require a team approach to develop an appropriate care plan. Team assessments provide challenges, such as structuring the assessment in a small space with one telehealth station and linking with rehabilitation specialists who are not at the same location. For example, a stroke rehabilitation consultation may involve a physician who specializes in physical medicine or rehabilitation (physiatrist), physical therapist and occupational therapist from a public-sector hospital; a private-sector orthotist at another site; a speech language pathologist at a specialized rehabilitation clinic; and the patient, patient's family and health providers at the local site.

Cross-discipline communication

As multiple healthcare disciplines could be involved in a telerehabilitation encounter, the potential for miscommunication increases. Differences in training and clinical experiences can lead to misinterpretation of assessment results. For example, depending on clinical training, clinicians could report the same ankle angle as $+5°$, $-5°$, or $95°$. Errors in interpretation can also occur from clinical procedures, such as differences when measuring hip range of motion in a seated or reclined position.

Solutions to challenges

To deal with these issues, telerehabilitation applications have taken advantage of many communication and information technologies. As with many telehealth applications, videoconferencing is a primary telerehabilitation tool. This is not surprising, as physical rehabilitation relies on understanding human body dynamics and three-dimensional body positioning. The subtleties of human motion are easier to convey visually than verbally. In fact, limited rehabilitation experience at the remote site could lead to misinformation being relayed over the telephone. Telerehabilitation research has shown that low-bandwidth connections (eg via a telephone modem) can be used to complete various clinical activities.[9,11] High-speed audio and video connections increase efficiency and the breadth of services that can be offered.

The need to deal with human motion has introduced various technologies that are not common in typical telehealth settings. Robotic devices have been designed to help people with disabilities perform movement-assisted therapy exercises while providing remote control and monitoring by a rehabilitation specialist.[12,13] Anthropomorphic robots have also been developed to encourage active play and therapeutic movements for children with disabilities.[14] Virtual reality (VR) research has provided a more entertaining patient environment for performing therapeutic exercises.[15–17] The VR approach also provides better opportunities for quantitatively assessing patient progress and interacting with other patients and caregivers. With VR systems that digitize the human body, movements can be automatically calculated and analysed to provide clinically relevant information. Data conferencing components, such as Whiteboards and Chat, have been used to enhance communication during online sessions.[9] Clinical prosthetists have also used application sharing for remote configuration of microprocessor-controlled prostheses.[18]

For paediatric telerehabilitation, the healthcare team must consider additional issues. As with any telehealth programme, a major objective is to reduce travel. This is an important factor in paediatrics, as each visit to an urban health centre is likely to involve one or more family members. In addition to the parents, the hospital trip may include siblings and other relatives or caregivers. Financial savings from reduced travel are well documented in the telehealth literature;[19–22] however, societal financial impact is not always mentioned. Most telehealth services are directed at small communities that do not have local rehabilitation specialty services. Lost workdays when accompanying children for clinic visits could have a large effect on small seasonal businesses. In addition, the local economy is affected, since funds spent in an urban centre for accommodation, meals, travel and other expenses are no longer available to be spent in the smaller community. Surprisingly, the cost and social benefits for the family and small communities have not received attention by decision makers – even in publicly funded health systems. An excellent testimonial for telehealth travel reduction benefits was provided in the early 1990s, when a parent in Thunder Bay, Ontario expressed her gratitude at no longer having to drive 37 hours for her child's five-minute follow-up appointment in Toronto (personal communication).

In addition to the economic and social effect of healthcare-related travel, children with disabilities can be at risk during long drives to urban specialist facilities. In cases in which a wheelchair user is resolving pressure sore problems, extended time sitting in a vehicle could undo weeks of healing. In addition, travel during cold winter months or during the extremes of summer heat can exacerbate respiratory problems in children. In cases where the clinic appointment is for a follow-up or pre-visit screening, telehealth provides a safer environment for the child.

Another aspect related to travel is lost classroom time. Limiting the number of in-person visits to the specialized rehabilitation centre could improve stability in the child's school life. It could also reduce the burden on teachers, who could be expected to maintain the student's academic progress with less classroom time. Integrating telehealth into schools is important for clinical follow-up and helping educators to deal with communication and environmental issues.[23–25]

The evidence

As with adult and elderly telerehabilitation applications, successful paediatric telehealth outcomes have been documented. Robinson et al reported high clinician satisfaction when comparing telemedicine services with the traditional clinic.[10] This study surveyed the paediatrician, physical therapist, occupational therapist, speech therapist, dietician and nurse psychoanalyst. Patient and family satisfaction was high on all issues except dealing with feelings of anger and frustration. The survey respondents considered face-to-face encounters as a better medium for addressing anger and frustration. The telerehabilitation programme was sustainable and continued to operate in Texas.

Sicotte et al and Scheidemann-Miller et al also reported positive results when implementing speech–language pathology telerehabilitation services (Fig. 22.1).[24,25] One study linked a paediatric tertiary care centre with a remote hospital, while the other linked specialized rehabilitation hospitals with schools. Clinician and client satisfaction ratings were high for both studies. However, Sicotte et al reported problems in dealing with agitated children who move constantly and shy children who speak softly. Parent satisfaction ratings were also high for technical and child–therapist contact quality. Sicotte et al reported improvements in speech fluency and reduction in stuttering frequency.

Problems in the Scheidemann-Miller et al study were mainly related to network bandwidth.[24] Peaks in bandwidth usage on the inter-school network created havoc with live video and audio content. This resulted in video image tiling, freeze frames and connection loss. Interaction between computer networks in hospitals, schools and other health service partners makes the delivery of telerehabilitation services complex. With any remote interaction, sustained data rates and quality of service guarantees are prerequisites for successful encounters. The multidisciplinary nature of telerehabilitation increases the potential of linking outside a well managed healthcare-only intranet.

The need for reliable cross-sector bandwidth can be addressed in different ways. Scheidemann-Miller et al installed a dedicated T1 line to the school;[24] however, this

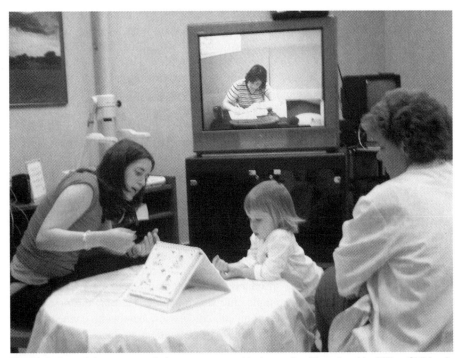

Fig 22.1. Speech language pathology assessment between the Bloorview MacMillan Children's Centre (Toronto) and Sault Ste Marie.

approach was not financially sustainable. In some regions, a common partner is used as the linking network. For example, the hospital and primary education networks could link through a local university. In North America, the SMART City approach brings together hospital, education, government and business to create regional data networks that provide large, managed, secure bandwidth between partners without using the public Internet.[26] As the distance to the remote telerehabilitation site increases, the likelihood of accessing a regional data network decreases. One high-capacity connection may be sufficient, however, to connect a small community to the large regional network environment.

Engbers *et al* also showed positive results when technical problems were avoided.[27] In this study, physiotherapists used a low-cost, personal-computer-based approach to provide physiotherapy consultations between hospitals. Sites communicated using Net-Meeting over a 56 kbit/s telephone line or ISDN connection. An important aspect of this study was that satisfactory results were obtained without a broadband network connection. The physiotherapists completed remote paediatric physiotherapy consultations by sending digital video clips of the child's motion by email to the specialist site and interacting by telephone or by desktop videoconference. A store-and-forward method was necessary for motion analysis, as a telephone modem Internet connection did not provide enough bandwidth for real-time videoconferencing at a clinically acceptable frame rate and image size. Although capturing and sending video clips added additional steps to the consultation process, the specialists benefited by being able to review the video and reply to the referring clinician at a convenient time. A therapist could also enhance clinical decision-making by using quantitative tools to help analyse the child's motion[28] and taking additional time to consider multiple views or critical moments in the gait cycle. The ability to slow down and step through a digital video clip was useful in improving the detection of gait problems.[8]

An interesting result from Engber's study was that physiotherapists considered the 10-second video clip used in the project too short to show the child's motion. This could be due to a child's very slow walking speed or extremely variable gait (ie many strides are necessary to understand the gait problem). As analysing motion is an important tele-rehabilitation requirement, paediatric telehealth providers should plan to deal with transmission of, access to and archiving of large video files. As a child grows, many gigabytes of video data may be collected to follow their progress. The task of deciding what data are stored varies, because many facilities do not include digital video as part of the patient's health record. Even if procedures are in place for archiving video tapes or disks, hospital networks may not be prepared to deliver multiple digital video files to the rehabilitation specialist's desktop for analysis and comparison.

Efficiency problems in the paediatric physiotherapy study were related to bandwidth or hardware. For example, file downloading, starting the system and connecting were too slow. Although clinicians can use low-bandwidth connections for decision-making, limited data transfer rates adversely affect productivity.

From a service perspective, appointment cancellations and no-shows were not affected by telerehabilitation.[10] However, modest improvements for patient visits and decreases in cancellations may be experienced in the novelty period when implementing a new treatment modality. The times to access traditional clinic and telehealth appointments were also the same. These results are not surprising, because, as telerehabilitation becomes a mature service and is integrated into day-to-day clinical practice, scheduling is a common issue. A case could be made that a successful telehealth programme does not need unique scheduling and appointment procedures. Telehealth administration procedures should be handled in the same manner as any other outreach or outpatient visit. Robinson *et al* reported an increase in the referral base because their telemedicine clinic improved screening for potential patients.[10] After the screening process, the presenting nurse could arrange for the appropriate referrals and provide local case management.

An important consideration for paediatric telerehabilitation encounters is accommodating accompanying people. These people may include therapists, family members, school personnel and community health workers. The physical location for a paediatric telerehabilitation encounter must accommodate the session participants and deal with the various characteristics of a rehabilitation service. A summary of facility recommendations is listed in Table 22.1.

Although most paediatric telerehabilitation studies have focussed on programmes and services, some work has been done on the technology required. Lathan and Malley developed a robot, disguised as a toy, that can be controlled by body movements, voice commands or a web interface (Fig. 22.2).[14] The combination of the 'gestural interface' and robotics allowed the researchers to develop protocols that combined active play

Table 22.1. Facility recommendations for paediatric telerehabilitation[18,19,21]

Item	Description
Seating capacity	Three to six adults
Room	Light blue walls
	90 cm doorway
	Adequate storage capacity
	Sink or sanitary wipes
	Dedicated room (ie a divider in a larger room may not reduce noise and other distractions)
Equipment	Examination table
	Floor mat
	Emergency box
	Tabletop workspace
	Telephone and fax machine
Communication	Videoconferencing system
	Document camera
	Auxiliary camera and camcorder
	Computer for data conferencing (eg whiteboard, application sharing, file transfer)
Setup	No distractions
	Detachable camera to capture motion (eg walking or wheeling)

and therapeutic movements to improve range of motion and cognitive development. The robot was capable of mimicking a child's movements, leading the child through exercises and providing movement analysis information that could be accessed remotely by a health professional.

There is potential for integrating robotic-assisted rehabilitation into a child's play time. Robot technology has the potential to represent a user in a virtual community for rehabilitation professionals who are looking to achieve physical capacity goals but only see the child during periodic follow-up appointments. A key element for such a programme is the therapist's ability to set the therapy rules and protocols easily and have intelligent software that can monitor the child's progress and report as critical indicators are reached. For example, a web-enabled robot could send data to a therapist when the child accomplishes the current therapy objective, the child's performance worsens or the child's activity level drops.

In comparison with the literature on adult telehealth, paediatric telerehabilitation has a very small evidence base. On the basis of current peer-reviewed studies, children have unique issues that can affect their clinical outcomes in a telerehabilitation setting. Unfortunately, this leads to uncertainty when applying research results from the general telerehabilitation literature to the paediatric population. Although the speech–language pathology area has produced two studies that support clinical applications, the areas of physiotherapy, occupational therapy, prosthetics and orthotics, psychosocial medicine, and physical medicine require additional research before evidence-based decisions about paediatric telerehabilitation programmes can be made. Research following children with cerebral palsy, amputations, spinal problems or head injury is also important, as these cases need continuing attention as the child develops.

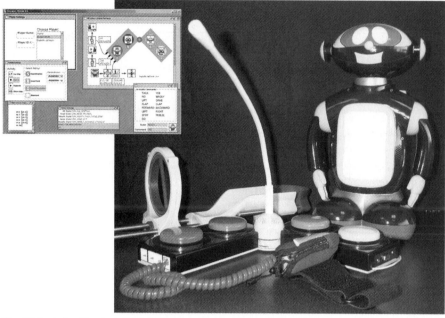

Fig 22.2. AnthroTronix telerehabilitation robot and the therapist control module screen (see http://www.atinc.com).

Paediatric telerehabilitation

Based on the literature and the existence of sustainable paediatric telerehabilitation programmes, it is clear that telehealth is a viable approach for remote paediatric rehabilitation services. The questions that remain are how can the service be best delivered and how should professionals be trained to deal with their young patients over a distance.

The case for paediatric telerehabilitation

Few paediatric telerehabilitation studies have been conducted, but all have reported positive clinical outcomes. As with almost all telehealth studies, patients and remote healthcare providers have high satisfaction ratings. This is not surprising, as these people are the main beneficiaries of reduced travel, better access to specialists and assistance with clinical decision-making. Specialists are also satisfied with telerehabilitation as a clinical modality, although satisfaction ratings are typically not as high as with face-to-face clinical encounters. This result is also not surprising, as the specialist must find ways to obtain the necessary information while working through a display monitor.

Many facilities throughout the world use telerehabilitation while not necessarily presenting outcomes data in the scientific literature. Websites that mention paediatric telerehabilitation can be found in many countries with active telehealth programmes.

Sustaining a healthcare programme is a good indication that consumers need the service and that the solution is viable.

Financially, cost savings have been reported for paediatric telerehabilitation.[10] These savings were attributed to travel time, although additional savings from increased staff productivity could be added. From a health institution's perspective, cost savings for paediatric telerehabilitation could be similar to adult populations. The costs to families and employers are much higher, however, as children typically are accompanied to their healthcare appointments.

Access to physical rehabilitation is a global problem. For complex disabilities, specialized rehabilitation care tends to be located in urban centres. In Ontario, Canada's most populous province, only 3 of 10 rehabilitation hospitals specialize in paediatric rehabilitation (Ontario covers over 1 million km^2 – an area larger than France and Spain combined). In many cases, rehabilitation is neglected because of distance problems, with the risk of more serious conditions developing.

As telecommunications spread throughout the world, telerehabilitation services become feasible in developing countries. A combination of clinical services and continuing education can help improve the quality of life for children with disabilities. More efficient and cost-effective contact between onsite visits enhances continuity, and potentially success rates, for health-aid programmes.

Differences between child and adult telerehabilitation

Most paediatric healthcare workers consider that a child should not be treated like a small adult: children have unique needs and characteristics that must be considered. A successful paediatric telerehabilitation programme will need to follow this principle. Areas for consideration are described below.

Attention and distractions

For some telerehabilitation installations, the videoconferencing equipment is located in the corner of a therapy area. Although this arrangement may be useful for examining motion or accessing rehabilitation equipment, visual or auditory distractions may make communicating with the child difficult. Setting up a secure telerehabilitation conferencing area that is relatively distraction-free is one way of dealing with attention problems. Other methods can involve use of the video medium and pacing the session to maintain the child's interest. Telepsychiatry studies have shown better retention of physician instructions if the specialist zooms in on their face when explaining things that they want the patient to remember. Similar techniques are used in television and film to signify an important moment or message. Television production methods may be an effective tool when working with children.

Conflict

An interesting finding from two of the paediatric telerehabilitation studies was the difficulties of dealing with anger, agitation and frustration over a videoconferencing link. These outcomes have not been reported in adult telerehabilitation studies. There may be various reasons for this difference. Children are not as experienced with conflict resolution and are often harder to reason with when they enter an agitated state than adults. Adults can discuss their concerns, but children may have more difficulty expressing their feelings using words. Children may be used to receiving information from a television and not interacting with the onscreen images. The videoconferencing system may reduce the level of control by removing the health provider's physical presence from the clinic room.

The second factor is the role of the family in the clinical encounter. A lack of experience with videoconferencing may leave parents feeling unable to communicate effectively during emotionally charged discussions about their child's healthcare. For both situations, clinicians involved with paediatric telerehabilitation should receive training in different approaches to conflict resolution over a videoconferencing link. Ideally, the rehabilitation specialist will learn to recognize signs of anger, agitation and frustration through the conferencing link and, working with the local health provider, take steps to help the child and family work through the screen (ie try to encourage the family to interact, move agitated family members closer to the screen when talking and use the camera zoom to control perceived distance).

Family

Children and frail elderly people are the main rehabilitation groups who are usually accompanied to their clinical appointment. The presence of family members affects how people interact during a remote encounter and how space is configured. As mentioned in the previous section, communication dynamics are different when discussing a child's care with a family and discussing treatment with an adult patient. The relatively small rooms used for telehealth in many community clinics may add to communication difficulties. If parents cannot be in the room during a physical rehabilitation consultation, they may feel removed from the clinical process and be more open to conflict situations. As rehabilitation specialists will not have control over the remote site setting, new strategies must be developed to create the optimum environment using a variety of technical and space configurations.

School

For adults, telehealth services from the clinic to the workplace have not received much attention; however, the need for telerehabilitation services in schools is well known. In many countries, rehabilitation is already provided in schools by speech–language pathologists, psychologists, therapists and nurses. Telerehabilitation provides a more efficient method of service delivery that can reduce the length of time that health professionals spend driving between schools and allow increased patient contact. As school-based telerehabilitation becomes integrated into clinic and school programmes, additional rehabilitation services could be provided, including assistive device follow-up appointments and technology access consultations.

A critical factor for successful school-based telerehabilitation is a reliable high-speed data connection. Dedicated broadband links between a clinic and a school have typically been unsustainable once the research project funding has ended. In urban settings, many school boards are installing broadband intranets for educational purposes. If a secure connection can be made from the rehabilitation hospital network to the school network, sustainability and reliability problems could be resolved.

However, this does not account for connections between an urban rehabilitation hospital and a rural school. In a rural setting, cooperation between healthcare, government and education sectors may be the only way to provide sustainable, reliable broadband access.

The future

Many new technologies and approaches have the potential to improve paediatric telerehabilitation services. Further research is needed to develop these ideas and verify the clinical value.

Wheelchair seating

For many children with disabilities, proper wheelchair seating is critical to their comfort, function and health (eg internal organs may be compressed by the ribs because of improper positioning). Issues that range from wheelchair prescription to customized seating would benefit from consultations with an occupational therapist, rehabilitation engineer or other seating specialist (Fig. 22.3). Access to the appropriate specialists should lead to the correct wheelchair prescriptions, correct configuration and correct decisions about customised seating and modifications. Little research has been done on telerehabilitation wheelchair assessments. In an ideal scenario, the specialist would be able to remotely analyse seating pressures, take measurements onscreen or visually lead the local health provider through the measurement process (eg using a whiteboard) and watch the client propel the wheelchair.

Whiteboard and application sharing

Most telerehabilitation programmes are limited to videoconferencing. However, data conferencing can also be a useful communication tool for online consultations. An interactive whiteboard is especially useful when trying to show the remote clinician where to take measurements or where to modify the device.[8] In these cases, the specialist can capture an image of the client with their wheelchair, prosthesis or brace and use the shared drawing tools to outline the areas for measurement or modification. Videoconferencing can still be used to verify that the correct measurements are being taken.

Application sharing allows the specialist to take remote control of any software running on the remote site computer. The system is based on the T.120 standard and works by sending a stream of program window images and all keyboard and mouse movements between sites. This gives remote users the impression that the software is running on their computer. For rehabilitation, the patient could connect their assistive device to the remote computer, start the device's configuration software, share the program over the data conferencing link and then allow the specialist to complete the assessment and configuration online. This approach can also be used with pressure monitoring or other diagnostic systems. Initial work with adults has shown positive outcomes for above-knee prosthetics and myoelectric arms.[18]

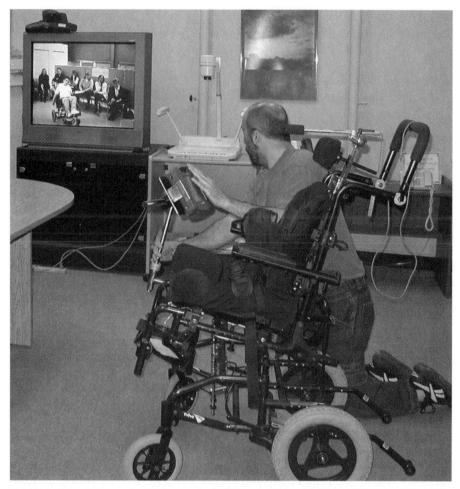

Fig 22.3. Wheelchair control system adjustment via videoconferencing (Bloorview MacMillan Children's Centre, Toronto).

Motion analysis

Motion analysis has become an important tool for clinical decision making for children with disabilities. It is especially important for cerebral palsy and conditions with spastic gait problems, where quantitative gait analysis is used by many orthopaedic surgeons, physiatrists and physiotherapists. Telerehabilitation is an ideal method for connecting between a central gait laboratory and the referring clinician to discuss results and review video analyses. Since gait analysis involves digital data, videoconferencing and data conferencing allows video, marker positions, electromyogram (EMG) and force information to be displayed between sites.

As well as traditional gait analysis, online motion analysis could be useful during a telerehabilitation encounter. Web-enabled software is being developed to provide onscreen measurement of distances, angles, timing and velocity.[28] These tools can bring simple quantitative analysis to the point of patient contact, whether onsite or online (Fig. 22.4).

Multipoint team consultations

Multipoint videoconferencing is typically used for continuing education. As more rehabilitation professionals are equipped for telehealth, the potential for multipoint clinical encounters increase. In rural communities particularly, rehabilitation care can involve many partners from different locations (eg hospital, clinic, private facility or school). More research is needed on the minimum technical requirements, optimum procedures, best administrative and scheduling methods, and etiquette for this approach. For example, uncertainty exists as to how the child and their family would react if the videoconferencing screen jumps from specialist to specialist during a team consultation.

Smart bandwidth monitoring

Most studies that use the public Internet or dial-up modem connections report variations in data transmission rates that can affect clinical decision-making. Telerehabilitation systems that run over the public Internet will need more

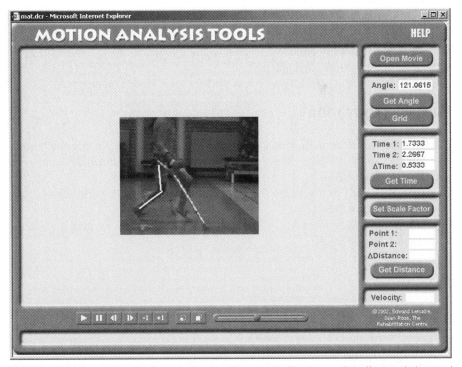

Fig 22.4. Web-based clinical gait analysis using Macromedia Shockwave (http://www.rehab.on.ca/cag/matshock/index.html). Video clip obtained from the Clinical Gait Analysis website (http://guardian.curtin.edu.au/cga/case.html).

sophisticated bandwidth monitoring so that clinicians are notified when they may be missing critical information. For example, degradation in audio quality because of automatic increases in compression may affect a speech–language pathology assessment.

Urban telehealth

The main objective in telehealth is to support clinicians and patients in rural and remote communities. For children, telerehabilitation has a place in urban centres. Telerehabilitation with schools has been described in this chapter. The larger number of children means that a much higher volume of online consultation could be expected in urban schools. The limited number of specialized paediatric rehabilitation facilities in most countries means that there may be a place for telerehabilitation interactions between cities. To increase efficiency, various members of the extended rehabilitation team could use telehealth to participate in clinics in the specialized rehabilitation hospital. For example, an orthopaedic surgeon or orthotist could connect remotely if they only had to see one client during a rehabilitation clinic.

Conclusion

Paediatric telerehabilitation is becoming a viable method of providing efficient health services; however, the scientific literature in this area is still sparse. Continued development and evaluation of telerehabilitation technology, protocols and administrative structures are required.

Further information

Institute for Rehabilitation Research and Development. Computer Applications Group – Motion Analysis Tools. http://www.rehab.on.ca/cag/matshock/index.html (last checked 8 August 2004).

Clinical gait analysis website. http://guardian.curtin.edu.au/cga/case.html (last checked 8 August 2004).

Gait and Clinical Movement Analysis (GCMA) Society. http://www.gcmas.org/ (last checked 8 August 2004).

References

1   Brown R, Pain K, Berwald C, *et al*. Distance education and caregiver support groups: comparison of traditional and telephone groups. *Journal of Head Trauma Rehabilitation* 1999; **14**: 257–268.

2   Brennan D, Georgeadis A, Baron C. Telerehabilitation tools for the provision of remote speech–language treatment. *Topics in Stroke Rehabilitation* 2002; **8**: 71–78.

3   Burns RB, Crislip D, Daviou P, *et al*. Using telerehabilitation to support assistive technology. *Assistive Technology* 1998; **10**: 126–133.

4   Dreyer NC, Dreyer KA, Shaw DK. Wittman PP. Efficacy of telemedicine in occupational therapy: a pilot study. *Journal of Allied Health* 2001; **30**: 39–42.

5   Hauber RP, Testani-Dufour L, Coleman K. Better care for low-level brain-injured patients and their families. *Journal of Neuroscience Nursing 2002*; **34**: 20–24.

6   Jerome LW, DeLeon PH, James LC, *et al*. The coming of age of telecommunications in psychological research and practice. *American Psychologist* 2000; **55**: 407–421.

7   Jin C, Ishikawa A, Sengoku Y, Ohyanagi T. A telehealth project for supporting an isolated physiotherapist in a rural community of Hokkaido. *Journal of Telemedicine and Telecare* 2000; **6** (suppl. 2): 35–36.

8   Lemaire ED, Jeffreys Y. Low-bandwidth telemedicine for remote orthotic assessment. *Prosthetics and Orthotics International* 1998; **22**: 155–167.

9   Lemaire ED, Boudrias Y, Greene G. Low-bandwidth, Internet-based telehealth for physical rehabilitation consultations. *Journal of Telemedicine and Telecare* 2001; **7**: 82–89.

10 Robinson SS, Seale DE, Tiernan KM, Berg B. Use of telemedicine to follow special needs children. *Telemedicine Journal and e-Health* 2003; **9**: 57–61.

11 Malagodi M, Schmeler MR, Shapcott NG, Pelleschi T. The use of telemedicine in assistive technology service delivery: results of a pilot study. *Technology: Special Interest Section Quarterly* 1998; **8**: 1–4.

12 Hesse S, Schulte-Tigges G, Konrad M, *et al*. Robot-assisted arm trainer for the passive and active practice of bilateral forearm and wrist movements in hemiparetic subjects. *Archives of Physical Medicine and Rehabilitation* 2003; **84**: 915–920.

13 Krebs HI, Volpe BT, Aisen ML, Hogan N. Increasing productivity and quality of care: robot-aided neuro-rehabilitation. *Journal of Rehabilitation Research and Development* 2000; **37**: 639–652.

14 Lathan CE, Malley S. Development of a new robotic interface for telerehabilitation. In *Proceedings of the 2001 EC/NSF Workshop on Universal Accessibility of Ubiquitous Computing: Providing for the Elderly 2001*. Alcácer do Sal, Portugal: ACM, 2001: 80–83.

15 Deutsch JE, Lewis JA, Boian R, Burdea G. Virtual reality telerehabilitation: an inter-disciplinary collaboration. In *Proceedings of the IEEE 29th Annual Northeast Bioengineering Conference.* Newark, New Jersey: IEEE, 2003: 281–282.

16 Gourlay D, Lun KC, Lee YN, Tay J. Virtual reality for relearning daily living skills. *International Journal of Medical Informatics* 2000; **60**; 255–261.

17 Sveistrup H, McComas J, Thornton M, *et al*. Experimental studies of virtual reality-delivered compared to conventional exercise programs for rehabilitation. *Cyberpsychology and Behavior* 2003; **6**: 245–249.

18 Lemaire ED, Fawcett JA. Using NetMeeting for remote configuration of the Otto Bock C-Leg: technical considerations. *Prosthetics and Orthotics International* 2002; **26**: 154–158.

19 Smith AC, Youngberry K, Christie F, *et al*. The family costs of attending hospital outpatient appointments via videoconference and in person. *Journal of Telemedicine and Telecare* 2003; **9** (suppl. 2): 58–561.

20 Crump WJ, Pfeil T. A telemedicine primer: an introduction to the technology and an overview of the literature. *Archives of Family Medicine* 1995; **4**: 796–803.

21 Specht JKP, Wakefield B, Flanagan J. Evaluating the cost of one telehealth application connecting an acute and long-term care setting. *Journal of Gerontological Nursing* 2001; **27**: 34–39.

22 Marcin JP, Ellis J, Mawis R, *et al*. Using telemedicine to provide pediatric subspecialty care to children with special health care needs in an underserved rural community. *Pediatrics* 2004; **113** (1 Pt 1): 1–6.

23 Artunian J. Rehab gets wired. *Rehabilitation Management* 1997; **10**: 54–6,58.

24 Sicotte C, Lehoux P, Fortier-Blanc J, Leblanc Y. Feasibility and outcome evaluation of a telemedicine application in speech–language pathology. *Journal of Telemedicine and Telecare* 2003; **9**: 253–258.

25 Scheidemann-Miller C, Clark PG, Smeltzer SS, *et al*. Two year results of a pilot study delivering speech therapy to students in a rural Oklahoma school via telemedicine. *Proceedings of the 35th Annual Hawaii International Conference on Systems Sciences.* In Sprague RH, ed. IEEE Computer Society Press, 2002: Los Alamitos, CA 9.

26 *Smart Communities*. Industry Canada. http://smartcommunities.ic.gc.ca/index_e.asp (last checked 18 March 2004).

27 Engbers L, Bloo H, Kleissen R, *et al*. Development of a teleconsultation system for communication between physiotherapists concerning children with complex movement and postural disorders. *Journal of Telemedicine and Telecare* 2003; **9**: 339–343.

28 Lemaire ED. A shockwave approach for web-based clinical motion analysis. *Telemedicine Journal and e-Health* 2004 (in press).

▶23

Telemedicine for Schoolchildren in Kansas

Pamela Whitten and Ryan Spaulding

Introduction

Schools are better able to meet their mission of education when they have classrooms full of healthy children. The National Health and Education Consortium reported that 'physical and mental health problems cause children to miss school, lack energy, be distracted, or have other problems which impair their ability to learn'.[1] Studies show that children who are physically fit tend to pay attention in class, complete their assignments and feel good about themselves.[1]

In the US, 53 million young people attend nearly 129 000 schools for about six hours of classroom time each day.[2] Because schools are the only institutions that can reach nearly all youth, they are in a unique and important position to affect the physical, emotional and behavioural health status of young people. Schools are good places to deliver health services for children who have difficulty in accessing health services because of lack of availability or transportation challenges. High-risk groups, such as children living in poverty, children from racial and ethnic minority groups, and children in remote areas, will particularly benefit from access to health services from their schools.

Fisher *et al* outlined 467 national health objectives, of which 107 were directed specifically toward school-age children.[3] Of those 107 objectives, 10 focused on the role of schools in improving the health of young people. Many schools already possess some infrastructure to offer health services in their facilities. According to the School Health Policies and Programs Study, more than 75% of schools have a part-time or full-time school nurse and more than half of schools have a recommended nurse-to-student ratio of 1:750 or better.[4] Almost 20% of American states require districts or schools to provide health services to students through collaborative arrangements with external healthcare agencies.

In addition to being a convenient and logical location for health-based services, schools are also excellent places to deliver health services for children. This is partly because they are the places in which physical, emotional and behavioural health problems frequently occur. For example, injuries often occur during physical activities. There are also various other health problems that call for school-based healthcare. Asthma is a prime example, as 6.3 million American children (8.7%) suffer from this chronic health condition. An estimated 14 million lost school days are attributed to asthma among school-age children.[5] One potential method for decreasing asthma-related or other disease-related absenteeism is to improve school-based health services. We launched a school-based telemedicine project in Kansas City, Kansas, in the late 1990s.

Starting a school-based project

Inner-city school-based telemedicine began in 1997 in Kansas. Other states have also begun school-based projects, such as Kentucky, which employed videoconferencing over ordinary telephone lines to conduct 150 telehealth consultations in 2000 and 2001.[6] In Kansas, the initial work was a collaborative effort between management of the telemedicine programme at the Kansas University Medical Center (KUMC) and healthcare coordinators at a Kansas City, Kansas school district. The KUMC housed an active telemedicine programme that had provided a wide range of services to rural Kansas since the mid 1990s. In 1997, school nurses in Kansas City reported an alarming trend among schoolchildren who were unable to access healthcare for routine acute conditions such as sore throat, ear infection, skin irritation and respiratory ailments. The problem extended well beyond these inner city children just missing a few days of school. These disadvantaged children were not receiving necessary healthcare interventions in a timely fashion, if at all.

In partnership with Unified School District (USD) 500, we developed urban school-based telemedicine. The USD 500 serves more than 20 000 students from lower-income and ethnically diverse families. For example, almost 75% of the student population participates in the federal free and reduced lunch programme. Half of the children are black, one-quarter are Hispanic and just over 20% are white. These children face a wide range of barriers to healthcare access, including language, inadequate transportation or economic resources, lack of familiarity with the medical community and citizenship status. Typically, healthcare for these children comes from the emergency rooms of the hospitals in the area.

Planning and logistical efforts were coordinated between the paediatric and psychiatry departments at the KUMC, the school district's central office and individual elementary schools in the district. Many hours were spent developing procedures, protocols and consent processes. The KUMC director and the executive vice chancellor for the medical school made several presentations to the school district's board of directors to obtain approval for the project. A wide range of legal issues were addressed as well. For example, the KUMC programme director had to submit a letter to the school district's liability insurer to obtain a waiver to launch the project. Training was carried out at each of the participating schools.

In 1998, personal computer-based videoconferencing systems (PictureTel) were installed at four schools (Fig. 23.1). The systems were equipped with a digital otoscope (AMD) and an electronic stethoscope (American Telecare Telephonic). Videoconferencing was based on ISDN lines operating at 128 kbit/s, which allowed real-time teleconsultation. The equipment was placed in the school nurses' offices, connecting them to the KUMC paediatric and psychiatry departments, and thus establishing a school-based telemedicine network, now named TeleKidcare.

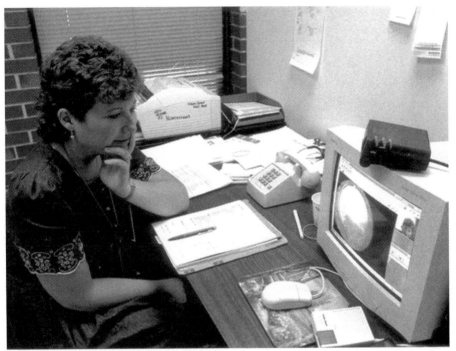

Fig 23.1. Paediatrician looking at an ear drum.

Utilization

During the pilot phase of the project, from March 1998 to May 1998, a total of 187 children received school-based telemedicine care. Table 23.1 summarizes the services provided during the pilot phase of the project. This showed that school-based telemedicine was effective at diagnosing ear infections and, with the aid of a rapid test, streptococcal infections could also be diagnosed. Rashes were more difficult to diagnose, especially if the student was dark-skinned. On the other hand, rashes are also difficult to diagnose in traditional, face-to-face consultations. Looking at a rash meant that the school nurse had to use descriptors such as papular (raised), macular (flat), scattered, wheals (elevated ridges) or erythematous (red-looking) for the physician. During the pilot phase – and subsequently – the most common problems were in ears, eyes, nose and throat. These problems accounted for almost 50% of the services provided. Table 23.2 summarizes the conditions treated from autumn 1998 to spring 2004.

Behavioural health for children was a common use of the telemedicine service. Some children received their first mental health evaluations through the telemedicine system, introducing them to much needed treatment and forging ongoing relationships with KUMC psychiatrists. These and other children were able to have follow-up visits for ongoing drug management, allowing the school nurse to be more involved in their

Table 23.1. Services provided during the three-month pilot phase

Diagnoses	Services
Ear, nose and throat	50 (28%)
Physical	36 (20%)
Dermatology	36 (20%)
Follow-up	23 (13%)
Upper respiratory	14 (8%)
Behavioural	11 (6%)
Miscellaneous	5 (3%)
Eye	3 (2%)
Total	**178 (100%)**

Table 23.2. Services provided from autumn 1998 to spring 2004

Diagnoses	Services
Ear, nose and throat	1176 (48%)
Behavioural	686 (28%)
Dermatology	343 (14%)
Respiratory	221 (9%)
Other	24 (1%)
Total	**2450 (100%)**

behavioural health and assist with treatment compliance. Some of these children also began receiving mental health therapy from two KUMC psychologists – a practice that continues to this day.

Surveys of physicians, school nurses, school administrators and families involved in the project suggest that users are satisfied with healthcare delivery provided by telemedicine and 98% of parents were 'satisfied' or 'very satisfied' with the services offered through TeleKidcare. Parents and family members explained that the school setting is a safe and familiar one, creating in many ways a better environment in which to receive healthcare.[7]

Factors in successful implementation

The TeleKidcare service is now provided to 31 schools; however, there were a number of growing pains during the first years. These problems had one thing in common – *they all stood in the way of the successful delivery of services*. The successful adoption of an innovation such as telemedicine depends on a successful implementation stage. Rogers stated that 'implementation usually follows the decision stage rather quickly unless it is held up by some logistical problem'.[8] Provision of telemedicine services to inner-city schools was no exception to this. We have addressed the problems one by one, and this has resulted in a successful school-based telemedicine programme. A number of research projects have been conducted to evaluate perceptions, cost issues and organizational challenges.[7,9–13] Through experience and research, we have learned that there are many issues to consider when implementing a school-based telemedicine service.

The excitement that surrounded school-based telemedicine overshadowed any early concerns about reimbursement. Although reimbursement for telemedicine in Kansas was available from Blue Cross, Blue Shield and Kansas Medicaid, the KUMC physicians and the school nurses were initially more focused on telemedicine and how it could improve access to healthcare for schoolchildren than on recovering fees. Early grants provided funding for research, but none provided direct support for physician services. An early cost study found that as the number of completed consultations at a site increased, the cost per consultation decreased.[12] The threshold – when the cost of a teleconsultation began to approximate the cost of a routine ambulatory paediatric care visit – was about 200 cases. This provided an economic justification for the use of the service.

In most telemedicine projects that involve multiple sites, a small number of locations account for the majority of the activity. In our case, two of the four schools accounted for nearly 90% of the consultations during the pilot phase in 1998. These two schools have continued to account for a significant proportion of all telemedicine activity as the number of schools in the network has grown over the years. There are a number of reasons for this. Both are elementary schools, and our experience shows that telemedicine is better at providing acute healthcare services for the common problems experienced by younger children. The two elementary schools are also relatively large, with populations of over 700 students. With a larger number of students, the nurses tend to see more sick children and, in turn, have more opportunities to become proficient with the telemedicine systems. These schools also have a high proportion of students (approximately 90%) in the federal free and reduced lunch programme. This reflects the underserved nature of the families. In addition, each school has a full-time school nurse. In contrast, many of the other schools have part-time nurses, so the availability of telemedicine is limited to the hours that they are present. We have learned that in urban areas, the most effective way to meet the needs of these families is to provide telemedicine in schools in which the participation in the federal free and reduced lunch programme is at least 70%.

As we began expanding the network to other schools, the significance of the role played by the school nurse became apparent.[10] The school nurse had to be a champion of telemedicine. In addition, the school nurse had to be an advocate for the health concerns of the students and to understand that telemedicine was an opportunity to use their medical training and education to the full. The role of the school nurse changed from one of distributing bandages for scraped knees to one of being a full participant in the medical care of a child. The nurse's role expanded to include working with the family to ensure compliance with the physician's treatment recommendations. School nurses who embraced this change in job description quickly adopted telemedicine.

However, a school nurse does not operate alone in a school. The endorsement and support of the building administrator is critical. At one school, the nurse complained that the principal seemed to be oblivious of the services offered by telemedicine. For example, he did not support the school nurse by allowing her time at 'meet the teacher' night to tell parents about the TeleKidcare service, nor did he encourage the faculty to take advantage of her medical expertise.

In summary, interviews with key stakeholders, such as school nurses, principals, teachers and parents, and trial and error suggested three specific strategies to improve adoption. First, telemedicine systems should be placed in elementary schools rather than middle or high schools. Second, telemedicine systems should be placed in elementary schools in which socioeconomic indicators, such as free and reduced lunch participation, show the underserved nature of the community. Finally, telemedicine systems should be placed in elementary schools in which there are enthusiastic full-time school nurses and building administrators.

Telemedicine is not a panacea

The lessons from the early years of telemedicine in schools in Kansas City suggest that it cannot solve every problem concerning the health and wellbeing of children. When telemedicine was first proposed, it was expected to be most helpful for students with special learning or physical needs. These children often missed a lot of school and the consensus was that telemedicine could help these students visit their doctors while reducing time away from school. Unfortunately, this did not occur. The special needs students almost never used telemedicine. Interviews with school nurses and parents suggested that when a family has a special needs child, they are already well integrated into the healthcare system, even before the child begins attending school. Instead, we found that the students who really needed school-based telemedicine were the children whose families struggle against the socioeconomic barriers encountered when attempting to access healthcare. These barriers include language, inadequate transportation or economic resources, lack of familiarity with the medical community, and citizenship status. When these children have acute medical needs, their parents often cannot get them to a doctor. This is important for telemedicine – a programme founded on technology is doomed to failure when the fundamental problems are not technological in nature.

Some services can be delivered via telemedicine technically but are perceived to involve significant challenges. One type of healthcare that was needed and tried early on was a complete physical examination service. Despite their best efforts to make physical examinations possible, the physicians and school nurses found that several important components of the examination could not be carried out satisfactorily. Physicians felt that it was imperative that their hands actually touch the patient during an abdominal examination. Providers were also concerned about the potential need to examine children's genitals and deemed this to be inappropriate to be done via telemedicine. After several months, it was decided to remove the complete physical examination from the list of possible telemedicine consultations. Telemedicine is excellent in some situations, but it cannot do everything.

In a perfect world, school districts should be responsible for educational issues and parents should tend to their children's medical needs; however, we do not live in a perfect world. Just as many schools in the US take advantage of federal breakfast programmes for their students (because educators have learned that a hungry child does not learn as efficiently), many schools now realize that a sick child cannot learn as well as a healthy child. Yet the role of a school as a health provider is still controversial in many school districts. Expansion of the project to rural Kansas communities began in 2000. The KUMC encountered one community divided in its attitude to education and healthcare. The school district administrators of this particular rural community submitted an application to be considered for the TeleKidcare network. Their application was accepted. However, when KUMC staff met the district's board of education, it was apparent that the board did not feel that healthcare had any place in its mandate. The board members felt strongly that their only area of focus should be education. In response to such attitudes, the KUMC designated TeleKidcare as a support service rather than a standalone programme. TeleKidcare in its present format is not designed to be a fully-fledged onsite clinic or medical home to students. Most Kansas community patrons do not want a school-based health centre on their school campuses. TeleKidcare can help with many acute or behavioural healthcare situations. Children can be diagnosed, receive treatment and get back into school. TeleKidcare is not an attempt by the school district to assume the responsibility for the healthcare of the student; rather, it is a tool at school to help parents access healthcare for their children.

TeleKidcare now and in the future

Although TeleKidcare was launched in 1998 and almost 2500 consultations have been conducted with children in Kansas schools, we still like to think of it as a new programme with tremendous growth potential. At the time of writing (2004), KUMC is working with 15 school districts (see Fig. 23.2) in the state, yet there are over 300 school districts in Kansas that could take advantage of this health delivery service. We continue to try and identify new districts to participate in Telekidcare on the basis on their needs and the manner in which telemedicine may help children to obtain care while in school. Although helping children is our primary goal, the school-based model also provides potential savings to the healthcare system.[12]

An exciting development in the expansion of the service in Kansas is the implementation of the Kan-Ed network in 2004. The network is designed to provide broadband Internet access to all schools, libraries, higher education institutions and hospitals in the state. If schools and hospitals in the state are connected to one another through a fast network, this may act as a catalyst for the expansion of school-based telehealth.

Another development is the possibility of offering increased paediatric behavioural healthcare to schools through telemedicine. During the 2003–4 school year, paediatric urgent care referrals decreased slightly and behavioural health referrals increased. This is not surprising. Many communities, especially rural ones, have at least one local physician to provide ambulatory medical care. However, very few rural communities have access to child psychologists or psychiatrists. Schools provide an excellent

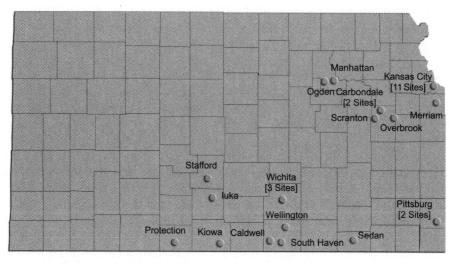

Fig 23.2. The Kansas TeleKidcare network.

access point for children to receive these services, so the KUMC will continue to monitor this trend and adapt the service accordingly.

Telemedicine for care of schoolchildren has been successful in Kansas, and in other states such as Kentucky. Using telehealth to bring care directly to the school offers an important opportunity to address the challenges of access for both urban and rural children.

Acknowledgements

TeleKidcare is a registered trade mark.

Box 23.1. Case studies

Early identification of a dangerous condition

Her son had been up all night 'breathing funny'. Even though she had called a nurse information line during the night, she was not reassured by what the nurse told her. She was familiar with telemedicine at school, because her son had received care for his attention deficit disorder through the programme, so she called his school nurse the first thing the next morning. The mother asked if her son could be seen that morning for his unusual breathing symptoms. The school nurse quickly arranged a telemedicine consultation.

Shortly after arriving at school, the student was examined via telemedicine by a paediatrician in the university paediatric clinic. The physician was alarmed by what he heard through the electronic stethoscope. He advised the student's mother to bring her son to the clinic immediately. After a quick taxi ride to the hospital, the student was treated in the intensive care unit for an acute asthma attack.

Before this incident, the student had no history of asthma. Although an emergency room visit would have been an alternative in this situation, school-based telemedicine provided the

---

family with an accessible, familiar and trustworthy healthcare option, allowing the student to be examined quickly and treated for a potentially dangerous medical condition.

Rapid examination without leaving school

A school nurse was in daily contact with a particular student who received nourishment through a feeding tube. One day, she observed the deterioration of the skin surrounding the feeding tube and contacted the parent to voice her concern. The parent reported that the surgeon was planning to replace the feeding tube in three or four months' time. The nurse accepted the parent's answer but remained apprehensive about waiting several months for the procedure.

When the student began to suffer a low-grade fever, the school nurse's worries escalated. She contacted the parent again, this time suggesting that the child be seen by telemedicine. The telemedicine physician could examine the area and offer an opinion in a timely manner. The mother agreed.

Using a video-otoscope, the school nurse showed the telemedicine physician the affected skin around the tube. The physician concurred with the school nurse – the skin condition would not improve until the feeding tube was replaced. Waiting three more months for this procedure would not be in the best interest of the child.

For a working parent, coordinating and attending a doctor's appointment for such a routine visit can be difficult, and the child would need to leave school to be seen. Instead, telemedicine provided a fast and convenient alternative, as well as enough professional advice for the mother to contact her son's surgeon. As a result, the procedure that was supposed to have waited for at least three more months was done in days. The student was back in class without suffering the complications that might have ensued.

Familiar environment for underprivileged families

Schools can be a trusted gateway for connecting families to healthcare services. In many inner-city communities, the neighbourhood school is perceived as a safe and nurturing environment for children. It is a place of immediate acceptance where the staff actively seek to meet the needs of students regardless of socioeconomic status, language barrier, cultural affiliation or citizenship. Many families know and trust the school nurse, and easing the entry into the healthcare system via telemedicine is a natural extension of the nurse's role.

The school nurse and the telemedicine consultation are excellent educational resources for families. The nurse often models effective interaction with a physician. Many parents feel uncomfortable in the presence of an unfamiliar healthcare provider, and questions that need to be voiced may never be asked. The school nurse is skilled at facilitating the discussion that needs to occur between patient and provider. We also know that the otoscope – which is a device used for looking into the ears and displays a large image of the inner ear on the television monitor – has frequently imposed a harsh reality onto surprised children and parents. This happens because they can actually see the red, bulging tympanic membrane that indicates otitis media, making it readily apparent why an ear infection is so painful. The presentation serves as an educational demonstration about the structure of the inner ear, and the visual effect reminds everybody about the need to comply with the medication orders given by the physician.

References

1   McCarthy AR, ed. *Good Health Means Better Learners*. Healthy Newsletters, Spring/Summer. Birmingham MI: Bridge Communications, 1998. http://www.bridge-comm.com/site/mgh_hn/ss98/learn.htm (last checked 13 August 2004).
2   Snyder TD, Hoffman CM, eds. *Digest of Education Statistics 2001. Publication 2002-130*. Washington DC: National Center for Education Statistics, 2002: Table 2. http://nces.ed.gov/pubs2002/2002130a.pdf (last checked 13 August 2004).

3   Fisher C, Hunt P, Kann L, *et al. Building a Healthier Future Through School Health Programs.* Atlanta, GA: Department of Health and Human Services, 2003. http://www.cdc.gov/nccdphp/promising_practices/ pdfs/SchoolHealth.pdf (last checked 13 August 2004).

4   Centers for Disease Control and Prevention (CDC), Department of Health and Human Services. SHPPS: School Health Policies and Programs Study 2000, *Journal of School Health* 2001; **71** (7). http://www.cdc.gov/HealthyYouth/shpps/index.htm (last checked 13 August 2004).

5   Mannino DM, Homa DM, Akinbami LJ, *et al. Surveillance for Asthma – United States, 1980–1999.* http://www.cdc.gov/mmwr/preview/mmwrhtml/ss5101a1.htm (last checked 13 August 2004).

6   Young TL, Ireson C. Effectiveness of school-based telehealth care in urban and rural elementary schools. *Pediatrics* 2003; **112**: 1088–1094.

7   Whitten P, Cook DJ, Shaw P, *et al.* TeleKidcare: bringing health care into schools. *Telemedicine Journal* 1998; **4**: 335–343.

8   Rogers EM. *Diffusion of Innovations.* 4th Edition. New York: Free Press, 1995.

9   Whitten P, Cook DJ. School-based telemedicine: using technology to bring health care to inner-city children. *Journal of Telemedicine and Telecare* 1999; **5** (suppl. 1): 23–25.

10   Whitten P, Cook D, Kingsley C, *et al.* School-based telemedicine: teachers', nurses' and administrators' perceptions. *Journal of Telemedicine and Telecare* 2000; **6** (suppl. 1): 129–132.

11   Whitten P, Kingsley C, Cook D, *et al.* School-based telehealth: an empirical analysis of teacher, nurse, and administrator perceptions. *Journal of School Health* 2001; **71**: 173–179.

12   Doolittle GC, Williams AR, Cook DJ. An estimation of costs of a pediatric telemedicine practice in public schools. *Medical Care* 2003; **41**: 100–109.

13   Cook DJ, Doolittle GC, Ferguson D, *et al.* Explaining the adoption of telemedicine services: an analysis of a paediatric telemedicine service. *Journal of Telemedicine and Telecare* 2002; **8** (suppl. 2): 106–107.

▶ 24

Telephone Helplines for Parents

Robert Ferguson

Introduction

The role of the telephone for non-medical information, support and guidance of new parents remains a promising but under-researched field. Anecdotal evidence from parents reinforces the benefits of child health call centres, while the literature strongly supports caller satisfaction with the services provided.

Paediatric telephone advice is a service that the community regards as essential. The high demand for telephone advice sought through hospitals, general practitioners, helplines, community nurses and paediatricians indicates that consumers value the ability to discuss health concerns with professionals. Estimates suggest that as many as 33% of all consultations in emergency departments occur via the telephone – and even more in the other fields of paediatric primary healthcare, such as maternal and child health nurse visits.[1–3] Australian and international data show that a large proportion of calls to call centres (up to 30%) relate to children aged 1–5 years.[4]

There is a long history of the use of the telephone as a means of providing services in paediatrics. This has generally been in response to parental uncertainty and worry about the care of their children. Research indicates that approximately 30% of parents worry about their children, even though they are growing and developing normally.[5] Not surprisingly, children younger than 5 years account for 45% of the total cost of medical services for children and young people aged less than 15 years. This represents a significant concentration of healthcare use and related cost in the first few years of an infant's life. The situation provides an opportunity for teaching and guidance from healthcare professionals, and parents welcome the opportunity to learn and be reassured.[5] In countries such as America, Sweden and the UK, primary healthcare–telenursing is a rapidly growing nursing specialty.[6]

Child health lines in Australia and New Zealand

Currently, eight Australian centres and one New Zealand centre provide primary healthcare services to parents via the telephone. The first centre was established in 1950. However, call centres are not immediately identifiable by their name. The names or titles chosen are rather colloquial, although they represent similar service provision. These include names such as 'Warmlines', 'Parent Lines', 'Parent Help Lines' and 'Child Health Lines'. Trying to identify call centres and the model of service delivery at a glance is thus not always possible.

An audit of 24-hour parent helplines in Australia was carried out in 1998. There is no standardized data collection set, so it is difficult to compare them. In general, the most frequent reason for parents or carers calling is infant feeding, while infant settling issues are also significant.[7] Most services have a cut-off point for providing services at the developmental ages of childhood or adolescence. Most calls are from female parents or carers calling about a child aged 0–5 years, which is similar to international trends.

All centres support the primary healthcare principle of equity to access services by providing low-cost services. The maximum call cost was a local call fee. In 80% of centres, callers remained anonymous, although most centres indicated that there were exceptions. Caller identifying information was collected to provide callback services (where the centre is unable to respond to calls, a message is left by the caller on the centre's answering machine) or in crisis situations (where child protection concerns were raised or thoughts of self-harm behaviour were reported). In all but one centre, the state government provided funding and most centres operate continuously. As interest in call centres is reasonably recent (particularly in Australia), it is not surprising that only 30% of services had designated managers. In addition, 80% of services indicated that even though they were fully staffed during their hours of operation, only 30% of the services were meeting consumer demand.

Many centres are understaffed. Common complaints by consumers of child health call centres are the inability to get through to a staff member and being placed in a queue or receiving an engaged signal. Callers will often abandon the call within a few minutes of queuing (eg in 2–3 minutes). Every time access is affected, confidence in the service diminishes, which may negatively affect future usage of the call centre. It is difficult to draw any conclusions about service demand. It is notable that in South Australia, the Parent Help Line provides services to more than 100 000 callers annually. This is the largest call volume among similar services, despite the state's birth rate being one of the lowest. Of the remaining centres, three provided less than 25 000 responses to calls annually and four provided between 50 000 and 74 999 services annually.

The allocation of resources varied among centres as did the number of employees. One-third of centres have fewer than five full-time-equivalent staff, while most have between five and ten staff.

Child health call centre staff provide information and support on well infants, children and young people – not advice about illness. Nonetheless, advice is provided to parents about illness, in particular fever management.[8] This is a complicated matter, as whether or not a condition is considered to represent illness depends on knowledge and experience. In future, child health call centres should consider a consistent approach to defining the model of service delivery and the objectives and scope in which staff practice.

The Child Health Line experience in Brisbane

The Riverton statewide call centre is a 24-hour, seven days a week telephone advisory service that operates across the state of Queensland. The telephone information and advice service became operational in 1991 at the Riverton Early Parenting Centre, although it had existed in some form since the 1980s. It was initiated in response to an increasing number of parents seeking telephone assistance from the Early Parenting Residential Service, particularly those from isolated rural communities. In 2000, the name was changed to 'Child Health Line' to more readily identify the service provided. Calls are received from Queensland and New South Wales. A local call cost applies to metropolitan callers, while a toll-free 1800 number is available for consumers outside the metropolitan area. Callers from other states in Australia, and those overseas, can also access the service – and are welcome to do so – but at their own expense.

The Child Health Line offers information and support on children and young (0–18 years) people's issues, such as behaviour management, crisis intervention, health of young people (immunization and illness), nutrition, safety and the availability of support services. The top five concerns of callers are listed in Table 24.1. Callers who request information, advice and support include parents, grandparents, carers, day care staff and health professionals. Most calls concern well babies.

Table 24.1. Top five reasons for calling the Child Health Line in Brisbane

Rank	Related health issue	Calls
1	Sleep or rest	10.8%
2	Breastfeeding	6.9%
3	Unsettled	6.1%
4	Formula feeding	5.9%
5	Parent support	4.6%

Service

Currently, the service provides approximately 50 000 occasions of service a year – or about 155 calls each day. In an attempt to estimate the potential for service demand, comparisons have been made between the South Australian Child and Youth Health Parent Line and the Queensland Child Health Line. In South Australia, the staffing level is sufficient to meet consumer demand, whereas the Queensland Child Health Line call volume and staffing levels have remained unchanged over the past six years and there is clear evidence that consumer demand is not being met. Nevertheless, anecdotally it continues to be a well respected resource.

Staff

Funding currently supports two staff daily to operate the centre. Additional staff are rostered onto the Child Health Line from other areas in the facility. Only staff experienced in child health are rostered to work in the Child Health Line. All staff have a general nursing qualification, and many have a midwifery certificate or child health certificate, or both. All new staff are supervised until they are evaluated as sufficiently skilled and experienced. Ongoing peer support and supervision is provided by the clinical nurse consultant, while monthly group supervision and regular staff development opportunities in child health issues are provided, including attendance at positive parenting programmes.

Database

A database (the Riverton Call Monitoring System) is completed electronically by the call centre staff or automatically by the telephone management information system. The Riverton Call Monitoring System software collects client demographic details, including the call subject's age and reason for the call. A number of drop-down menus simplify call recording. At present, the system does not have the ability for call staff to add clinical documentation. The aim of the software is to assist with monitoring call activity and evaluate staffing requirements and performance.

Currently, the name and contact details of the caller are not collected. If a query is made about a call then it is not possible to track back to the exact call, especially if there are two operators working in the call centre at once (unless the caller volunteers identifying information). As with most similar services, calls are not documented unless the call is in relation to an emergency or a child protection issue.

Age of call subject

In a 12-month period, most calls to the Child Health Line were about infants aged 0–12 months. The second largest group involved children aged 1–2 years, and there was a gradual reduction in calls as children got older (Table 24.2). Although this is consistent with the findings from Australian child health call centres,[7] it differs from findings in the literature, where children aged 1–5 years are more highly represented.[4] The most likely explanation is the marketing of the Child Health Line. Marketing essentially is limited to the personal health record or 'baby book' that all new parents receive from the maternity hospital. This information relates to the first 12 months of life, so it may be assumed by consumers that the Child Health Line is limited to this developmental stage. In addition, agencies such as maternal and child health clinics that refer callers to the Child Health Line have a stronger focus on the first 12 months of life.

Telephone call activity

Registered births (since most calls concern young infants) and service call volume have been used as yardsticks to estimate the potential for service demand. As discussed above, South Australia was the only state in which community demand was being met. In 2002, South Australia had 17 665 births,[9] and approximately 100 000 calls were recorded. In comparison, Queensland had 47 771 births,[9] yet only 50 000 calls were recorded that year. Using the South Australian rate of call traffic to births, it can be estimated that the demand in Queensland should be closer to 270 000 calls per year. A number of reasons may explain why the Queensland Child Health Line call rate is low. These relate to resource availability, which includes limited marketing, low staff numbers, and limited technology and services offered.

Table 24.2. Age of callers to the Child Health Line (survey from 1 July 2002 to 30 June 2003)

Age	Callers
0–2 weeks	3618 (8.6%)
2–6 weeks	5951 (14.2%)
6 weeks–3 months	5552 (13.3%)
3–6 months	8013 (19.1%)
6–9 months	5913 (14.1%)
9–12 months	3981 (9.5%)
1–2 years	5419 (12.9%)
2–3 years	1910 (4.6%)
Pre-school	843 (2.0%)
School age	485 (1.2%)
Adolescents	106 (0.3%)
Antenatal	100 (0.2%)
Total	**41 891 (100%)**

Call activity in the Child Health Line begins to increase after 06:00, peaks in the middle of the day and noticeably reduces at about 21:00 (Fig. 24.1). This pattern is similar to other reports in the literature. The centre has five telephone lines, one of which is the 1800 free-call number. Currently, the system has a queuing facility that allows four calls to be queued. The average length of a call is approximately four minutes, with most calls being made by the mother. A crude cost analysis indicates that the cost of each call is approximately A\$6. For comparison, the approximate cost from HealthDirect (WA Department of Health) was \$20 per triage call.

Callers in the queue receive a greeting message and a message about emergencies. The option of broadcasting health messages and other sources for health information (such as a child health website) is being explored. The current call management software is relatively old and has many limitations, which reduces the likelihood that a successful connection can be made via the 1800 number. This is a concern, as there are areas of Queensland where there are fewer child health services (regional and rural centres) and children from such areas would most benefit from this service. In the UK, the targets set by the National Health Service are less than 0.1% of calls engaged and less than 5% of calls abandoned.[10] In comparison, the Child Health Line has room for improvement.

Call centre quality assurance

For too long, experiential learning has been the only preparation for nurses entering the call centre workforce. It should not be assumed that hands-on, face-to-face clinical expertise is a skill directly transferable to telephone nursing (although it is certainly of benefit) or that telephone nursing is a natural ability.[11] Specific training and education are required to develop the skills of effective verbal and aural assessment and problem solving over the telephone. The quality indicators in Boxes 24.3 and 24.4 and Table 24.3 are a guide to the ways that other services measure the quality of the service they provide.[4,10,12]

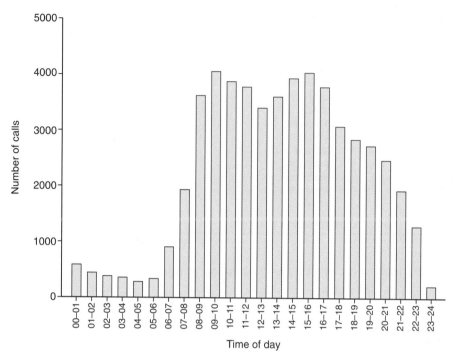

Fig. 24.1. Child Health Line call traffic (survey from 1 July 2003 to 30 June 2004).

The use of decision-making support software to ensure the consistency of accurate advice and information provided to callers is inconclusive.[11,13–15] Appropriateness of advice and information is disputed among experienced clinicians. As previously noted, research suggests that the appropriateness of information depends on the experience of the call centre staff and the assessment information available to them at the time of decision making. There is a mass of knowledge and information pertaining to call centre targets, and standards are being developed by HealthDirect in Western Australia, NHS Direct in the UK and the Telephone Helplines Association, also in the UK. In particular, NHS Direct, in partnership with the Royal College of Nursing and Institutes of Higher Education, has vigorously pursued the development of research, education, information technology, performance management strategies, quality frameworks, memoranda of understanding and local service agreements.[10] This body of knowledge provides insight into the complexities of call centre development and is a sound starting point for the Australasian context.

Conclusion

Call centres are undergoing an analysis to confirm their position in the healthcare delivery system. The organizational diversity in which centres operate and the varying

---

Box 24.1. Performance management

- Operational 24 hours a day, 7 days a week
- Access for people with hearing impairment and from non-English-speaking backgrounds
- Call interaction documentation
- Advice supported by a clinical decision support system
- Patient confidentiality maintained
- Activity and performance reporting
- Ability to link with other services and transfer calls
- 80% of calls answered in the first 20 seconds
- Call abandonment rate <5%
- Call time (talk time and after call work) 550 seconds
- Call audits: 1% of calls monitored daily against call standards
- Shadow shopper: monthly
- Caller surveys: monthly

Box 24.2. Individual performance indicators

- Opening, closing, transferring and holding
- Establishing caller needs
- Rapport and conversation control
- Attentive listening
- Capturing relevant data
- Data entry accuracy
- Use of approved resources and information
- Primary assessment
- Interpretation of presenting problem
- Choice of guideline
- Determining first pertinent positive and disposition
- Need to override disposition
- Provision of understandable solution
- Lack of bias
- Management of difficult calls
- Group supervision: access to group supervision once a month
- Coaching: access to coaching once a month
- Performance appraisal and development: performed with line manager 6-monthly
- Practice knowledge updates: at least four times per year

Table 24.3. Quality control

Action and input	Monitoring
• Staff recruitment informed by competencies required in role	• Monitor competence and staff retention
• Induction establishes awareness of organisational objectives, knowledge of own role and its contribution and skills and knowledge to do the job	• Monitor performance
• Protocols establish the basis of best and safe practice	• Monitor adverse incidents
• Preceptorship and mentoring establish good standards of practice	• Monitor standards
• Cross sectional audit monitors compliance with protocols established to ensure good practice	• Benchmarking compares performance against organizational standards
• Reflective audit enables individual staff to assess quality of own performance	• Measure time out for reflection
• Group supervision supports professional development and awareness of own practice	• Measure time out for supervision
• Shadow shopper, complaints, accolades and professional feedback	• Feed into coaching and review
• Coaching enables supervisory feedback on performance and supportive inputs – remedial or praise	• Monitor coaching activity and keep written records for individuals. Feed issues into training programme
• Performance appraisal and development review brings together inputs, sickness and all aspects of individual's performance. Identifies development and input needs in performance appraisal and development plan	• Monitor performance appraisal and development review for individuals. Feed issues into training programme

methodological approaches and standards, however, mean that comparisons and generalizations are difficult to make.[16,17] The many studies undertaken are unsuitable for meta-analysis, and clinical conclusions derived from the provision of telehealth remain speculative for call centres.

Questions of cost-effectiveness are generally unanswered. Establishing a body of methodologically sound research that allows legitimate comparison of service models is of highest priority if call centres are to be evaluated objectively. In addition, research into the healthcare system needs to explore how families with children connect with the health system. What opportunities are available to guide healthy childhood development? What services are best delivered by the different technologies, how frequently and how much? What are the financial, cultural and ethnic barriers to service access?

The UK continues to lead the way in call centre utilization. NHS Direct has expanded across the UK, with the implementation of an online Internet enquiry service and exploration of the use of digital interactive television healthcare services. It has been suggested that digital TV, which promises faster, easier access to health information, will allow people to book appointments with their general practitioner and even have conversations with NHS Direct nurses on screen. Whether or not this ever comes into routine service, increased collaboration and integration among primary healthcare providers should bring both consumer and organizational benefits.

References

1   Bristol S. Telephone advice for parents of newborns. *Nebraska Nurse* 1993; **26**: 8–9.
2   Delichatsios H, Callahan M, Charlson M. Outcomes of telephone medical care. *Journal of General Internal Medicine* 1998; **13**: 579–585.
3   Oberklaid F. Paediatric telephone advice: a major gap in quality service delivery. *Journal of Paediatrics and Child Health* 2002; **38**: 6–7.
4   Turner V, Bentley P, Hodgson S, *et al*. Telephone triage in Western Australia. *Medical Journal of Australia* 2002; **176**: 100–103.
5   Glascoe FP, Oberklaid F, Dworkin PH, Trimm F. Brief approaches to educating patients and parents in primary care. *Pediatrics* 1998; **101**: 1–8.
6   Valanis B, Tanner C, Moscato SR, *et al*. A model for examining predictors of outcomes of telephone nursing advice. *Journal of Nursing Administration* 2003; **33**: 91–95.
7   Sheehan A, Barclay L. An audit of 24 hour parent help lines across Australia. http://www.goodbeginnings.net.au/files/library_publications/10.pdf (last checked 13 August 2004).
8   Andrews JK, Armstrong KL, Fraser JA. Professional telephone advice to parents with sick children: time for quality control! *Journal of Paediatrics and Child Health* 2002; **38**: 23–26.
9   Australian Bureau of Statistics. *Births Australia 3301.0 Issue 2002 Table 7.1 Births Registered*. Canberra: Australian Bureau of Statistics, 2002: 44.
10 Department of Health UK. *NHS Direct Commissioning Framework April 2004-05. Guidance for Primary Care Trusts on Commissioning NHS Direct Services from 1 April 2004*. http://www.nhsdirect.nhs.uk/misc/fGatewayfeb04.pdf (last checked 13 August 2004).
11 Marklund B, Silfverhielm B, Bengtsson C. Evaluation of an educational programme for telephone advisers in primary health care. *Family Practice* 1989; **6**: 263–267.
12 Butcher A, ed. *Telephone Helplines Association. Guidelines for Good Practice*. 3rd Edition. London: Telephone Helplines Association, 1999.
13 Edwards B. Telephone triage: how experienced nurses reach decisions. *Journal of Advanced Nursing* 1994; **19**: 717–724.
14 Williams S, Crouch R, Dale J. Providing health-care advice by telephone. *Professional Nurse* 1995; **10**: 750–752.
15 Cariello F. Computerized telephone nurse triage an evaluation of service quality and cost. *Journal of Ambulatory Care Management* 2003; **26**: 124–137.
16 Mair F, Haycox A, May C, Williams T. A review of telemedicine cost-effectiveness studies. *Journal of Telemedicine and Telecare* 2000; **6** (suppl. 1): 38–40.
17 Lobley D. The economics of telemedicine. *Journal of Telemedicine and Telecare* 1997; **3**: 117–125.

▶ 25

A National Telephone and Online Counselling Service for Young Australians

Wendy Reid and Debra Caswell

Introduction

The Kids Help Line (KHL) is Australia's only free national telephone and online counselling service for children and young people aged 5–18 years. The service began in 1991 and operates from a single site in Brisbane, Queensland. The telephone service is available 24 hours a day from anywhere in Australia by toll-free number. After launching a website in 1996, requests from children and young people led to the introduction of email counselling in 1999 and real-time web counselling in 2000. These developments reflect the increasing use of computers and online technologies by young people, with an attendant demand by clients for communication choices when seeking help. The KHL service is primarily funded by lotteries that are run by the charity organization, BoysTown. Additional funds are derived through donations, fundraising activities, government and corporate sponsorship.

Mission and goals

The core mission of the KHL is to help young people develop strategies and skills that enable them to manage their own lives more effectively. As part of this, the KHL provides free and accessible national services founded on the principles of empowerment and child centred practice. The objectives are to:

▶ provide free, confidential counselling services for all people aged 5–18 years in Australia that meet the highest standards of professional practice and management

▶ collect, analyse and disseminate non-identifying information that contributes to research and reflects the issues and problems of KHL's clients

▶ advocate on behalf of KHL's clients where their interests are ignored, minimized or unrepresented

▶ assist young people to have a direct voice on policies or issues that affect them

▶ use existing technological and professional expertise to develop services to other groups in the community.

The KHL has adopted the following operational principles:

▶ all callers are treated with respect

▶ callers are free to choose the sex of the counsellor to whom they speak

▶ callers are able to access the same counsellor if they wish to call back

▶ callers are encouraged to give feedback about the service they receive

▶ confidentiality and anonymity are respected unless there is a 'duty of care' requirement.

Confidentiality is an important consideration for young people when accessing help, and callers may choose to withhold their name, particularly when talking about highly personal or sensitive issues. If young people reveal they are being harmed or are at risk of being harmed, or they intend to harm another, counsellors explain the limits of confidentiality and the meaning of duty of care.

Research and evaluation

Non-identifying information is collected about all telephone and online contacts, and recorded in a database. This provides a unique source of information about the issues and concerns of young Australians and forms the basis of the KHL research agenda and advocacy platform. It also provides valuable information for policy development at a number of levels in government and non-government sectors. It is used to highlight possible gaps in service delivery, assist in the planning and targeting of scarce resources and support funding or grant applications for service development. Access to this information is available on request for a fee. The data are also used to ensure continuous quality improvement by informing staff training and providing a baseline for ongoing service evaluation.

Counsellor training

The KHL service is staffed by more than 100 paid, professionally trained and supervised counsellors. More than 90% have tertiary qualifications in psychology, social work or related disciplines. Counsellor selection depends on successfully completing a one-week, full-time skills-based training course, as well as successfully completing a 250-hour probationary period. The KHL expects counsellors to take on a programme of professional development, including the achievement of competency levels that result in a balanced, effective and accountable style of practice.

Counsellor supervision

All counsellors are supervised regularly and submit their practice to routine monitoring and continuous evaluation. A two-tier system of supervision ensures that counsellors are provided with direct supervision while on counselling shifts, plus at least one hour per month working on professional development with a personal supervisor or in a group with their peers. Shift supervisors are available for most counselling shifts. Shift supervision allows access to timely support and advice for counsellors about responding to difficult calls, feedback about calls, information about organizational procedures and policies, and debriefing for calls that the counsellors find challenging. Supervision and performance reviews ensure that clients' needs are being met adequately and help to maintain the quality of service delivery and manage risk.

Child-centred practice and empowerment

The KHL promotes a non-judgmental, confidential service where no problem is too small, too embarrassing or too 'out of bounds' to talk about. Counsellors apply the central principles of empowerment and child-centred practice in accordance with the service's mission statement. Empowerment involves assisting each caller to clarify their concerns, formulate options, develop strategies for positive change, and identify and understand the consequences of particular courses of action. Callers are encouraged to believe in themselves and recognize their personal strengths. Respect is accorded to each caller's individuality, feelings and the right to make personal decisions. At the same time, productive relationships with parents, teachers, peers and other people of significance are encouraged.

Child-centred practice commits counsellors to viewing the young person's situation from the young person's perspective, examining the consequences of professional practice on children and young people and making explicit the ideology and ethics on which decisions are based. It demands that the interests and welfare of the child be paramount, allowing them to challenge adult interpretations of their experience and interests, and to express their own perceptions and beliefs.

Telephone counselling

An average of 20 000 children and young people call KHL each week, with 50% successfully connecting to a counsellor. Between 1999 and 2003, there was a steady increase in answered calls: from 400 000 in 1999 to 522 825 in 2003.

Operational considerations

Callers have direct access to counsellors and can choose to speak to a male or female counsellor. They can also call back and speak with the same counsellor in order to work through issues over a period of time. The length of calls varies from only a few minutes for enquiries and questions to an hour or longer for serious issues such as self-harm and mental health. The average length of calls across all problem types in 2003 was 18 minutes.

Over 60% of callers report that they have used the service before. The service is busiest between 15:00 and 21:00 on weekdays, and during weekends and school holidays, reflecting school attendance hours in Australia. At these busy times, callers may have to wait for some time in a queue before getting through to a counsellor. In 2003, half of the calls made to the KHL were from children and young people living in rural and remote regions of Australia.

Client profile

Figure 25.1 shows the pattern of usage by age and sex. As is the case across most human service agencies, girls make almost three-quarters of calls to the service (72%). More than half (54%) of those who seek help by telephone are younger than 15 years.

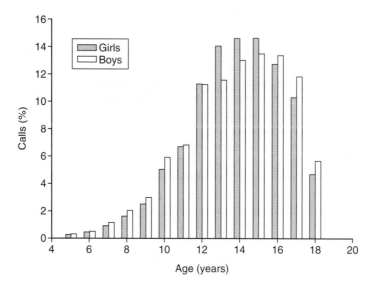

Fig 25.1. Telephone calls by sex and age.

Why young people call the Kids Help Line

Calls are logged into one of 36 problem categories. Figure 25.2 shows the main reasons that children and young people called the service during a three-year period from 2001 to 2003. Most calls concerned relationships with family, friends or partners – a consistent trend across the 13 years that the service has been operating. Over the past few years, the proportion of calls regarding bullying and mental health has increased, while concerns about child abuse and peer relationships have decreased slightly.

Online counselling

The KHL has maintained an online presence since 1996, when its website was launched. Email counselling commenced in 1999, and real-time web counselling in 2000. Each week an average of 415 young people contact the service by email, and 260 make contact via real-time web counselling. All email messages are responded to, and half of those who contact by web counselling successfully connect with a counsellor.

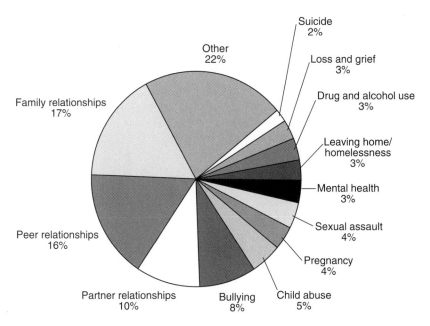

Fig 25.2 Top 12 problem categories during the three-year period 2001–3.

Operational considerations

As is the case with the telephone counselling service, those who contact the service using online modalities (web and email) have direct access to counsellors, can choose the sex of their counsellor and can make contact with the same counsellor again to work through issues over time. Applying these operational principles had a direct effect on software development for online services.

Online counselling is more resource-intensive than telephone counselling, with the average length of contact in 2003 being 46 minutes for real-time web sessions and 25 minutes for email messages (with a turnaround period averaging five days). This difference from telephone sessions is due to several factors. Written communication is more time-consuming than spoken communication. Those who use online options are older, and the types of problems they seek help for tend to be more complex and severe. At times, delays in connecting speeds or young people multitasking (doing homework or listening to music) while participating in the session can also slow the interaction.

Of the 12 256 web counselling contacts and 15 746 email contacts that were completed between 2001 and 2003, three-quarters were from metropolitan areas and one-quarter from rural and remote regions of Australia.

Client profile

The age and sex of young people who use online counselling differ from those who use telephone counselling (Fig 25.3). Two-thirds of the clients using online options are aged between 15 and 18 years compared with 46% of telephone clients. Of particular interest is that boys are more likely to use the telephone than online options in comparison with girls. In 2003, boys made 12% of online contacts. In contrast, boys made 28% of calls to the telephone service.

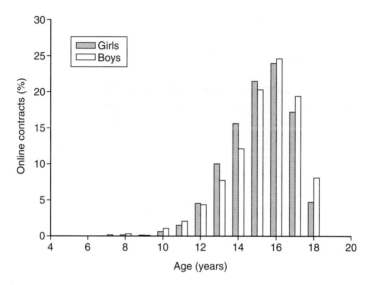

Fig 25.3 Online contacts by sex and age.

Why young people contact Kids Help Online

Most online contacts are about relationships with family and peers (Fig. 25.4). This is similar to telephone counselling. The proportion of online contacts about mental health, suicide and eating behaviours, however, is three times higher than contacts made by telephone, while emotional and behavioural management and self-image contacts are made at twice the rate.

Trends in demand and response

On average, growth in demand for online counselling has risen by 43% each year since 1999, despite a lack of advertising and limited media exposure (Fig. 25.5). This growth in demand indicates the relevance that online modalities offer young people in terms of options for seeking help.

An online feedback survey conducted by the KHL in 2002 and 2003 found that one-third of online clients were new clients. Of the 227 respondents to the survey, half used email only (51%); one-third used web only (31%), and the remainder (18%) used both web and email. Twenty-four percent of respondents stated that they would not seek help elsewhere if KHL's online access was not available. Of those participants who would not have sought help elsewhere, 69% had previously had face-to-face counselling.

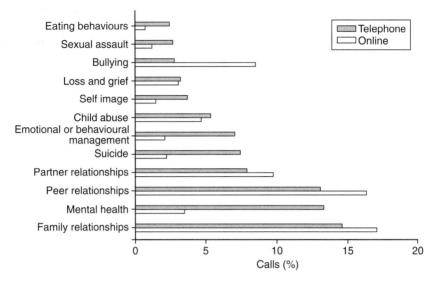

Fig 25.4. Telephone and online problem categories during the three-year period 2001–3.

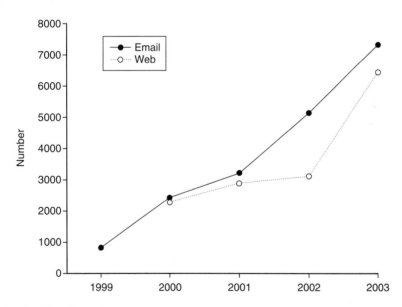

Fig 25.5. Online demand.

Response times were of concern for 45% of email clients who were dissatisfied with the time taken to receive a reply (more than four days in 57% of cases). In spite of long response times, however, 64% of online clients gave positive assessments of the service.

Developmental differences

As young people develop, the issues about which they contact the KHL change. Table 25.1 shows the main reasons at various ages in rank order (telephone data, 2003). Families are the most important issue for young children and continue to be so throughout childhood and the teenage years. Peers become increasingly important to children as they move towards adolescence, however, until at about 14 or 15 years, relationships with partners become a key focus.

Bullying is a particular concern for younger children and those in their middle years, as is child abuse. Interestingly, young children also seek help for managing their emotions and behaviours, developmental concerns, and loss and grief (most commonly associated with family breakdown). As children move into adolescence, issues related to sexuality (and for older girls, pregnancy) arise. For boys, drug and alcohol use becomes a concern. For older clients aged 15–18 years, mental health,

Table 25.1. Main reasons that clients contact the KHL

Client's age (years)		
5–9	10–14	15–18
Female callers		
• Family relationships	• Peer relationships	• Partner relationships
• Bullying	• Family relationships	• Family relationships
• Peer relationships	• Bullying	• Peer relationships
• Child abuse	• Partner relationships	• Pregnancy
• Emotional or behavioural management	• Child abuse	• Emotional or behavioural management
• Loss and grief	• Emotional or behavioural management	• Mental health
• Developmental issues	• Developmental issues	• Leaving home or homelessness
• Life skills	• Pregnancy	• Child abuse
• Physical health	• Loss and grief	• Suicide
• School-related authority	• Sexual activity	• Drug and alcohol use
Male callers		
• Family relationships	• Family relationships	• Partner relationships
• Bullying	• Bullying	• Family relationships
• Peer relationships	• Peer relationships	• Sexual activity
• Emotional or behavioural management	• Child abuse	• Drug and alcohol use
• Child abuse	• Partner relationships	• Peer relationships
• Loss and grief	• Emotional or behavioural management	• Leaving home or homelessness
• School-related authority	• Sexual activity	• Emotional or behavioural management
• Physical health	• Drug and alcohol use	• Sexual orientation
• Developmental issues	• Leaving home or homelessness	• Mental health
• Leaving home or homelessness	• School-related authority	• Bullying

suicide and leaving home (or homelessness) become concerns. The following section explores some of these issues in more detail.

Issues for young people – telephone and online

The main issues raised by telephone – family, peers and partners – are similar to those raised online apart from bullying (ranked fourth for telephone counselling) and mental health (ranked second for online counselling), which reflects the different ages of telephone and online users.

Family relationships

During 13 years of operation, family relationships have consistently been the most common reason that children and young people contact the KHL, with one in every five contacts being about family issues. These figures do not include contacts about other types of family-related problems such as child abuse, domestic violence, the physical or mental health or death of family members, or being forced out of home. This highlights the crucial role that families play in the wellbeing of children and young people. Children and young people who contact the KHL about family relationships are 40% more likely to have parents who are separated or divorced and less likely to have parents who are married or living together than all clients. In 2003:

- 13% of contacts concerning families were from young people experiencing family breakdown, separation or divorce; these young people frequently express distress, confusion and grief

- 42% were from children and young people experiencing major or frequent family conflict and disruption

- 28% were from children and young people experiencing occasional family conflict or disruption

- 12% were from children and young people concerned about family members.

The nature and severity of young people's concerns relating to family conflict and disruption vary widely. These concerns can be loosely grouped into the following issues:

- fighting and arguments between parents

- sibling disputes over sharing resources or responsibilities

- issues around discipline

- the need for acknowledgment, time or affection from parents

- 'getting into trouble' for various misdemeanours

- teenagers seeking greater independence

▶ the myriad other issues that arise in families over affections, responsibilities, resources and privacy.

Case studies

▶ A 13-year-old girl called because she was worried about her mother, who was suffering from depression. The girl wanted to help her mother but did not know how. She also wanted to talk to her mother about her own worries but was fearful that she would make things worse by burdening her.

▶ A 13-year-old boy rang to let the counsellor know that he was spending Christmas with his father for the very first time. He was happy that the KHL had helped him come to terms with his relationship with his father and wanted to express his gratitude to the counsellor in a 'major way'. He also wanted to speak to a supervisor to say that he was 'over the moon'.

Peer relationships

Relationships with peers and friends play an important role in the social and psychological development of young people. Peers provide adolescents with a reference group for information and also with opportunities to explore new roles. Dating, social events, types of dress, drinking, drug use, sport and hobbies all take place largely in the company of others of a similar age. Peers are a critical part of the adolescent's transition to independence from the family. As such, issues of friendship consistently receive high ratings of importance from teenagers.

Since the KHL began operating nationally in 1993, the proportion of contacts relating to peer relationships has increased steadily, highlighting the importance that friends and peer groups play in young people's lives. The largest proportion of callers (67%) were aged 10–14 years, and girls made 85% of these contacts.

Contacts about peer relationships include problems about issues concerning a friend's wellbeing, peer group pressure, choosing and making friends, jealousy and friendship breakdowns, and feeling shy, lonely or excluded. Peer pressure to conform to various activities, such as smoking, drug or alcohol use, running away from home, dangerous play, or sex, are common problems in calls concerning relationships with friends. Trust and communication are also significant issues for young people in their friendships with each other. Honesty and openness are highly valued – lies, betrayal of trust and breaking of confidences are regular aspects of these calls.

Case study

▶ A 13-year-old boy called, concerned for his older friend, who had begun using drugs on a daily basis – in large quantities and potentially dangerous combinations. He had expressed his concerns to his friend, but this had the effect of his friend becoming more secretive about his behaviour. The boy was worried that he had not handled the situation properly by raising it, and called the KHL for advice.

Partner relationships

Relationships with partners are a greater concern for older teenagers. A peer relationship is the most frequent reason that young people aged 15–18 years seek help from the KHL. Issues include problems between the caller and their partner or intimate friend, as well as sexual issues in significant or established relationships, including opposite- and same-sex relationships.

Young people telephoning about intimate relationships are most likely (61%) to be concerned about establishing or negotiating a relationship. These calls involve uncertainty about telling someone that they 'like' them, trust issues and uncertainty about what to do after having an argument with their partner. A further 32% of these contacts relate to significant relationship difficulties or relationship breakdowns. The most common reasons for seeking help are:

▶ the need to process and understand why a partner has broken up with them

▶ uncertainty about how to break off a relationship

▶ coping with a partner who has cheated

▶ discussion of trust and faithfulness issues

▶ violence or the fear of violence in the relationship

▶ the effect that their partner's drug or alcohol use has on the relationship.

A small proportion (7%) of concerns are from young people feeling uncertainty or pressure to have sex in a significant or already-established relationship.

Case study
An 18-year-old boy called, to talk about difficulties he was having with his girlfriend. He loved her and wanted to become engaged. However, her response was to ask for 'some space'. He was scared that in giving her 'space' she would meet somebody else and their relationship would end. The counsellor encouraged him to explore his feelings and to discuss the link between his feelings and his present behaviour. Together, they reviewed the appropriateness of using alcohol as a crutch, and he agreed that he should cease this behaviour and determine other methods of dealing with his feelings. At the end of the call, the boy had determined to find a quiet time to open up communication about his feelings with both his girlfriend and his parents.

Bullying
Bullying is the fourth most common reason that young people seek help from the service. The proportion of calls concerning bullying has increased from 5% of all calls in 1999 to 8% in 2003. Bullying is ranked as the third most common reason that children younger than 15 years telephone the service. In general, boys make about one-quarter of all calls to the KHL; however, in the case of bullying, boys make almost

40% of calls. This difference is not surprising given that boys are reported as being bullied more often than girls.[1]

The young people who call the KHL about bullying identify a variety of reasons for their victimisation. These reasons include:

- ethnicity (the rate of bullying calls from indigenous and non-English-speaking callers is higher than for other callers)
- resistance to pressure to behave in a certain way
- physical differences
- high achievement
- being new
- sexual orientation
- socioeconomic background.

Ninety-four percent of callers had been bullied at least once, with 37% of these young people experiencing frequent incidents or continual harassment. A further 44% reported episodic incidents, while 19% telephoned about an isolated instance of bullying.

Child abuse

During 2003, KHL counsellors responded to 3398 contacts from children and young people with concerns about child abuse. This represents 6% of all counselling contacts across telephone, web and email counselling. More than 80% of these contacts concern physical (45%) and sexual (36%) abuse. However, emotional abuse, neglect and sexual offending are also significant issues for children and young people. For some children, multiple types of abuse were occurring in their home.

The largest proportion (56%) of both telephone and online clients reporting physical abuse stated that they were the victims of ongoing abuse (either occasional or regular). The nature of severity of physical abuse contacts is summarized in Fig. 25.6. Across both media, 6% of young people stated that they were at risk of injury at the time of their call. A further 16% of children reported an isolated incident, while for 9% of young people the abuse was no longer occurring but they were seeking support with unresolved issues. The remaining 13% were seeking information.

Sexual abuse is defined as the exploitation of a child by a family member for sexual gratification or stimulation, characterized by secrecy and distortion of the adult-and-child relationship. Of those who sought help for sexual abuse in 2003, most (74%) had been abused at least once. The nature and severity of sexual abuse contacts is summarized in Fig. 25.7. Across both media, 18% of these young people reported ongoing (occasional or regular) sexual abuse to their counsellor, while a further 9% reported an isolated instance of abuse. For 44% of clients, the abuse was no longer current, but issues resulting from the abuse were unresolved. The remaining young people were reporting a current risk of sexual abuse (16%) or were seeking information (13%).

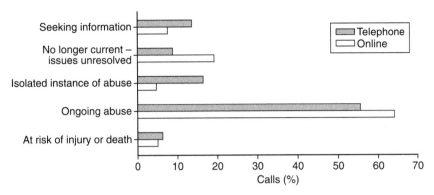

Fig 25.6. The nature and severity of physical abuse contacts.

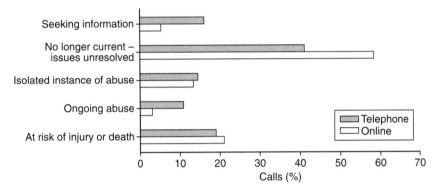

Fig 25.7. The nature and severity of sexual abuse calls.

Case study

A female (14 years old) was abused by her father from 2 years of age to 8 years of age, and he is currently being charged. She suffers from anxiety and suicidal thoughts – she blames herself for the abuse.

Mental health issues

KHL counsellors respond to nearly 3500 telephone, web and email contacts concerning mental health each year (4% of counselling calls). Furthermore, mental health issues are frequently subsumed under other problem types, including eating behaviours, substance use, emotional and behavioural management, and suicide. This represents a growing problem.

The National Survey of Mental Health and Wellbeing was the first study to investigate the incidence of mental health problems among children and adolescents at a national level in Australia.[2,3] The study found that 14% of children and young people in Australia have mental health problems that are comparable in severity to problems seen in children actually attending mental health clinics. The proportion of calls to the

KHL's telephone counselling service about mental health concerns has been steadily increasing over the past 10 years: 1.3% of calls in 1993 to 3.1% of calls in 2003. Most (74%) of the young people who contact the KHL about mental health issues are aged 15–18 years.

Young people who contact the KHL about mental health concerns using online options are more likely to report experiencing mild or occasional mental health concerns, but less likely to make contact about a significant other, seek information or report having a clinically diagnosed mental health problem than those who contact by telephone (Fig. 25.8). Although discussing symptoms and behaviours is the most common type of contact from all age groups, younger callers are more likely to be seeking information or have concerns about a significant other. Older callers contact the service more often about having a mental health diagnosis or are severely distressed because of a mental health problem.

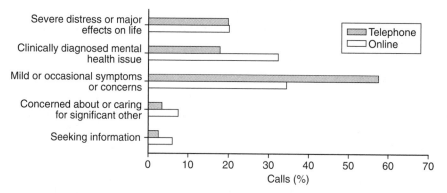

Fig 25.8. Telephone and online mental health contacts.

The significance of an immediate (or near immediate) counselling service is evinced by the fact that apart from presenting at a large public hospital for possible treatment, services such as the KHL provide a unique on-demand service for young people with possibly serious mental health issues or child abuse.

The KHL fulfils a vital early intervention role in helping young people with a range of mental health problems to access further support. Counsellors also play a vital part in reducing young people's exposure to potential causal factors such as child abuse and neglect by connecting them with statutory child protection authorities. A number of young people who contact the KHL with mental health concerns do so as a part of an agreement or safety plan they have with an existing support service.

Case study

A 15-year-old girl telephoned with immediate suicide intent. She had suffered bullying and harassment from students at school over the past year and tried to commit suicide a few months previously by cutting her wrists. This became known to the other students, and their comments were making her life unbearable. Her parents had arranged for her to have counselling, but the first appointment was not scheduled for another two weeks. She was desperate to change schools and make a fresh start. After talking through various options, she agreed to have a good talk with her mother and father about what was happening at school and how serious her self-harm feelings were. She indicated that she would like to keep in regular contact with the same counsellor.

Special populations

Special populations of callers include those categorized as:

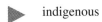 indigenous

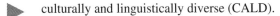 culturally and linguistically diverse (CALD).

The KHL defines CALD callers as any caller whose first language is not English or whose cultural background, or immediate family, is derived from a non-English-speaking tradition. This does not include callers from English-speaking nations such as the UK, US or Canada.

Indigenous callers

The proportion of calls received each year from children and young people from indigenous backgrounds has steadily increased from 2.2% in 1996 to 4% of all counselling calls made in 2003. In 2002, indigenous use peaked at 7% of all calls. Ten issues stand out as the major concerns for indigenous callers. Together, these 10 problems account for more than three-quarters of the calls from young indigenous Australians. The proportion of calls from indigenous and non-indigenous young people (as represented by the proportion of calls from each group) is shown in Fig. 25.9.

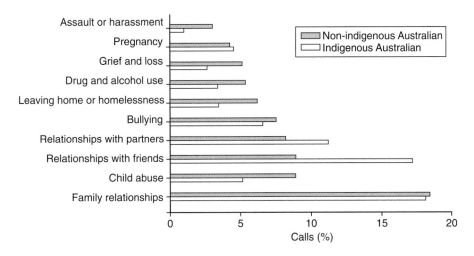

Fig 25.9. Calls from indigenous and non-indigenous young people.

As is the case with non-indigenous children and young people, relationships with parents and family are the major concern for indigenous young people. They account for 19% of calls. Almost half of callers (46%) report experiencing frequent or major family conflict or disruption. A further 25% report occasional family conflict, while 10% are experiencing issues related to family breakdown, separation or divorce. The remaining 19% of callers have worries about a family member. Indigenous callers are more likely to be worried about a family member and less likely to telephone about occasional family conflict or disruption than non-indigenous callers.

Although child abuse is a common reason why both indigenous and non-indigenous children telephone the KHL, the proportion of calls relating to child abuse is 75% greater for indigenous callers. These calls relate to neglect and to emotional, physical and sexual abuse, with physical and sexual abuse making up the majority. Although peer relationships are the third most common reason why young people from indigenous backgrounds contact the KHL, this group makes a significantly smaller proportion of calls than their Anglo-Australian counterparts – 9% compared with 17%.

Young people from indigenous backgrounds are twice as likely to be experiencing violence (verbal harassment, physical assault, domestic violence, sexual harassment and sexual assault), accounting for 6.3% of indigenous calls compared with 3.2% for non-indigenous callers. The proportion of calls from indigenous young people about drug or alcohol concerns, or both, is 60% greater, and drug and alcohol use is more frequent and severe. Such statistics relating to grave events in young indigenous lives should not, of course, be construed as being representative of the lives of all indigenous people.

Like callers from other social and cultural groups, many calls from indigenous clients are young people 'checking out' the service. The KHL policy of treating all clients with respect provides these callers with a positive experience of contacting the service, thereby increasing the likelihood of them calling again, if needed.

Case study

A male indigenous caller was about 14 years old. He had quite a few friends with him at the phone, chatting and laughing away. He talked about the Australian Football carnival that was happening the following week, and a band that was coming to town, which he was excited about. I explained that he could call the KHL to talk if he wasn't feeling too good inside or if he just wanted to chat. He started telling me about how he'd been to Uluru and seen an old man. I'm not sure I understood the full significance of this experience, as he was talking to his friends in the Aboriginal language, at the same time as he was talking to me. He also said that a friend at the phone was sniffing petrol. Another friend of his had died from this. He said he doesn't sniff petrol.

Culturally and linguistically diverse callers

The proportion of calls received each year from children and young people of CALD backgrounds has steadily increased from 4.1% in 1995 to 8% of all counselling calls made in 2003. For issues such as bullying, study, self-image and relationships with partners, callers of CALD backgrounds make higher proportions of calls than their

Anglophone counterparts. Problems concerning pregnancy, sexual activity, drug use and developmental issues account for a significantly lower proportion of calls from this group. Of the CALD young people, girls make the majority (73%) of calls.

Like their indigenous and non-indigenous counterparts, relationships with parents and family are the biggest concern of CALD callers, accounting for one-quarter of all calls. Almost 60% of these children and young people report experiencing frequent or major family conflict or disruption. The CALD callers are more likely to seek help about frequent or major family conflict and disruption and less likely to be telephoning about family breakdown, separation or divorce than their Anglo-Australian peers. In addition, conflict in CALD families is more likely to be intergenerational conflict, caused by the merging of cultures, as opposed to marital conflict or disruption caused by separation or divorce.

About one-third (30%) of CALD callers report significant or ongoing friendship problems, which are often related to cultural and language differences. Similarly, language and cultural differences are the major themes in calls related to making and maintaining friendships. Significant peer relationship issues may also be linked to parental restrictions on friendships, study commitments and being different in a new school. Children and young people of non-English-speaking backgrounds make 40% more calls concerning bullying than their Anglo-Australian counterparts. Furthermore, the bullying that CALD callers report is more severe and often based on racial or cultural differences.

Case study

A girl aged 17 years has grown up in Australia, but her family is very strongly connected to its Egyptian cultural history. She is now entering an arranged marriage and feels that all the control she has over her life is being taken away.

Client outcomes

Counsellors in the KHL service have access to a computerized referral database. The database contains details about some 8000 agencies around Australia that provide various services to children and young people. It allows callers to be referred to services in their own locality, where appropriate, either by providing contact information or via a direct, three-way telephone link. Most referrals are for child protection, legal assistance, emergency accommodation, pregnancy and contraception, and drug and alcohol counselling. The database is reviewed and updated constantly, both through client feedback and by regular interagency contact.

Telephone counselling

During 1999–2003, 11% of callers were referred to other support services (including crisis response and three-way linkups). For 77% of callers, no referral was made. In 7% of calls, counsellors were unable to give a referral because either no appropriate service was available or the caller terminated the call. For the remaining 5% of callers, the nature of the issue did not require a referral. During 2003, one in seven (14%)

young people who contacted the KHL made an agreement to reconnect with their counsellor again at a specific date and time. Duty-of-care actions, such as contacting an emergency service or child protection agency, were required for 4% of calls.

Online counselling

During 2001–2003, 4% of online clients were referred to other support services and 9% were referred to their doctor, school or guidance counsellor or mental health worker or received other non-specific referrals. In 14% of contacts, either counsellors were unable to give a referral or the client was referred to KHL telephone or web counselling. For the remaining 73% of clients, the nature of their issue did not require a referral. Thirteen percent of young people who contacted the KHL via web counselling made an agreement to reconnect with their counsellor again at a specific date and time.

Conclusion

The service offered by the Kids Help Line highlights the importance of new technologies in assisting children and young people who are seeking help. The benefits of providing contact through more than one medium are as follows.

▶ Ease of use: many young people are familiar with computers and online techniques.

▶ Ease of access: young people are not required to travel to attend a face-to-face counselling session.

▶ Control over access: young people can choose when to connect and disconnect from a counselling session, they can choose the counsellor they would like to interact with, they do not need to make an appointment and, with regard to online counselling, young people can take a break from the session, if required, to regain their composure.

▶ Privacy and confidentiality: the KHL operates under strict guidelines to protect the privacy and confidentiality of young people accessing the service – for example with online counselling no record of the session remains on the young person's personal computer.

▶ Safety and trust: the counselling environment offered by KHL operates under child-centred practice and empowerment principles.

The KHL is committed to integrating technological advances across telephone, email and web counselling services. Underpinning this commitment is the further empowerment of young people in Australia to develop and enhance the skills needed to experience rich and fulfilling relationships in a changing society.

Further information

Kids Help Line. http://www.kidshelp.com.au (last checked 12 August 2004).

Kids Help Line. Peer skills. http://www.peerskills.com.au (last checked 12 August 2004).

Parentline. http://www.parentline.com.au (last checked 12 August 2004).

References

1   Rigby K. What children tell us about bullying in schools. *Children Australia* 1997; **22**: 28–34.

2   Raphael B. *Promoting the Mental Health and Wellbeing of Children and Young People: Discussion paper No.1: Key Principles.* Canberra: Department of Health and Aged Care, 2000. http://www.health.gov.au/hsdd/mentalhe/resources/reports/pmhcyp_paper.htm (last checked 12 August 2004).

3   Sawyer MG, Arney FM, Baghurst PA, *et al. Mental Health of Young People in Australia.* Canberra: Commonwealth Department of Health and Aged Care, 2000. http://www.health.gov.au/hsdd/mentalhe/resources/young/index.htm (last checked 12 August 2004).

Section 3: Education

▶26

Grand Rounds at the Royal Children's Hospital in Brisbane

Robert McCrossin and Niall Higgins

Introduction

A teaching hospital should be a source of specialized knowledge that permits the shared care of patients throughout its region of responsibility. Clinical care should be a mixture of direct delivery by the primary carers and tertiary consultants, and virtual consultation by the same groups. This approach betrays two biases: to multidisciplinary medicine, as opposed to solo medical consultation, and to education as a key part of clinical care delivery. One-way education is no more appropriate than one-way consultation. With this in mind, videoconferencing of the grand rounds at the Royal Children's Hospital (RCH) in Brisbane began in 1997.

Reports on grand rounds show some heterogeneity, eg multiple centres presenting an organ-specific round and single centres presenting departmental rounds.[1,2] Some problems reported included the diffidence of some contributors to make presentations and severe scheduling difficulties with multiple departments reluctant to change schedules.

Grand rounds are essentially a medical exercise, although other disciplines may attend. The RCH grand round is a whole-of-hospital round, with all medical departments of the teaching hospital and all provincial centres expected to participate. Peer review operates and is widely regarded as a valuable part of the process. The major ongoing issue is quality control. The RCH allocates four slots in a 44-week programme to presentations by allied health disciplines. As there is a major local thrust in nursing research, currently a further one or two slots are devoted to nursing research topics.

Literature review

The literature shows that virtual grand rounds are being conducted in Canada,[2-5] the US,[1,6,7] Australia[8,9] and Argentina.[10] They cover general medicine and a range of specialty areas, such as geriatrics, pathology and oncology. The only report of paediatric grand rounds by videoconference is from Australia, although it may be assumed that such activities take place elsewhere in the world.[8] Most hospitals running virtual grand rounds do so to improve access to medical education. They also find it a cost-effective means of providing this education.[9,10] The audience, outside the main provider hospital, tends to be located in rural or remote areas (or even developing countries), where access to tertiary centres and resources may be limited. A combination of ISDN and IP videoconferencing is used. Hospitals predominantly use ISDN lines at present.

Seven of the 10 providers conducted grand rounds with multiple sites – for example, in Alberta, Canada, grand rounds in geriatric medicine were conducted each week with up to 23 sites, both urban and rural, participating.[3] One provider in Nova Scotia, Canada conducted point-to-point videoconferencing between a tertiary hospital and one regional hospital. Over five months, they conducted 29 grand rounds in both medicine and cardiology.[2] One of the remaining providers used a website and one did not make reference to site numbers. Virtual grand rounds have become an increasingly popular, cost-effective and appropriate means of improving access to medical education worldwide.

Grand rounds at the Royal Children's Hospital

For a long time, the grand round at the RCH, which lasts for approximately one hour, has begun at 07:45 hours on Wednesdays. The starting time was presumably chosen so that visiting medical officers (VMOs) and visitors from nearby hospitals could attend and still reach their hospitals, clinics and consulting rooms at a reasonable hour. Attendance by full-time staff and junior staff from the RCH is variable. There has been an occasional flurry of guilt or concern about local attendance, and various other possible times, generally lunchtimes, have been proposed as being more convenient. However, the current scheduling has not been changed for several reasons described below.

Attendees at regular meetings have the event imprinted into their unconscious, so that their attendance is part of their normal activity. Thus changing a time is fraught with danger, as regular attendees may be lost, without attracting new attendees. This is why, for example, 'regular' meetings at greater than weekly intervals frequently do not work: the imprint appears to fade exponentially after one week. In the late 1990s, there was an undercurrent of opinion that the needs of VMOs were of little consequence. However, the RCH will rely on VMOs for the foreseeable future, and their availability is necessarily constrained by having to earn an honest living in the real world.

As 19 sites currently participate in grand rounds, a change of time would have considerable consequences. This potential impact is reinforced by the demographics of the audience. The local audience at the RCH comprises 20–40 people, mainly medical staff (including students), unless the meeting concerns one of the other disciplines. The outside centres contribute up to 90 attendees: about 80% doctors, 10% medical students and 10% other disciplines. The provinces thus have the majority. The total audience of up to 130 people is very pleasing, if a little daunting. For a variety of reasons, the RCH has in the last few years developed a more vigorous academic culture, and lunchtimes are now used for research meetings, journal clubs, audit and clinical standards meetings, so these times are no longer available. Thus the early morning timing will not be easily changed.

Growth of the network

The grand rounds in Brisbane are conducted by multisite videoconference using sites connected by a single ISDN line at 128 kbit/s. We currently use two multiport bridges, which allow a total of 21 sites to be connected. Currently up to 20 sites participate – 18 in Queensland and 2 in New Zealand – and at least once a year we link to a guest speaker from an additional overseas location. The network has grown from 12 sites participating in Queensland just three years ago. Further possible growth in New South Wales will depend on bridge availability.

Grand round attendance by RCH subspecialists continues to be a problem. A few subspecialists do attend, because they are curious folk who value breadth of knowledge. Most have no real interest outside their own discipline, and it is of course easy to consult their colleagues, providing they recognize that a patient has a problem in another system. Provincial specialists, on the other hand, have to have broad skills. Their thirst for knowledge is humbling and the grand rounds have evolved to meet their needs. It follows that in designing the technical aspects of videoconferencing, their needs are paramount. If grand rounds are designed appropriately for the distance audience, they will inevitably be appropriate for the locals.

Designing the programme

The grand rounds programme must accommodate a variety of sessions. These include specialties at the teaching hospital, our associated district services and city hospitals, and the provincial centres, and the telecast of some regular special events. The list of participants is shown in Table 26.1. This adds up to a total of 57 topics. In a typical year, 44 Wednesdays are available. Furthermore, it is obvious that some of these areas (eg radiology, general paediatrics and neonatology) need more than one slot per year. It is also inevitable that a teaching hospital will attract some 3–5 'visiting firemen' per year, who will also need a slot. In addition, we are attracting an increasing number of visiting fellows on sabbatical. All of this leads to a scheduling problem of some complexity.

A particularly pleasing feature has been the readiness of the provincial centres to coordinate a presentation. The nature of these sessions has changed with our increasing familiarity with the technology. Initially, the sessions tended to cover issues such as acute resuscitation, transport to major centres and such like. Now the sessions are often interactive, with a local case and expert comment from the city subspecialist. We are getting quite adventurous. One successful session was chaired from the Gold Coast, with a visiting fireman lecturing in Brisbane and discussion from everywhere. There is also occasional participation from outside agencies. For example, a meeting on the deleterious effects of ultraviolet radiation involved the physics department of the University of Southern Queensland in an interdisciplinary session run from the RCH.

Table 26.1. Participants in the RCH grand rounds

Provincial centres (18)
Centres/Units/Services
- Royal Women's Hospital neonatal unit
- Queensland Clinical Genetics Service
- Sir Albert Sakzewski Virus Research Centre
- Prince Charles cardiology unit
- Community Child Health Service
- Child Advocacy
- Child Development
- Mental Health
- Dentistry
- Radiology
- Nuclear Medicine
- Intensive Care
- Rehabilitation
- Clinical Epidemiology
- Clinical Pharmacology
- Toxicology and Envenomation

Medical Subspecialties
- Endocrinology and Diabetes
- Metabolic Medicine
- Respiratory
- Haematology and Oncology

- Gastroenterology and Hepatology
- General Paediatric Medicine
- Neurology
- Nephrology
- Immunology
- Infectious Diseases
- Dermatology

Surgical Subspecialties
- Paediatric Surgery
- Ophthalmology
- Ear, Nose and Throat
- Neurosurgery
- Orthopaedics
- Burns
- Plastics
- Transplantation

Allied Health
Nursing
Medical Ethics
Events
- RCHF Visiting Professor (2 weeks)
- Research Fellow presentations (2 weeks)

Registrar participation

One area that has been squeezed because of the lack of programme slots is general paediatrics at the RCH. This has led to reduced registrar participation, both in presenting cases and in presenting researched (and hopefully even research) information. Although this is still common from the provincial sites, the more precious time devoted to subspecialties at the RCH has led to subspecialists tending to monopolize the presentations. This is an area for further improvement.

Complaints

Generally, the shortcomings of any session are painfully apparent to the local audience. Recurring themes over the years form the bulk of the consumer feedback complaints. These involve the content, the platform and the delivery.

Content

▶ Microscopic text

▶ Poor colour contrast

▶ Slides too busy

▶ Graphs and diagrams too busy

Platform

▶ Poor sound

▶ Poor lighting

▶ Poor staging, so that the presenter cannot face the distant audience, the local audience and the screen simultaneously

Delivery

▶ Every known technical glitch (and some previously unknown).

A similar list has been reported elsewhere.[2] All these problems can be solved by the combination of good design and full-time technical support and backup.

Education of presenters

Some initial concerns were that doctors would not take kindly to having to conform to rules to minimize the presentation problems. This is nonsense. No one wants to do a bad job, and doctors as a profession take their responsibility to educate their peers, and in particular junior staff, very seriously. Once technical support for presenters was available at the RCH, it was heavily used. It is partly a matter of peer pressure. Once a high standard has been reached, no one wants to be upstaged. There was initially, however, a well-founded scepticism about, and some fear of, the technology. It is not fair to expect the occasional lecturer to operate the audiovisual and videoconferencing equipment unaided, and we think that early efforts to try and force senior people to do so without much help were misguided. This just produces stubborn and uncooperative behaviour. Anecdotally, this is a common cause of failure. The uptake of technical help, once available, has led to excellent performance by senior staff.

Presenters are encouraged to produce the basic text and diagrams for their lectures as PowerPoint files, and the technical staff then format them before the presentation. This has proved highly successful. In principle, more formatting might be done by presenters, but if it is performed by our own technical staff, it is easier to maintain a consistent quality, as well as to market the hospital with our corporate format.

Design

The RCH slide template that has evolved has a number of subtle features (Fig. 26.1). The colour scheme is simple and functional. Dark text on an off-white background is the clearest combination possible. The margin has a picture of the hospital and a corporate identifier, which are constant from slide to slide. The bottom right hand corner is kept free for a live transmitted picture-in-picture of the presenter. This is the place where the eye comes to rest after scanning the slide. The amount of room left when the normal font size is used is small, which prevents overbusy slides. There is now widespread acceptance of this corporate format, which thus produces a consistent standard.

Presentation has been helped greatly by the auditorium design. The monitor placement allows the presenter to face both the local and remote audiences, and the slides, at the same time (Fig. 26.2). The sound system required considerable planning. Questioners in the audience often freeze when asked to follow simple protocols, and roving microphones are an unqualified disaster in practice. The ceiling microphones and audience camera have been very successful, as long as the floor manager and technician work as a team. This produces excellent three-way interaction between both audiences and the speaker. It is recommended that any auditorium used for this purpose should have these features. Allen *et al* also found that the sound quality during question time is the weak link, and this will be a focus of our next upgrade.[2]

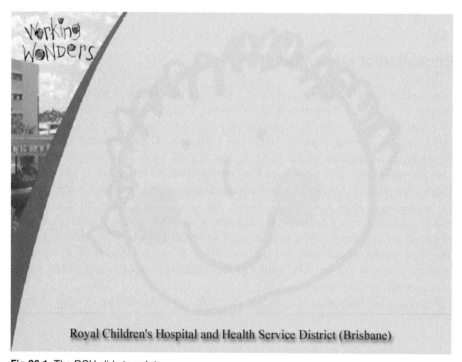

Royal Children's Hospital and Health Service District (Brisbane)

Fig 26.1. The RCH slide template.

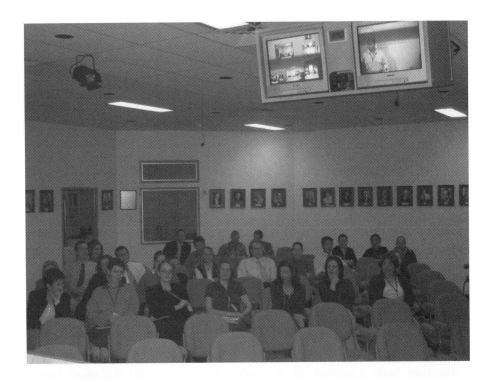

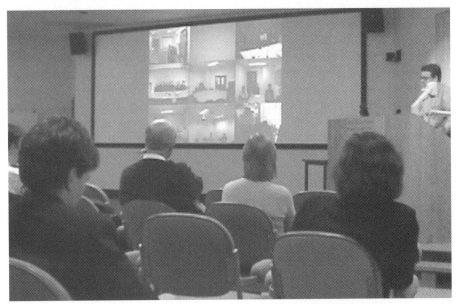

Fig 26.2. (a) Auditorium from the viewpoint of the presenter; the presenter's monitors are mounted in the ceiling over the heads of the local audience. (b) Multipoint conference in progress. The split screen is shown from the viewpoint of the audience; the audience camera is to the left and above the presenter's head.

Factors in success

Executive sponsorship is often touted as critical in the success of any organizational endeavour. Unfortunately this is true. Although health departments pay lip service to the importance of education, the crushing weight of delivering clinical services with inadequate funding means that it requires a degree of intestinal fortitude for hospital management to direct adequate funds to other areas. Education is a sacred cow that tends to be shipped to the abattoir when the inevitable annual funding crisis arises. Education in general, and tele-education in particular, has been sponsored personally by the executive group at RCH, and progress is very favourable compared with like institutions that have not had that direct support. Most of the workforce in a hospital is nursing, and the technician position at RCH was provided by nursing. The incumbent thus combines technical skills with the clinical knowledge necessary to interact easily with the clinical presenters.

Involvement of the provincial centres as true partners in content delivery is likewise crucial. The RCH has a genuine commitment to a multidisciplinary model of education and practice, and this will be the next focus of growth.

Synergies

There have been a number of successful associations with the grand rounds programme. The entire paediatric community in Queensland is comfortable with the technology. They use it every week. There is thus increased likelihood of using the technology for clinical service delivery.

Queensland is the most decentralized state in Australia, and recruitment and retention of staff to provincial centres has been made easier because of the extensive tele-education programme. With the established skills and technology, any educational session can be videoconferenced without undue difficulty. The Royal Australasian College of Physicians lecture programme and critical appraisal journal club are now broadcast widely. Junior staff now take part in network study groups, so that provincial trainees are not disadvantaged in the most critical training hurdle of their medical careers.

Is it a success?

Can grand rounds by videoconferencing be considered successful, either in Queensland specifically or elsewhere in general? We believe so. In 1947, George Orwell observed that:

> 'Ultimately there is no test of…merit except survival, which is in itself merely an index of majority opinion.'[11]

In the case of the RCH grand rounds, every week up to 130 busy health professionals in two countries and 19 centres tune in outside normal working hours. They do not have to, and they would not do so if the grand rounds were not valuable to them. Hippocrates might have said:

'The need is great, the scope wide, growth inexorable and timing difficult.'

In our setting, the challenge is to continue to improve and to justify the interest of the participants and their loyalty.

References

1 Laochamroonvorapongse D, Johnson E, Foong HB, Elpern DJ. A Brave New World: virtual grand rounds in dermatology. *Seminars in Cutaneous Medicine and Surgery* 2002; **21**: 232–236.

2 Allen M, Sargeant J, MacDougall E, O'Brien B. Evaluation of videoconferenced grand rounds. *Journal of Telemedicine and Telecare* 2002; **8**: 210–216.

3 Sclater K, Alagiakrishnan K, Sclater A. An investigation of videoconferenced geriatric medicine grand rounds in Alberta. *Journal of Telemedicine and Telecare* 2004; **10**: 104–107.

4 Sargeant J, Allen M, O'Brien B, MacDougall E. Videoconferenced grand rounds: needs assessment for community specialists. *Journal of Continuing Education in the Health Professions* 2003; **23**: 116–123.

5 Gagliardi A, Smith A, Goel V, DePetrillo D. Feasibility study of multidisciplinary oncology rounds by videoconference for surgeons in remote locales. *BMC Medical Informatics and Decision Making* <electronic resource> 2003; **3**: 7.

6 Ellis DG, Mayrose J. The success of emergency telemedicine at the State University of New York at Buffalo. *Telemedicine Journal and e-Health* 2003; **9**: 73–79.

7 Ruskin KJ, Palmer TE, Hagenouw RR, *et al.* Internet teleconferencing as a clinical tool for anesthesiologists. *Journal of Clinical Monitoring and Computing* 1998; **14**: 183–189.

8 McCrossin R. Successes and failures with grand rounds via videoconferencing at the Royal Children's Hospital in Brisbane. *Journal of Telemedicine and Telecare* 2001; **7** (suppl. 2): 25–28.

9 Faoagali J, Coles W, Price L, Siebert D. Telepathology. *Journal of Telemedicine and Telecare* 2001; **7** (suppl. 2): 71–72.

10 Altrudi R, Eurnekian A, Gandsas A, *et al.* Videoconferencing as a medical educational tool: first experience in Argentinean public hospital. *Studies in Health Technology and Informatics* 1998; **50**: 364–365.

11 Orwell G. Lear, Tolstoy and the Fool. In *The Collected Essays, Journalism and Letters of George Orwell*. Orwell S, Angus I, eds. London, Penguin: 1970.

▶27

Educational Videoconferences for Parents in the Bronx

Marina Reznik and Philip O Ozuah

Introduction

Parental health education is important for many reasons. First, parents play a critical role in managing their children's disease.[1] Second, effective management of a paediatric illness, whether acute or chronic, requires involvement of both children and their families. Lack of parental knowledge about their child's illness leads to lower adherence to the drug and management plan,[2] underestimation of severity of illness and delayed seeking of medical care.

A close partnership between children, their families and healthcare providers is an important component of successful management of any disease. Paediatricians used to spend more than a third of their patient care time on patient education and counselling.[3] Evidence suggests that physicians today face multiple pressures to see a greater number of patients and have less time for each visit.[4] Such pressures on clinicians tend to leave little time for patient education. Despite these changes, however, the relationship between patients and physicians remains fundamental to high-quality care.

Previous studies have shown that racial and ethnic disparities persist in many aspects of primary care delivery.[5,6] Asthma, for example, is a common childhood illness, with increasing prevalence and morbidity among underserved and minority children.[7] Several reports have shown that in comparison with white children, black and Latino children had worse asthma status, less use of preventive asthma drugs and fewer office visits for asthma, which suggest inadequate use of preventive services.[8,9] In addition, minority children whose parents are less educated are at a higher risk for under use of preventive asthma drugs.[10]

Studies have shown that language barriers are largely responsible for racial and ethnic disparities in healthcare.[11,12] The Bronx district in New York is unique, since more than half of its residents speak a language other than English.[13] Effective strategies for bridging the language barrier and educating parents about their child's illness are needed to improve the immigrant population's access to healthcare, quality of care and health status. Videoconferencing can address these gaps by providing linguistically appropriate health services and delivering health education to a large immigrant population.

Background – brief literature review

Videoconferencing has been used in other countries as a means of educating people in rural areas.[14,15] However, the use of videoconferencing to deliver health education to children or their parents has not been widely applied in the US. Although there is a growing literature related to telemedicine in general,[16] only a few reports describe the role of videoconferencing in providing health education to parents.

A telemedicine programme, 'Baby CareLink', has been developed in the Neonatal Intensive Care Unit at the Beth Israel Deaconess Medical Center in Boston, Massachusetts.[17] The object is to provide information, education and emotional support to families of premature infants throughout their hospital stay and after discharge.[18] Videoconferencing and the web are used to enhance interactions between families, staff and community providers. Baby CareLink allows families to have increased access to the healthcare team and educational information and, most importantly, to have virtual visits with their hospitalized infant from home using the videoconference equipment. A randomized trial of Baby CareLink showed that it significantly improved family satisfaction with inpatient care, provided educational and emotional support for families and facilitated earlier discharge to home of very low-birthweight infants.[17]

The Telemedicine In-Home Monitoring Evaluation Pilot project was developed in Hawaii to show that Internet-based interactions between patients and their healthcare providers achieve a level of compliance with medical treatment plans equal to or better than that achieved by in-person visits. Another goal of this pilot project was to examine the impact of patient education on the use of peak flow meters and metered-dose inhalers (MDI) with spacers for asthma management.[19] Furthermore, this project aims to decrease future hospitalizations and avoid unnecessary increases in drug dosage by educating the children and their parents on proper use of MDIs and spacers.[19]

Videoconferencing in the Bronx

The Children's Hospital at Montefiore located in the Bronx serves a large immigrant community. In 2000, Hispanics or Latinos comprised 48% of the total population in the Bronx and blacks or African–Americans comprised 36%.[13] Asthma is the major health problem for children in this community.[20] Asthma is also the most common cause of childhood disability in the US.[21] The prevalence of asthma among children from the Bronx is at least twice that seen in the US as a whole,[22] and the Bronx is the New York City borough with the highest rates of both asthma hospitalizations and deaths.[20]

Effective management of paediatric asthma requires the involvement of both children and their parents. Some reports suggest that asthma education programmes for inner-city children improve asthma knowledge and self-management behaviour.[23–25] However, such programmes for inner-city immigrant parents of asthmatic children are not widely available in the US.[26–29] A needs assessment, carried out by the Center for Immigrant families located in the South Bronx, identified asthma as one of the topics parents would like to learn more about. We began videoconferencing sessions to deliver health education in the Bronx in March 2003. This was designed to bridge the gap between inner-city immigrant parents and the healthcare system. We wanted to test the feasibility and effectiveness of videoconferencing in delivering health education to a large immigrant population.

A total of three videoconferencing sessions were conducted in 2003. To test knowledge gain, we employed a before–after study design for each videoconference. We administered a questionnaire consisting of true and false statements at the beginning and end of each videoconference. Ethics permission for the study was not required. An English–Spanish interpreter was present in the classroom during the videoconferences and provided translation as needed. Both sites were supported by technical coordinators, who ensured the proper functioning of the equipment. The videoconferencing units (Intel TeamStation System) were connected via three ISDN lines at a bandwidth of 384 kbit/s.

Videoconference 1: Asthma overview

The first videoconference was held in March 2003.[30] We created an asthma curriculum on the basis of information provided in the brochure for the New York City Childhood Asthma Initiative, the Open Airways for Schools curriculum and *Protecting Our Children's Environment: An Educational Outreach Guide on Asthma*.[31–33]

We used an interactive videoconferencing session to deliver an asthma education programme to a convenience sample of mainly Latino immigrant parents who attended a class on English as a second language at the Center for Immigrant Families in the South Bronx. This session was the first in the two-part videoconference series on asthma and focused mainly on asthma triggers and the prevention of asthma exacerbations. Most of the videoconference time was dedicated to questions from the participants (Figs 27.1 and 27.2).

A total of 60 people participated. The mean age of the participants was 36 years. Sixty-nine percent of the participants were women, 54% were born in the Dominican Republic and 21% were born in Mexico. As a group, they had lived in the US for a median of six years.

Asthma knowledge improved significantly after the videoconference. More participants responded correctly to the following statements at the post-test (Fig. 27.3):

▶ Children with asthma can run and play like their friends who do not have asthma (49% correct at pre-test versus 96% correct at post-test, $p < 0.001$)

▶ Children with asthma have to miss a lot of school (31% correct at pre-test versus 59% correct at post-test, $p < 0.001$).

Most participants asked questions and commented on their personal experiences with asthma. Their questions included:

▶ Why is the asthma prevalence so high in the Bronx?

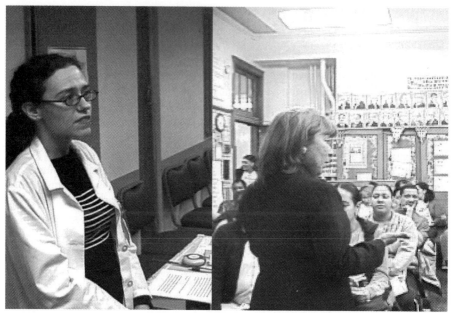

Fig. 27.1. Videoconference on asthma overview.

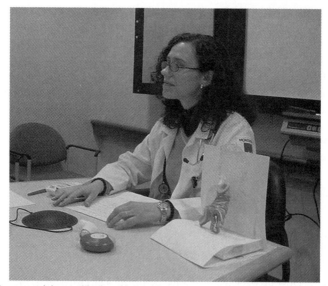

Fig. 27.2. Airway models used in the videoconference.

▶ Is asthma a genetic condition?

▶ What causes asthma?

▶ How does one access medical care?

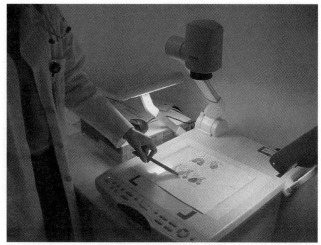

Fig. 27.3. Diagram of airways used during the videoconference.

We assessed the same participants three months later for knowledge retention from the first videoconference. Participants showed a high level of knowledge retention. On the two questionnaire items asked again, the proportions of participants answering correctly were still high: 76% for 'Children with asthma can run and play like their friends who do not have asthma' and 49% for 'Children with asthma have to miss a lot of school'.

Videoconference 2: Asthma drugs

The second videoconference was held in June 2003 and was the last in the two-part series on asthma.[30] This videoconferencing session was delivered to the same audience as the first session and addressed the topic of asthma drugs and their proper use (Fig. 27.4). Fifty-six participants returned for the second videoconference. After the videoconference, more participants responded correctly to the following statements:

▶ Some children with asthma need to take a medicine every day to prevent their asthma attacks from starting (62% correct at pre-test versus 80% correct at post-test, $p = 0.013$)

▶ Children who take asthma medicine everyday become addicted to it (63% correct at pre-test versus 84% correct at post-test, $p = 0.002$).

As in the first videoconference session, most of the videoconference time was dedicated to questions from the participants. Some of the questions raised included:

▶ How do I manage an acute asthma attack at home?

▶ What are the side-effects of asthma drugs?

▶ Can asthma be cured?

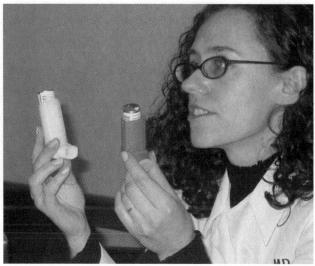

Fig. 27.4. Explaining the difference between the preventive and quick-relief drugs used in asthma.

As in the first session, these questions stimulated an interactive and dynamic dialogue between participants and the presenter.

Videoconference 3: Summer safety

The third videoconference was held in July 2003 with the goal of improving knowledge about summer safety for children.[34] We created a 'Summer Safety Tips' curriculum based on the American Academy of Pediatrics (AAP) summer safety tips and advice from the AAP Committee on Environmental Health, as well as information from a group of parents called KidSource Online. Our curriculum included information on insect repellent usage, sun protection and bicycle, water, backyard and car safety (Fig. 27.5).

We delivered the videoconference from the Children's Hospital at Montefiore in the Bronx. Thirty-three people participated. They represented a convenience sample of immigrant parents who attended a class in English as a second language at the Center for Immigrant Families in the South Bronx, where the videoconference was held. Of the participants, 74% were women and 70% were from the Dominican Republic. Their mean age was 39 years.

After the videoconference, participants showed significant knowledge gains by responding correctly to the following two statements (Fig. 27.6):

▶ To protect children from mosquitoes, use insect repellent that adults use and reapply it every hour (75% correct at pre-test versus 97% correct at post-test, $p = 0.039$)

▶ Children do not need to wear sunglasses during summer (66% correct at pre-test versus 94% correct at post-test, $p = 0.004$).

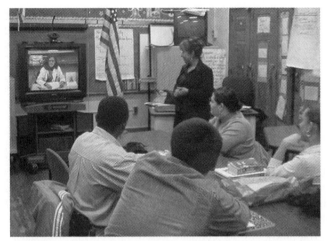

Fig. 27.5. Participants and an interpreter (standing) during one of the videoconferences.

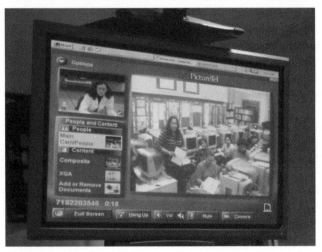

Fig. 27.6. Videoconference monitor.

Educational videoconferences for parents

We believe that educational videoconferencing for parents has an exciting future. To date, the participants in our videoconferences have been mainly Latino immigrants in the Bronx. It is not yet known if videoconferencing will be as effective an educational tool in a non-Latino immigrant population. Future videoconferencing sessions may be extended to different groups of immigrants as well as non-immigrants.

In our study, all three videoconferences were led in English. Although the sessions were translated into Spanish by a bilingual interpreter, it is possible that some information was misinterpreted by participants. Future work may involve videoconferences led by a bilingual healthcare professional who is fluent in the native language of the participants. Also, while we used a single videoconferencing site, multi-site videoconferencing would reach a larger audience. We plan to use this modality for future educational videoconferencing for parents. In addition, we plan to create curricula on other topics that are of interest to our community.

Future research directions

There are many possibilities for future research in the area of educational videoconferencing for parents. The series of two videoconferencing sessions that we led focused mainly on a general overview of asthma. It is not known if a curriculum that focuses on more specific aspects of asthma would be as successful. Furthermore, our study did not compare videoconferencing with other educational tools. A study that compares videoconferencing with other educational modalities thus would be helpful in determining the most effective strategy for parental health education.

Until recently, the only way paediatricians provided health information and education to families was during healthcare maintenance visits. Now, with the evolution and increased popularity of telemedicine in educating parents about health issues, we may need to explore further if the use of videoconferencing for providing health information is as effective as in-person education provided by a physician in the office.

There are only a few reports of consumer satisfaction with educational videoconferencing.[15,35] Evaluation of parental satisfaction with both the material presented and its method of transmission is necessary if telemedicine is to become a routine method for delivering community education. In addition, the needs of communities must be assessed, so the health issues that are of interest to these communities should be incorporated into future videoconferencing sessions if possible.

Conclusion

We have explored the feasibility of videoconferencing in delivering health education to inner-city immigrant parents. We found that videoconferencing improved knowledge of several health education topics, and, moreover, it led to knowledge retention. We conclude that interactive videoconferencing is a useful tool in delivering health education to a large immigrant population.

It is possible that, in the future, educational videoconferencing will completely replace face-to-face education provided by a physician in the office, but until that time comes, videoconferencing remains an essential supplement to it. Given the increasing constraints on physicians' time, educational videoconferencing can provide a solution for the delivery of health education to parents.

Further information

Asthma Society of Canada. This website provides information about asthma, its triggers and its treatment. It also has a link to a website where parents and children can learn about asthma together by using games and helpful facts, as well as sharing stories with other families of children with asthma. http://www.asthma.ca/adults/ (last checked 3 August 2004).

National Heart, Lung, and Blood Institute. Diseases and Conditions Index: Asthma. This website provides the general public with facts (in English and Spanish) about asthma, its signs and symptoms, and its treatment and prevention. http://www.nhlbi.nih.gov/ health/dci/Diseases/Asthma/Asthma_WhatIs.html (last checked 3 August 2004).

My Asthma – part of the MyHealthyLife Network. This website is dedicated to assisting people with asthma in managing their asthma and allergies by providing them with information about asthma, its treatment options and better symptom control. In addition, people with asthma can read real-life stories about others with asthma and receive personalized education and answers to questions about asthma from MyAsthma health team. http://www.myasthma.com (last checked 3 August 2004).

Department of Health and Human Services. Centers for Disease Control and Prevention. This website provides basic facts about asthma, such as a definition of asthma, its diagnosis, epidemiology, triggers and treatment. http://www.cdc.gov/ nceh/airpollution/asthma/faqs.htm (last checked 3 August 2004).

The Skin Cancer Foundation. This website is committed to educating parents and children about protecting themselves against the harmful rays of the sun. It provides facts about sun safety as well as basic information about different types of skin cancer and its early detection. http://www.skincancer.org/children/ (last checked 3 August 2004).

American Academy of Pediatrics. Keeping Skin Safe and Healthy. This website provides the news release from the American Academy of Pediatrics on sun safety tips and the dangers of long-term sun exposure. http://www.aap.org/advocacy/ archives/tanning.htm (last checked 3 August 2004).

Department of Health and Human Services. Centers for Disease Control and Prevention. This website provides facts and statistics about skin cancer, a sun safety guide for parents and a question and answer section. http://www.cdc.gov/ chooseyourcover/guide.htm (last checked 3 August 2004).

References

1 Fadzil A, Norzila MZ. Parental asthma knowledge. *Medical Journal of Malaysia* 2002; **57**: 474–481.
2 Milgrom H, Bender B. Nonadherence to asthma treatment and failure of therapy. *Current Opinion in Pediatrics* 1997; **9**: 590–595.
3 Bartlett EE. Effective approaches to patient education for the busy pediatrician. *Pediatrics* 1984; **74**: 920–923.
4 Levinson W, D'Aunno T, Gorawara-Bhat R, *et al.* Patient–physician communication as organizational innovation in the managed care setting. *American Journal of Managed Care* 2002; **8**: 622–630.
5 Stevens GD, Shi L. Racial and ethnic disparities in the quality of primary care for children. *Journal of Family Practice* 2002; **51**: 573.

6   Buescher PA, Horton SJ, Devaney BL, *et al*. Differences in the use of health services between white and African American children enrolled in Medicaid in North Carolina. *Maternal and Child Health Journal* 2003 **7**: 45–52.

7   Mansour ME, Lanphear BP, DeWitt TG. Barriers to asthma care in urban children: parent perspectives. *Pediatrics* 2000; **106**: 512–519.

8   Lieu TA, Lozano P, Finkelstein JA, *et al*. Racial/ethnic variation in asthma status and management practices among children in managed Medicaid. *Pediatrics* 2002; **109**: 857–865.

9   Akinbami LJ, LaFleur BJ, Schoendorf KC. Racial and income disparities in childhood asthma in the United States. *Ambulatory Pediatrics* 2002; **2**: 382–387.

10   Finkelstein JA, Lozano P, Farber HJ, *et al*. Underuse of controller medications among Medicaid-insured children with asthma. *Archives of Pediatrics and Adolescent Medicine* 2002; **156**: 562–567.

11   Weech-Maldonado R, Morales LS, Spritzer K, *et al*. Racial and ethnic differences in parents' assessments of pediatric care in Medicaid managed care. *Health Services Research* 2001; **36**: 575–594.

12   Timmins CL. The impact of language barriers on the health care of Latinos in the United States: a review of the literature and guidelines for practice. *Journal of Midwifery and Women's Health* 2002; **47**: 80–96.

13   United States Census 2000. http://www.census.gov/main/www/cen2000.html (last checked 17 March 2004).

14   Faulkner K. Successes and failures in videoconferencing: a community health education programme. *Journal of Telemedicine and Telecare* 2001; **7** (suppl. 2): 65–67.

15   Faulkner K, McClelland L. Using videoconferencing to deliver a health education program to women health consumers in rural and remote Queensland: an early attempt and future plans. *Australian Journal of Rural Health* 2002; **10**: 65–72.

16   Wootton R, Yellowlees P, McLaren P (eds). *Telepsychiatry and e-Mental Health.* London: Royal Society of Medicine Press, 2003.

17   Gray JE, Safran C, Davis RB, *et al*. Baby CareLink: using the internet and telemedicine to improve care for high-risk infants. *Pediatrics* 2000; **106**: 1318–1324.

18   Phillips M. Telemedicine in the neonatal intensive care unit. *Pediatric Nursing* 1999; **25**: 185–189.

19   Murphy JC. Telemedicine offers new way to manage asthma. *American Journal of Health-System Pharmacy* 2001; **58**: 1693,1696.

20   City of New York Department of Health. *Asthma Facts.* http://www.nyc.gov/html/doh/pdf/asthma/facts.pdf (last checked 17 March 2004).

21   Newacheck PW, Halfon N. Prevalence, impact, and trends in childhood disability due to asthma. *Archives of Pediatrics and Adolescent Medicine* 2000; **154**: 287–293.

22   Crain EF, Weiss KB, Bijur PE, *et al*. An estimate of the prevalence of asthma and wheezing among inner-city children. *Pediatrics* 1994; **94**: 356–362.

23   Christiansen SC, Martin SB, Schleicher NC, *et al*. Evaluation of a school-based asthma education program for inner-city children. *Journal of Allergy and Clinical Immunology* 1997; **100**: 613–617.

24   Bartholomew LK, Gold RS, Parcel GS, *et al*. Watch, Discover, Think, and Act: evaluation of computer-assisted instruction to improve asthma self-management in inner-city children. *Patient Education and Counseling* 2000; **39**: 269–280.

25   Wolf FM, Guevara JP, Grum CM, *et al*. Educational interventions for asthma in children. *Cochrane Database of Systematic Reviews* 2003; (1): CD000326.

26   Stevens CA, Wesseldine LJ, Couriel JM, *et al*. Parental education and guided self-management of asthma and wheezing in the pre-school child: a randomized controlled trial. *Thorax* 2002; **57**: 39–44.

27   Fadzil A, Norzila MZ. Parental asthma knowledge. *Medical Journal of Malaysia* 2002; **57**: 474–481.

28   Peterson-Sweeney K, McMullen A, *et al*. Parental perceptions of their child's asthma: management and medication use. *Journal of Pediatric Health Care* 2003; **17**: 118–125.

29   Kieckhefer GM, Ratcliffe M. What parents of children with asthma tell us. *Journal of Pediatric Health Care* 2000; **14**: 122–126.

30   Reznik M, Sharif I, Ozuah PO. Use of interactive videoconferencing to deliver asthma education to inner-city immigrants. *Journal of Telemedicine and Telecare* 2004; **10**: 118-120.

31   City of New York Department of Health. *Childhood Asthma Initiative.* http://www.nyc.gov/html/doh/html/asthma/asthma.html (last checked 17 March 2004).

32   American Lung Association. *Open Airways for Schools Program.* http://www.lungusa.org/events/astopen.html (last checked 17 March 2004).

33   National Safety Council. *Asthma.* http://www.nsc.org/ehc/asthma.htm (last checked 17 March 2004).

34   Reznik M, Sharif I, Ozuah PO. Improving immigrant health education using videoconferencing. *Journal of Telemedicine and Telecare* 2004; **10**: 60–61.

35   Yip MP, Mackenzie A, Chan J. Patient satisfaction with telediabetes education in Hong Kong. *Journal of Telemedicine and Telecare* 2002; **8**: 48–51.

▶ 28

Paediatric Websites for Healthcare Professionals

Michael South

Introduction

Over the last decade, work-related use of the Internet has become a regular part of the life of most medical professionals. This development has affected those involved in the healthcare of children as much as those in most other areas of medicine. Very wide variation in the computer and Internet skills of child health professionals, however, remains.

Paediatricians and other healthcare professionals now find themselves accessing the Internet for many different purposes. There has been substantial growth in the quantity of paediatric information available on the Internet, and many interactive resources have become readily accessible.[1] Studies of the information-seeking behaviour of paediatricians have shown significant variation in the use of electronic resources but an increasing trend to Internet use. Simple interventions have been shown to increase Internet use and efficiency in information retrieval.[2] It is now common to find computers with Internet connections available in consulting rooms, ward areas and emergency departments. All of these changes have resulted in increasing professional use of the Internet and such use has also moved closer to the point of patient care. Internet resources are now quite frequently used as an integral part of the paediatric consultation.

Currently, many medical professionals use websites produced by others, while a smaller number are producing websites of their own. The sites vary in their purpose and sophistication. Finding good-quality websites, evaluating their content, managing the links to this information to keep it readily available and incorporating the information into daily practice effectively all pose a number of challenges. Using Internet information during remote telepaediatric consultations provides an additional technical challenge.

Existing websites as resources for professionals

How they may be helpful

Most medical professionals use the Internet for a wide range of purposes, some of which are outlined in Table 28.1. Professionals find themselves using the Internet both at home and at work, during personal study time, and increasingly at the time of patient care. Although the Internet is an enormously useful resource, it can also lead to significant time wasting if the required information is difficult to access.

Table 28.1. Most medical professionals use the Internet for a wide range of purposes. This table, with active links, can be downloaded from http://www.wch.org.au/genmed/resources.cfm?doc_id=5999

Purpose	Example sites

Searching medical literature	• Pubmed
	  http://www4.ncbi.nlm.nih.gov/PubMed/
	• Ovid
	  http://www.ovid.com/
	• Cochrane Collaboration
	  http://www.update-software.com/clibng/cliblogon.htm

Abstracting services	• Medscape
	  http://www.medscape.com
	• Journal Watch
	  http://pediatrics.jwatch.org/
	• MS-Paed-List
	  http://www.rch-ms-lists.org

Electronic table of contents alerts	• *Journal of Pediatrics*
	  http://www3.us.elsevierhealth.com/jpeds/
	• *Archives of Disease in Childhood*
	  http://adc.bmjjournals.com/
	• *Journal of Paediatrics and Child Health*
	  http://www.blackwell-synergy.com/rd.asp?code=JPC&goto=journal
	• *British Medical Journal*
	  http://bmj.bmjjournals.com/
	• *Lancet*
	  http://www.thelancet.com/

Guidelines, policies and disease-specific information	• American Academy of Pediatrics
	  http://www.aap.org
	• Royal Australasian College of Physicians
	  http://www.racp.edu.au/
	• Isabel UK
	  http://www.isabel.org.uk
	• Royal Children's Hospital, Melbourne
	  http://www.rch.org.au/clinicalguide
	• EMedicine
	  http://www.emedicine.com/ped/search.htm

Continuing medical education	• Medscape
	  http://www.medscape.com
	• ADHDcme
	  http://www.ADHDcme.com

Patient management tools	• Royal Children's Hospital, Melbourne http://www.rch.unimelb.edu.au/genmed/clinical.cfm?doc_id=2399

Drug information	• MIMS
	  http://www.mims.com.au
	• Therapeutic Guidelines
	  http://etg.hcn.net.au/
	• ePocrates
	  http://www.epocrates.com
	• Drug Doses – Shann
	  http://www.rch.org.au/clinicalguide/forms/drugDoses.cfm

Professional society contact	• Royal Australasian College of Physicians
	http://www.racp.edu.au/
Parent or child information	• Royal Children's Hospital, Melbourne
	http://www.wch.org.au/kidsinfo
	• Child and Youth Health, South Australia
	http://www.cyh.com/
	• Great Ormond Street Hospital, London
	http://www.gosh.nhs.uk/factsheets/
Paediatric discussion lists	• Ped-Talk (General Paediatrics)
	http://www.pcc.com/lists/pedtalk/
	• Ped-Lung (Respiratory Paediatrics)
	http://www.resp.paediatrics.ubc.ca/index.htm

Finding good websites

The Internet contains a very large amount of information on child health topics. Simply typing the word 'pediatric' into the Google search engine will produce at least 3.5 million potential sites, and the English spelling 'paediatric' will produce a further 500 000 sites.

Most users will rely on search engines (eg Google, Yahoo and AltaVista) to find appropriate websites. This is often a successful strategy, but it can also be frustrating and inefficient. It is worth users taking the time to become familiar in detail with at least one of these search engines, taking the time to learn the search syntax and understand how the engine presents sites that it indexes. Google will usually present a long and fairly comprehensive list of relevant websites for most topics. Its main strength is that it gives priority to sites that have most links from other sites (and again weights these sites according to their own linking status). This method means that it is more likely that popular and respected sites appear near the top of the listing. Inclusion of additional and specific terms can help to narrow search results. Professionals used to searching Medline will be familiar with the trade-off between sensitivity and specificity that can occur during the compilation of a search strategy.

An alternative search engine method is the use of 'groups' or 'directories'. For example, Yahoo and Google have children's health directories (http://dir.yahoo.com/Health/, http://directory.google.com/Top/Health/Child_Health/) that each concentrate a large amount of relevant material into one searchable location.

There are many portals or gateways for paediatric information on the Internet. These essentially are websites in which the administrators have collected together many links on the topic of interest. One of the biggest sites, with links to over 6000 resources, is 'Harriet Lane Links' (http://derm.med.jhmi.edu/poi/); the site is maintained by staff at Johns Hopkins University. Other useful portals include General Paediatrics.com (http://generalpediatrics.com/), Hardin MD (www.lib.uiowa.edu/hardin/md/ped.html) and MedlinePlus (www.nlm.nih.gov/medlineplus/childrenshealth.html).

Another useful strategy for finding good-quality sites is to look at the 'Links' page provided on sites that you already respect. The site authors will usually have given some thought to which sites they are prepared to endorse when including links from their own material.

Evaluating websites

The lack of a requirement for peer review, or supervision by a publishing house, means that anyone with an Internet connection can publish material on the web. Health professionals will usually not have too much difficulty in judging the quality of material they find on the Internet, but for patients and their families this can be a difficult task. Health professionals will probably use the same criteria as they do when assessing the validity of material published in printed media, including knowledge of the qualifications, experience and authority of the authors.

Various authors have suggested criteria for assessing the quality of websites, one set of which is given in Table 28.2.[3] Although the use of such criteria can be helpful, they should not be applied unthinkingly. Some excellent resource sites on the web will fail some or all of these criteria.

Table 28.2. Criteria for assessing the quality of websites (after Nesbitt *et al*[3])

Criteria	Question
Accessibility	Can the site be found using common search engines?
Attribution	Are references and sources for all content provided?
Authorship	Are authors and their affiliations and credentials provided?
Content	Is the information provided valid? (Critically appraise using the same methods as for printed resources)?
	Are linked sites valid?
Currency	Are the dates of posting and last update provided?
Disclosure	Is the 'ownership' of the website clear?
	Are advertising, underwriting and other conflicts of interest made explicit?
Ease of use	Is the site easy to navigate?
	Does it load quickly?
	Do features work properly?
Innovation	Is the information delivered in a way that exploits the potential of multimedia without 'overdoing it'?
Readability	What is the reading age level?

The Health On the Net Foundation (HONF) is a non-government agency concerned with ethical and quality issues for websites that contain health information. Their code of practice provides an excellent structure for website evaluation (http://www.hon.ch/HONcode/Conduct.html), and their own search engine provides a means of searching a large collection of sites that the foundation has certified as meeting their code (http://www.hon.ch/MedHunt/). Again, many excellent sites fall outside the code of practice. However, users can be assured that those sites produced through a HONF search will be reputable and authoritative.

Producing your own professional website

Reasons for producing your own website

At the most basic level, a web page can be helpful purely as a means of organizing frequently needed links to web content elsewhere on the Internet for personal use. My own such 'personal' page is at http://www.wch.org.au/genmed/ clinical.cfm?&doc_id=5915. Producing such a page is a very simple undertaking and can be done in most word processors such as Word (Microsoft). Using a web page format can be much more useful than relying on the book-marking systems in most browsers. These can be inherently difficult to organize.

The web version of Table 28.1 includes live web links. It was generated in Word, and can be downloaded for readers to experiment with (http://www.wch.org.au/genmed/ resources.cfm?&doc_id=5999). A simple organizational web page such as this can be kept on the user's own computer, or if they have the requisite facilities, can be uploaded to a web server. The former method will be useful only if access is required from the user's own computer, while the latter will allow access from multiple sites and for many users.

Beyond producing simple web pages for personal use, professionals may have many other reasons for producing a website. Many of these overlap with the aims of users outlined in Table 28.1. In addition, there may be more commercial motives, such as practice marketing to potential patients or referrers.

Website content

It is common to hear of websites produced with considerable effort and financial expense that have disappointingly low volumes of traffic. Often these sites contain static material that could just as easily have been published in print and provide nothing innovative or interesting to attract users. While their own curriculum and publication list might fascinate individual professionals, other users of the web may be less interested.

When designing a website, it is critical for the producers to consider exactly who their audience might be (eg other professionals, patients or families) and to think about what these users might be searching for on the Internet. The use of surveys or focus groups can help inform such planning and avoid considerable wasted effort. Duplication of resources found elsewhere on the web is best avoided – adding links to external sites is much easier than reinventing the wheel. The HONF guidelines are a useful resource, and website producers should consider the use of disclaimers and obtaining legal advice if their site provides treatment advice.

Too many health-related websites suffer from the fact that the producers had a rush of enthusiasm during the initial phases of production, which was not maintained for the much more difficult task of long-term maintenance and updating. Leaving out-of-date material on such sites can be both frustrating and potentially misleading, or even dangerous, for users.

Content management

Many software tools may be employed in website management. Again, it is worth the effort of considering this in detail before embarking on site production.

 How many authors will be involved?

▶ Who will maintain the site?

▶ Will the whole of the site be available on the Internet or will some be on a private Intranet?

▶ Will a commercial website production or management company be involved or will all the work be undertaken in house?

Some excellent content management systems are available that allow authors to generate web material with little training, allowing them to concentrate on their content knowledge. One or more individuals with additional technical training can then undertake the overall site management. Such systems can be expensive, but they are often worth consideration because of the greatly increased efficiency of site management. Comparative reviews of content management systems are available on the Internet (http://www.pcmag.com/category2/0,1738,4803,00.asp).

Integrating website use into clinical practice

Internet use is rapidly getting closer to the point of patient care. The presence of computers in clinical areas and the availability of appropriate resources on the web are major driving factors in this development. Web-based technology is also becoming the standard for many clinical information systems, including pathology and radiology reporting. The future lies in the convergence and integration of all of these systems through a single web interface. This has many technical advantages as well as being more efficient for users who can find all their information in one place without the need for multiple system logon and the need only to learn the use of a single interface.

Many institutions recognize the great benefit provided by Internet access for staff, while others see it as expensive, unnecessary and a potential means for staff to waste time on activities unrelated to their work. With appropriate and well-published guidelines for usage, providing Internet access to clinical staff should have many benefits. An example of the use of well-integrated web technology in direct clinical practice is shown in Fig. 28.1.

Internet use during the consultation

Many health professionals have become familiar with using computers during a patient consultation. Such use may include accessing pathology reports, electronic prescribing or updating an electronic patient record. Internet use can also be valuable during the session. Various resources (eg symptom diaries or written disease-specific information) might be accessed for printing, or online tools such as body mass index (BMI) or growth velocity calculators may be used. Some examples of online tools are given in Table 28.3.

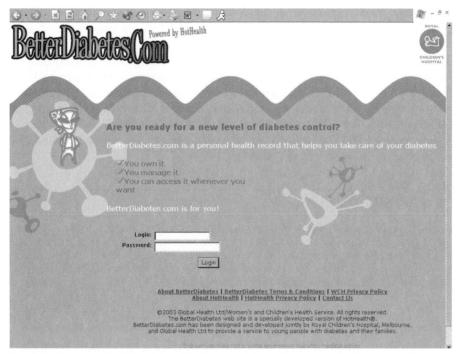

Fig. 28.1. An example of close integration between information, web technology and patient care (http://www.betterdiabetes.com).

Table 28.3. Online tools

Tool	URL
Sleeping diary	http://www.rch.org.au/emplibrary/genmed/sleepcrydiary.pdf
Child health information for parents	http://www.wch.org.au/kidsinfo/factsheets.cfm?doc_id=3664
Online medical calculators	http://www.emedhome.com/resources_calculators.cfm
Body mass index calculator and curves	http://www.rch.org.au/genmed/clinical.cfm?doc_id=2603

Sometimes it is helpful to show material to patients or their families on the computer screen. This requires the consulting room to be set up appropriately, so that the screen can be seen easily. There may be technical challenges if the clinician wishes to show on-screen Internet material during a telemedicine consultation.

Both the clinician and the patient or family may access web-based information before or after the consultation. A large amount of medical information is freely available on the Internet, which inevitably has led to patients and families accessing this material themselves. In many Western countries, more than 50% of homes have computers and most of these have an Internet connection.[4] Accessing health-related information is a very common reason for use of the Internet and seems to be on the increase.[5]

The quality of information available is very variable, and patients or families may not be able to recognize reliable information without some guidance. Families may access high-quality information, as most of the resources available to medical professionals can also be accessed freely by others. This can lead to the situation where families may have as much, or in some cases more, information about their child's problem as the professional whom they are consulting. Some professionals see this as a threatening change to the 'balance of power' during a consultation.[6,7] Others readily embrace the concept that families will seek this information and have modified part of their role during the consultation so that they now assist families in interpreting information that they have found through the Internet. Clinicians can also have a role in directing families to high-quality information and other resources such as the online presence of many support groups (see Chapter 29).

Box 28.1. BetterDiabetes.com

BetterDiabetes.Com was designed by staff of the Royal Children's Hospital Diabetes Service in Melbourne to improve the care of patients with diabetes who attend clinics at the hospital. The system generates a computerized personal patient record available to both the treating team (eg physicians, nurses, educators and dieticians) and the child or family. As long as they have Internet access at home, patients or their family can:

- create a lifelong health record

- have an accurate summary of their diabetes history, including summaries of all clinic visits

- have an up-to-date record of current diabetes status, including current issues, test results and insulin dosage

- keep a personal health journal including non-diabetic issues

- upload glucose readings directly from a glucometer into their online health record

- track and graph all measurements and test results – glucose, height, weight and haemoglobin A_{1c}

- send secure messages to diabetes educators asking for advice on how to best manage their diabetes and receive secure messages in reply

- have access to the online system 24 hours a day from anywhere in the world

- maintain precise control over the security and access to their online information

- access educational material on diabetes.

The treating team can access all of this information and use the database of information for audit and research purposes (with appropriate consent).

Detailed clinical guidelines are available for junior staff who may have to manage diabetic clinical situations, eg in the emergency department. Guidelines are available for the care of a newly diagnosed diabetic, for diabetics needing surgery and for dealing with telephone calls from diabetic patients or family members seeking advice about acute problems. Junior staff who are not members of the diabetes service but who take phone calls out of hours have their own interface to enter information about the advice given to individual callers. This is sent securely to the diabetes educators who can follow up with the family and provide feedback about the advice given to the junior staff.

The system is very popular with staff, patients and families.

The users' site may be found at: http://www.betterdiabetes.com, and the clinical guidelines at http://www.rch.org.au/clinicalguide under 'Diabetes'.

Conclusion

The practice of medicine is steadily becoming more dependent on computers. In certain areas, such as the switch to electronic medical records in hospitals, the progress has been slower than some had predicted. The growth of the Internet and the integration of web-based technologies, however, are progressing rapidly. These changes bring the potential for major improvements in information and knowledge management, which should improve the quality of healthcare. There should also be improvements in efficiency, but some people are worried about the pace of medical practice and the risks to the doctor–patient relationship.

References

1   Kim GR, Lehmann CU. The impact of the Internet on pediatric medicine. *Paediatric Drugs* 2003; **5**: 433–441.
2   D'Alessandro DM, Kreiter CD, Peterson MW. An evaluation of information-seeking behaviors of general pediatricians. *Pediatrics* 2004; **113**: 64–69.
3   Nesbitt TS, Jerant A, Balsbaugh T. Equipping primary care physicians for the digital age. The Internet, online education, handheld computers, and telemedicine. *Western Journal of Medicine* 2002; **176**: 116–120.
4   Australian Bureau of Statistics. *Use of the Internet by Householders, Australia, November 2000*. Cat. no. 8147.0. Canberra: Australian Bureau of Statistics, 2001.
5   Baker L, Wagner TH, Singer S, Bundorf MK. Use of the Internet and e-mail for health care information: results from a national survey. *Journal of the American Medical Association* 2000; **289**: 2400–2406.
6   D'Alessandro DM, Dosa NP. Empowering children and families with information technology. *Archives of Pediatrics and Adolescent Medicine* 2001; **155**: 1131–1136.
7   Trevitt R, Smitherman R, Fitzgerald L, *et al.* Internet use by patients – a shift in power? *EDTNA ERCA Journal* 2001; **27**: 28–30.

▶ 29

Internet Sites for Parents, Children and Young People

Judy Barbour

Introduction

Since the mid-1990s, the expansion of the Internet has made it very easy for people to obtain information quickly and free of charge. The availability of health information on the Internet has grown rapidly, but the effect of this on healthcare outcomes is uncertain.[1] The Internet is clearly a very useful professional tool, but many practitioners have concerns about the use of health information from the Internet by patients and their families. Well-informed patients can be more successful at managing their health problems, but many believe that patients are best served if the information that guides their self-care is selected by experts – people who have been trained to know where to look for information and how to judge its quality and relevance.

Nevertheless, families are increasingly obtaining information from the Internet, especially for 'second opinions', making judgements about that information and expecting their knowledge to be respected in decision-making. Although not all Australians have access to the Internet, which raises issues of equity, the proportion with access is increasing and most families can access the Internet at home, school or work or in community centres such as libraries. People in remote areas may have greater access to the Internet than other less isolated people through special initiatives. Families can obtain the information they want at times that suit them, particularly at times when other healthcare services are closed.

This chapter focuses on websites that are available to parents, young people and children – primarily sites that are free and unrestricted. The discussion is not limited to sites specifically designed for patients, however, as ready access is available to many sites primarily intended for health professionals. Any review of sites on the web must acknowledge that there is a huge range of very high-quality health information on the Internet – and a vast amount of information that is of low quality.

Publishing on the Internet

The Internet is in many ways an ideal medium for a publisher of health information who does not need to recover publication costs through sales of a product, such as a journal or book. Text and graphical information can be published on the Internet quickly, in an attractive and concise format, and updated rapidly in response to new health issues arising, or changes in treatment or management practices. Although the presentation and quality of information on websites varies greatly, the Internet has become a publishing medium for almost everyone. Many free or inexpensive tools are available for constructing web pages, and such pages can be made available to the community at large at low cost to the individual.

This ease of publication raises concerns, however, because it is easy to publish information that is of questionable quality. Non-orthodox practitioners may publish recommendations that seem unwise, ineffective, sometimes dangerous or unreasonably expensive. Some sites carry unrepresentative personal experiences, while others, which seem to provide authoritative health information, are primarily commercial enterprises. There are concerns that such sites could lead patients to make harmful choices about their health or demand treatments that are not available or in their best interests.

Quality of health information on the Internet

Access to a range of health information of varying quality on the Internet has raised a number of potential concerns: for example, that people will be less likely to seek professional help when they need it, that they may follow incorrect and potentially dangerous advice, that they may seek out or demand inappropriate treatments or even that they are more up to date with the international literature than their doctor. These concerns are not new, nor specific to the Internet, as pointed out by the author of a rather enjoyable 'Editor's choice' in the *British Medical Journal* about the 'dangers' of talk.[2] People have always chatted to family, friends and neighbours about their health problems and received unreliable advice.

One of the most frequently mentioned concerns that professionals have about the Internet relates to the quality of the information available and if people without professional training are able to judge whether or not what they find is appropriate or correct.[3] Many apparently reputable websites have provided advice that did not match best practice standards (although this does seem to be improving[4]), and there have been some anecdotal reports of people experiencing adverse health outcomes after following advice found on the Internet. The numbers of people who have not come to harm or who have benefited from information on the Internet can never be known (and single case studies of success are rarely published). The challenge for healthcare professionals is to help parents, children and young people to identify high-quality sources of health information on the Internet and to use them to improve their health outcomes.

Recognising high quality websites

For people to gain from information on the Internet, the information needs to be of a high standard and well presented. Much effort has gone into determining the principles for the development of high-quality health site content and ways of assessing the quality of a website. The Health On the Net (HON) Foundation has developed a set of principles that has been adopted widely.[5] Health site developers who agree to conform to these principles may be awarded 'HONcode' accreditation and be able to display the HONcode logo on their site.

The HONcode principles include:

▶ authority (any medical advice is only provided by trained and qualified professionals)

▶ complementarity (the information supports, and does not replace, the relationship between the visitor and their existing physician)

▶ confidentiality (is respected; the site honours or exceeds legal requirements)

▶ attribution (clear references are given to sources of data)

▶ justifiability (claims are supported by evidence)

▶ transparency of authorship (including contact addresses being provided)

▶ transparency of sponsorship (support for the site is clearly identified)

▶ honesty in advertising and editorial policy.

Principles developed by other organizations tend to be similar, with differences related to the purpose of the accreditation (eg INASP,[6] principles relating to authority, coverage, presentation, currency, cost and freedom of use, and CHIQ,[7] principles relating to accuracy, clarity and relevance).

Problems with quality markers

Although adherence to website accreditation principles gives some assurance to users that the information on the site is of high quality, there may be problems with the use of such quality assurance tools. It is not possible for the organization awarding the quality accreditation to examine all pieces of information on each site that is accredited. These codes of practice cannot be policed thoroughly. Even so, it seems that the quality of health information on some sites is improving, which may be due in part to application of these quality principles.[4,8]

Even if information meets a recognized quality standard, it may not be useful. Much of the health information published on the Internet is poorly written when judged by readability and comprehension criteria: it may use medical jargon, scientific words that are not commonly understood, and complex words and sentence structure.

In contrast, many sites that may be very useful for parents, children and other non-professionals will not meet all of the 'quality' principles. Sites developed by parents (eg chat rooms and information portals), which can be of great support to other parents, will not meet all HONcode principles, although they may have their own high quality standards that are carefully applied.[9] There is a role for 'popularizers' of scientific or medical information, both in print publication and on the Internet. The authors of such content may not necessarily be medically qualified experts (and hence their material may not be accredited by some standards). However, the content of such sites can be well written, derived from recognized research sources, fully referenced, credible and reliable.

Using information of variable quality

It is a fact of modern life that we are all exposed to a huge volume of information of variable quality that we sift through. We develop skills at selecting what information is useful and refine our views as we are presented with new information. Information comes from many sources, including friends and family, the 'media', advertising, and professionals with differing views.[10]

Most young parents will have developed some skills in finding and assessing material on the Internet during their schooling, and many will have considerable critical thinking skills. They will have been taught to locate multiple sources of data, compare conflicting information and make some judgements about the credibility of the sources, although they may not use all of these skills systematically. In a family, the most 'net savvy' person is likely to be asked to search for information. Adept searchers of the Internet will tap into networks to find others who can guide their searches and help them assess what they find. Research by Ferguson and colleagues found that patients were unexpectedly very competent at 'telling the good from the bad'.[3]

Children are being taught these skills but are less experienced in this sifting process, so they need more guidance to sources of high-quality information. The assessment of information by young people involves an additional hurdle – that of cynicism. It seems that young people are often reluctant to accept information that appears to have been written by older people. The goal for content authors is to ensure the quality of health information, while maintaining their credibility with the age group concerned. The youth section of the Child and Youth Health site (see below) was written by youth workers, and stories submitted by young people are published as aids to establishing its credibility and relevance.

Supporting families in their use of the Internet

Although it is reasonable to assume that parents and young people have some knowledge and skills in finding and assessing information, it is also clear that people continue to come to health professionals because they value that professional person's expertise and the human contact. The challenge for health professionals is to use patients' knowledge to complement their relationship, supporting families in finding information they want through the Internet and helping them make the best use of that material.

Some ways that health professionals can assist families to access, evaluate and use such information include:

▶ ensuring that high-quality information is available on the Internet (eg by professionals publishing their own information on the Internet)

▶ referring families to websites of value

▶ assisting families with information search strategies

▶ assisting families to evaluate information that they have found via the Internet.

The rest of this chapter focuses on these activities.

Ensuring high-quality information on the Internet

If practitioners or organizations have resources to publish on the Internet, then developing a website is now easy, using readily available and inexpensive software. (Note, however, that developing a high-quality, useful and respected site is neither simple nor cheap.) Having their own site enables organizations or practitioners to publish information that is of specific interest to their own patients, as well as possibly being valuable to many more families.

Development of the Child and Youth Health website

Child and Youth Health is a statewide community child and youth health service funded by the South Australian Government. The Child and Youth Health website (http://www.cyh.com) was launched in May 1998, with about 130 parenting and child health topics written primarily for parents. The site aimed to provide a broad range of referenced, evidence-based information written by experts. It was also intended to support the Child and Youth Health Parent Helpline (a 24-hour call centre). The site currently has more than 600 topics in three sections ('Parenting and Child Health', 'Youth Health' and 'Kids Only'). It is visited by people from all over the world, used for teaching in several health professional courses and supports the work of several other Australian health services. Although there are now many Internet sites for child and youth health problems, few cover the parenting and wellbeing issues that are a feature of this website (Fig. 29.1).

Before the launch of this site, Child and Youth Health provided information for parents in a range of pamphlets and booklets. Using the Internet was seen as a cheaper way of providing information to parents, with the potential to reach greater numbers of families as access to the Internet becomes more widespread. Alternatives such as standalone 'kiosks' using information on CD-ROM had been explored, but it was realized that the Internet provided potentially much greater accessibility and that information could be quickly and continuously updated. Of course, the initial setup costs for a large information website were substantial, with the need to purchase site design and database development, as well as ongoing server and maintenance costs. There are also substantial ongoing costs related to staff resources for writing, editing and reviewing topics. Still, for the number of client contacts provided by the website, the cost per item of service is very low compared with all other Child and Youth Health

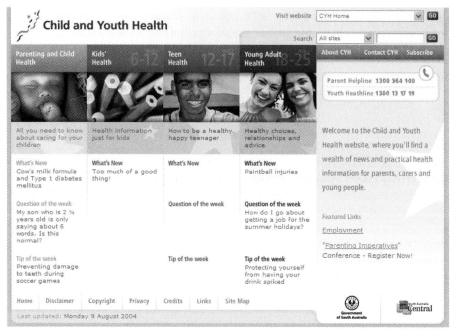

Fig. 29.1. The Child and Youth Health website home page.

services. The number of other contacts that Child and Youth Health provides through its traditional services has remained similar over the years. The Child and Youth Health website provides additional services that could not otherwise have been done within budget constraints.

The use of the site has grown rapidly. In early 2004, there were about 4000 page loads from the site per day. Traffic to the site has nearly trebled in the two years to March 2004. Some of this growth may be due to the gradual expansion in the use of broadband Internet services by families. There were 50 000 page loads from the Parenting and Child Health section of the site in March 2004, more than 41 000 page loads from the Kids Only section, and more than 23 000 from the Youth section. (A 'page load' is the display of a topic or 'chunk' of information via a website, similar to viewing a page of a book). These are very high visitor numbers – in the 'top ten' health sites in Australia. About half of the site visitors come from Australia, and the rest from more than 100 different countries.

To ensure the quality of the website:

▶ The topics are written by experts in child and youth health, child development and child behaviour and edited by experts in specific topic areas.

▶ The language is pitched (for the Parenting and Child Health section) at a reading age of 12 years (similar to general articles in the popular press).

▶ The content is evidence-based, up to date and provided with references.

▶ The site is designed to make it easy for parents to find what they are looking for, and the layout of each topic enhances readability (eg by use of dot points, space between sections, font and colour choice).

▶ All links are checked for source (eg government, academic and parent support) and relevance to topic, and are non-commercial.

▶ Criticism and corrections are invited for continuous quality improvement.

Important features included in the topics are contact information for local resources (including Internet links if available). References are included, many of which are for publications available on the Internet, so that parents can follow them up and learn more about an area of interest. Although the organization provides direct services only to families in South Australia, the Internet site is also used by many people outside South Australia. Links are provided to local, national (Australian) and international resources and references.

Evolution of the Parenting and Child Health section of the site

Since the launch of the Child and Youth Health website, many new parenting and child health topics have been added. There are currently more than 360 topics, and this section of the site continues to be the largest. Topics have been selected based on:

▶ relevance to the core business and areas of expertise of the organization (such as care of infants, child development and child behaviour)

▶ requests from parents (often coming via the Child and Youth Health Parent Helpline)

▶ topicality.

The Parenting and Child Health section includes topics that cover areas such as infant and child development and behaviour, parenting, infant and child care, infections and other medical conditions, mental health issues, safety, child protection, nutrition, and a wide variety of social issues (Fig. 29.2). The topics have been tested with groups of parents to ensure that the language is easy to read and that the topics are of interest and relevance to parents.

A feature of the Internet is the ability to prepare material and publish it very rapidly. When necessary, information can be published in a day (eg immediately after 11 September 2001, when a topic was published about the impact of disasters on children). Existing web topics can be updated very quickly, when required, to reflect the latest research, guidelines or practices. With print-based information, it can be difficult to ensure that all pamphlets containing out-of-date information are taken out of circulation, particularly in outlying clinics or healthcare centres. Books, being more highly valued, tend to remain in circulation even when many years out of date. The greatest challenge with the Parenting and Child Health section of the site is ensuring that all topics continue to be regularly reviewed and are up to date.

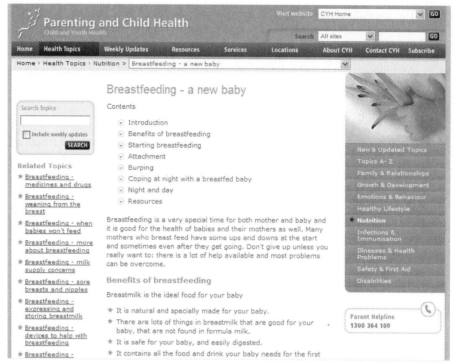

Fig. 29.2. A topic on the Parenting and Child Health section of the Child and Youth Health website.

Development of the Youth Health section of the site

Child and Youth Health includes a major division focusing on youth health and wellbeing (12–24 years). Youth workers in Child and Youth Health conducted interviews and focus groups with young people to find out what information they wanted. Topics were written by youth workers, and grouped into broad categories of:

▶ drugs and alcohol

▶ relationships

▶ healthy body

▶ healthy mind

▶ sexual health

▶ society and you.

The youth site was launched in March 1999 and now has about 130 topics (Fig. 29.3). This section of the site will be reviewed, in recognition that the information needs of people aged 12–17 years are different from those aged 18–24 years. Topic selection and writing style will also be reconsidered.

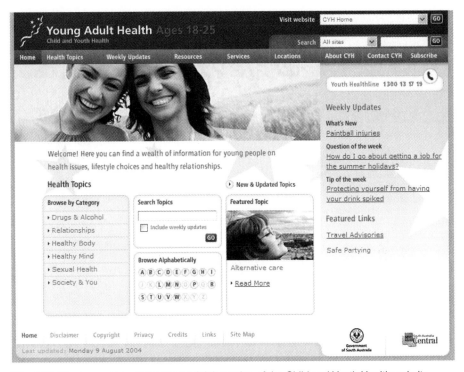

Fig. 29.3. The home page of the Young Adult section of the Child and Youth Health website.

Sites for primary school-aged children

There are relatively few health and wellbeing information sites for children of primary school age, yet such children use computers and the Internet as part of their everyday learning. We recognized the importance of a safe and reliable source of information for this age group, and have established a partnership with primary school education authorities in South Australia. This has resulted in a website called Kids Only. One feature of the Kids Only site is that when children visit it (see Fig. 29.4) they cannot get to other parts of the Child and Youth Health site – this is because material in many topics in the parent and youth sections of the Child and Youth Health site is not suitable for primary school-age children. For similar reasons, there are also no links to external sites on the Kids Only site.

All of the topics (now over 160) on the Kids Only site have been written by a primary school teacher with input from primary schoolchildren and illustrations produced by the schoolchildren. The topics are again evidence-based, and all have been edited by medical and other staff with expertise in the topic area, but do not, in this instance, have references shown on the topic. This section of the site has proved enormously successful and is being used in an increasing number of schools. It can also be useful for children who are looking for information outside school. Links to the Kids Only topics are being added to many of our Parenting and Child Health topics, as

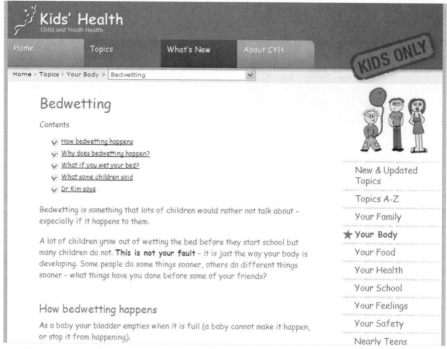

Fig. 29.4. A topic on the Kids Only section of the Child and Youth Health website.

they can be used by parents to help them to explain health and wellbeing issues to their children.

Developing your own site

Although there are many high-quality sites on the web, it is likely that specialist sites with up-to-date information and local resources will be valuable alternatives to publishing material such as books, magazines or pamphlets.

Design and content

Many criteria affect how useful a website will be to its audience. Some of them have been referred to in the section about quality above. The input of trained developers to design and navigation is important to a website's credibility, as people are unlikely to stay long on a poorly designed site. The design needs to suit the abilities of the intended users, especially if they have disabilities that affect their access to information. The Crippled Children's Association of South Australia has a site that is an excellent demonstration of ways in which accessibility can be maximized in line with World Wide Web Consortium guidelines.[11]

In the US, the National Cancer Institute developed excellent guidelines for improving the communication of cancer research.[12] These guidelines are applicable to all health topics and are highly recommended. Chapter 15 of the guidelines, on writing web content, is essential reading.

Understandable content is crucial to any website. Although health education relies heavily on written material, little has been done to ensure that patients can actually understand what is written.[13] Not only do words need to be readable, but the way that sentences are structured can clarify or completely obscure meaning. Care also needs to be taken to find out what families want to know. Often content is determined by what practitioners think is important, and this may not always be useful for families.

There are many guides to assist writing for non-medical people, including those published by the Centre for Literacy (Quebec, Canada)[13] and the Treadwell Library (Massachusetts General Hospital)[14] and a free online book *Writing for Change*.[15] There are also 'readability' guides, such as 'Bobby', to help authors test web pages and improve clarity.[16]

When designing and building websites, it is sometimes tempting to use a variety of multimedia and other technologies to add colour and movement – but these features usually require greater computing power and Internet bandwidth than your target audience (eg families) can be assumed to have, since they may be using older computers with slow Internet connections. Technologies such as Flash animation have their place, but their implementation without considering alternative ways of getting to your information may mean that some visitors cannot get beyond your home page. A lot of graphics can be a problem for users with slow Internet connections.

Powerful search engines are available, which can be integrated with a site's design. On large sites, which may contain many hundreds of pages, indexing of page content and search capabilities are important for ease of use. As well as targeted searches based on keywords, many sites offer different ways to browse their content, including displaying alphabetical listings of topics by title and displaying topic titles grouped by categories. These can help people to get an idea of the range of information held on the website and may lead them to useful information that they were not directly seeking.

Referring families to websites of value

So many excellent websites are available through the Internet that any list that is compiled is bound to be idiosyncratic. The following information is affected by some of the disadvantages of printed material as compared with material on the web, including that:

▶ the list of sites may already be out of date (organization names and web addresses may change, so site lists need regular checking and updating)

▶ the list may be incomplete (the sites given later reflect the work of the author of this paper, rather than what your practice might need).

A good way to start a list of useful parenting, youth and child health sites may be to ask parents, young people or children for sites that they have found helpful; these may not always be the sites that seem most valuable to practitioners. Local sites that have limited content may be valued over large international sites.

Finding some sites that address the topic of interest is easy. Try simple searches using a search engine such as Google, combining the disease or topic name with your location. For example, the keywords 'breastfeeding' and 'Australia' bring up, as the first site listed, Breastfeeding Australia (formerly Nursing Mothers Association; http://www.breastfeeding.asn.au/). Similarly, 'diabetes' with 'Australia' brings up Diabetes Australia (http://www.diabetesaustralia.com.au/home/index.htm).

Most of these sites then will have links to more local (state), national and international sites, which can be excellent sources of information for professionals, as well as parents and young people. For example, the Diabetes Australia site has links to:

▶ Diabetes Australia – South Australia (http://www.diabetessa.com.au)

▶ Diabetes Australia – Multilingual Website (http://www.diabetesaustralia.com.au/multilingualdiabetes/index.htm)

▶ National Aboriginal Community Controlled Health (http://www.naccho.org.au)

▶ Children With Diabetes (US) (http://www.childrenwithdiabetes.com): an excellent site for families even though it contains a lot of advertising.

There are many other ways to find good Internet sites, such as using portal sites that compile directories of other sites (eg Health*Insite*, an Australian government portal), clearinghouse sites, special interest compilations (such as disability or drug information networks) and sites for professionals. Some examples of these are listed below.

Assisting families with search strategies

Search engines such as Google can yield a lot of highly relevant sites, but people may not use search terms that increase the likelihood of getting what they want. The keyword 'diabetes', for example, produced more than 13 million results (in April 2004); 'diabetes child' reduced this to more than 2 million and 'diabetes child Australia' to about 140 000. In research about how people search the Internet, it was noted that searchers usually did not look beyond the first screen of the Google search results (and many did not seem to know that there were more screens with additional options).[17] Provision of some sites to begin searching on may help to get users started; this can be followed by encouragement to follow links, suggestions about search terms and contact information for local support groups.

Assisting parents to interpret what they have found

Along with the concerns of health professionals about what people may find on the Internet is the problem of being overloaded by the information that parents may bring to a consultation. Parents and young people coming to see a medical practitioner usually do so because they value the opinion of that practitioner.[1] The interpersonal skills of the practitioner in receiving and using the information are critical, but there are some skills that parents and others can apply to assist them in sifting through information, making the task of their medical adviser simpler. For example:

▶ checking whether or not the site has a quality accreditation (eg the HONcode)

▶ reviewing the site information using quality criteria such as those of the HONcode, INASP or CHIQ (see below for references)

▶ seeking information from other sites for comparison (you may need to provide a list of some reliable sites)

▶ seeking information from local associations (eg Diabetes Australia or Asthma Australia).

This not only will give the practitioner time but will also show respect for the parents' ability to find out information about something that is of critical interest to them – the health of their child or themselves.

Conclusion

There is little doubt that families will increasingly obtain much of the information that they use in decision-making from the Internet and seek support from others who have experienced similar health problems. Practitioners will be increasingly faced with the challenges of helping families to evaluate information and decide how to use it. When patients' knowledge is accorded respect, there is a greater likelihood that they will continue to seek the opinions of health professionals and that their health outcomes may benefit.

Acknowledgements

I am grateful to Paul Christie, Manager Web Services, Child and Youth Health, for editing and support.

Further information

Disclaimer: the inclusion of a website in this list should not be construed as an endorsement of it.

Directories of quality sites and information

Health*Insite* (Australian Government) http://www.healthinsite.gov.au/

Medical Library Association (US) http://www.mlanet.org (MLA lists, for example, their 'Top Ten' most useful websites at http://www.mlanet.org/resources/medspeak/topten.html)

Medicine on the Net (COR Health, US) http://www.corhealth.com/motn/

Large sites with topics on many areas

Child and Youth Health http://www.cyh.com

Children's Hospital of Philadelphia (one of thousands of hospital sites, but a well-structured site with a large amount of information for parents) http://www.chop.edu/consumer/index.jsp

Mayo Clinic http://www.mayoclinic.com

MEDLINEplus (for consumers) http://medlineplus.gov

Clearinghouses

Australian Indigenous Health*InfoNet* (at Edith Cowan University, WA) http://www.healthinfonet.ecu.edu.au/

Australian Youth Facts and Stats, Australian Clearinghouse for Youth Studies http://www.youthfacts.com.au

Special subject compilations

Australian Drug Information Network (ADIN) http://www.adin.com.au

Auseinet: Australian Network for Promotion, Prevention and Early Intervention for Mental Health http://www.auseinet.com

Canadian Organisation for Rare Disorders http://www.cord.ca/

Genetics Home Reference, National Library of Medicine (US) http://ghr.nlm.nih.gov

NSW Multicultural Health Communication Service http://www.health.nsw.gov.au/health-public-affairs/mhcs/

Organizations and support groups

Asthma Foundations of Australia http://www.asthmaaustralia.org.au/

Autism Association of South Australia http://www.autismsa.org.au/

Beyondblue; National depression initiative http://www.beyondblue.org.au

CanTeen; Australian organization for young people living with cancer (12–24 years) http://www.canteen.org.au/

Diabetes Australia http://www.diabetesaustralia.com.au/

Enablenet, for information on disability and a meeting place for people interested in disability issues (individuals, families, professionals) (published by a peer support group, DIRC) http://www.enable.net.au/

Headroom, mental health information for children, young people, parents and friends, professionals, and service providers http://www.headroom.net.au/

Kids Help Line http://www.kidshelp.com.au/

Sexually Transmitted Diseases Service (South Australia), Clinic 275 http://www.stdservices.on.net (large amount of information for students)

Siblings Australia, services for siblings of children with special needs
http://www.siblingsaustralia.org.au/

Yarrow Place, rape and sexual assault service (South Australia) http://www.wch.sa.gov.au/
services/az/other/yarrowplace/files/

Young Media Australia http://www.youngmedia.org.au/

Sites for professionals that can be accessed by consumers

British Medical Journal (and associated journals) http://bmj.bmjjournals.com/

Centers for Disease Control and Prevention (US) http://www.cdc.gov

Child Health and Paediatrics Specialist Library, National Electronic Library for
Health, NHS, UK http://www.nelh.nhs.uk/

INASP: International Network for the Availability of Scientific Publications (UK)
http://www.inasp.info/

'Informedhealthonline', Health Education and Research Foundation Ltd (Melbourne),
information based on Cochrane Reviews http://www.informedhealthonline.org/

National Institute of Mental Health (US) http://www.nimh.nih.gov

National Library of Medicine (US) http://www.nlm.nih.gov

National Library of Medicine (US) 'PubMed' site http://www.ncbi.nlm.nih.gov/
entrez/query.fcgi (access to Medline and other research journal information).

References

1 Murray E, Lo B, Pollack L, *et al*. The impact of health information on the Internet on the physician-patient relationship. *Archives of Internal Medicine* 2003; **163**: 1727–1734.
2 Editor's choice. The invention of talk. *British Medical Journal* 2002; **324**: http://bmj.bmjjournals.com/cgi/content/full/324/7337/0/j
3 Ferguson T. From patients to end users. *British Medical Journal* 2002; **324**: 555–556.
4 Pandolfini C, Bonati M. Follow up of quality of public orientated health information on the world wide web: systematic re-evaluation. *British Medical Journal* 2002; **324**: 582–583.
5 Health On Net Foundation. HONcode of Conduct (HONcode) for medical and health websites. http://www.hon.ch/HONcode
6 INASP: International Network for the Availability of Scientific Publications (US) http://inasp.info/health/links/info.html (last checked 7 June 2004).
7 CHIQ: The Centre for Health Information Quality. Help for Health Trust (UK). http://www.hfht.org/chiq (last checked 7 June 2004).
8 Kunst H, Groot D, Latthe PM, *et al*. Accuracy of information on apparently credible websites: survey of five common health topics. *British Medical Journal* 2002; **324**: 581–582.
9 Purcell GP, Wilson P, Delamothe T. The quality of health information on the Internet. *British Medical Journal* 2002; **324**: 557–558.
10 Shepperd S, Charnock D. Against Internet exceptionalism. *British Medical Journal* 2002; **324**: 556–557.
11 Crippled Children's Association of South Australia Web accessibility. http://www.cca.org.au/access.asp?pvalue=51 (last checked 7 June 2004).
12 US Department of Health and Human Services. Usability.gov. http://usability.gov/ (last checked 5 August 2004).
13 Atkinson T. *Plain Language and Patient Education: a Summary of Current Research*. Centre for Literacy (Canada). http://www.nald.ca/province/que/litcent/health/briefs/no1/1.htm (last checked 7 June 2004).
14 Treadwell Library. *Writing in Plain Language*. Health Literacy Resources online, Massachusetts General Hospital. http://www.mgh.harvard.edu/library/default.asp?page=plain_language (last checked 7 June 2004).
15 International Development Research Centre. *Writing for Change*. (Free interactive book about effective writing). http://web.idrc.ca/IMAGES/books/WFC_English/WFC_English/ (last checked 7 June 2004).

16   Watchfire Corporation. *Bobby Online*. http://bobby.watchfire.com/bobby/html/en/index.jsp (last checked 7 June 2004).
17   Eysenbach G, Kohler C. How do consumers search for and appraise health information on the world wide web? Qualitative study using focus groups, usability tests, and in-depth interviews. *British Medical Journal* 2002; **324**: 573–577.

► 30

Conclusion

Richard Wootton and Jennifer Batch

Introduction

The challenges in the provision of health services for children and young people are considerable – and continue to grow. Everyone knows that that there are huge inequalities between rich and poor countries around the world – perhaps no more so than in the health of their children. In rich countries, 6 in every 1000 children die before their fifth birthday. In the poorest countries, 120 per 1000 die before their fifth birthday. There are nearly 11 million child deaths each year in the world (41% in sub-Saharan Africa; 34% in south Asia) (Fig. 30.1).[1] In Australia and other affluent countries, the burden of healthcare for children must include the new morbidities related to lifestyle, lack of education and social factors. Many conditions that cause health problems in adults have their genesis in childhood. Aggressive, violent behaviour in adults may be traced to conduct disorders in childhood.[2] Physical and sexual abuse of children, if untreated, leads to intractable mental health problems and a cycle of continuing abuse in later generations.[3] Obesity in childhood predisposes to adult obesity, type 2 diabetes and premature cardiovascular morbidity and mortality.

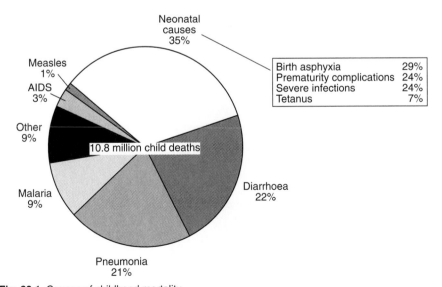

Fig. 30.1. Causes of childhood mortality.

Child morbidity and mortality is a multifactorial problem. Child health cannot be considered in isolation and, in all countries, health is one factor that interacts with wealth, employment, education and social structure. To treat a child's illness, or to save a child's life, requires both an effective intervention, eg an antimalarial drug, and an effective delivery mechanism, eg via community health workers. Although much is known about interventions, relatively little is known about delivery mechanisms. Telemedicine (telepaediatrics) may prove to be an effective method of delivering healthcare and education to children, families and health professionals (Fig. 30.2).

As the work reported in this book shows, telepaediatrics is an important and developing part of the range of healthcare services available to isolated or remote children and families. As well as delivery of clinical care, educational aspects of telemedicine have the potential to provide essential health information to children, families and healthcare practitioners. Despite this significant and emerging role, a number of problems and unresolved issues remain. Principal among these is the lack of evidence from research or programme evaluation to support the quality of clinical care provided by telepaediatrics compared with face-to-face contact.[4] Such research and evaluation should lead to the development of standards of telepaediatric care that would be available to guide the development of new programmes and the maintenance of clinical quality. Many telepaediatric programmes are currently run as research programmes or as part of new initiative grants. The cost-effectiveness and economic sustainability of telepaediatric programmes independent from research or other grants needs to be studied carefully. Reimbursement remains an unresolved issue, as do some of the medicolegal aspects of the delivery of healthcare at a distance.

Spooner and Gotlieb have suggested that telepaediatrics could create a two-tiered system in which patients who are able to pay are granted access to healthcare in person while poor children are treated by telemedicine.[5] Conversely, without appropriate funding for telepaediatrics, a telepaediatric consultation may only be available to those who can pay, while poorer patients must wait for a face-to-face encounter.

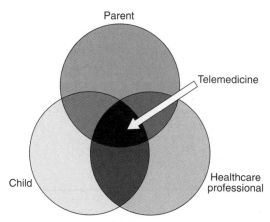

Fig. 30.2. Telemedicine may have a place in the delivery of health services for children and families.

What do the users think of telepaediatrics?

An early concern in the development of telemedicine was whether or not distance interaction in medicine would be acceptable to the users – whether the patient or the doctor. This led, in the latter half of the 1990s, to a rash of studies of patient and doctor satisfaction, not all of first-class scientific quality. Nonetheless, studies of a wide range of general telemedicine applications showed that, on the whole, users of telemedicine like it.[6] Neither clinicians nor patients report major dissatisfaction with telemedicine. In our own experience, the same applies for telepaediatrics. Although there have been fewer studies of user satisfaction in telepaediatrics, all attest to its popularity.[7–11] Whatever other barriers to the diffusion of telepaediatrics exist, consumer resistance is not one of them.

The place of telemedicine in paediatrics

What then is the place of telemedicine in paediatrics? We are not blind advocates for the use of telepaediatrics (nor for telemedicine in general), and, in particular, we do not suggest that telepaediatrics will completely replace physical outreach services or that patients will never need to be transferred between hospitals in future. Rather, we have tried to present the current and potential applications of telemedicine in a disinterested way, at the same time highlighting the limitations and unresolved issues. As this book shows, telemedicine seems to have great potential in the paediatric field, and its many applications deserve careful investigation. One hopes that telepaediatrics will not fall victim to the hype that surrounds much of information technology in healthcare. Our best guess about the place of telepaediatrics in future healthcare is that when used intelligently, it will supplement conventional delivery techniques, not replace them.

The future

Successful use of telepaediatrics allows clinical services to be redesigned. The scarce (and expensive) subspecialists can be concentrated in tertiary centres, where they can work more efficiently as a group, rather than attempting to practise in isolation in the regions. Using telemedicine, they can apply their expertise across the country and reduce the travelling required of patient or doctor. Telemedicine can also provide educational benefits for children, families and health professionals alike.

Future research into telepaediatrics should include evaluation of its use and its cost-effectiveness compared with traditional physical outreach services and care provided at major centres for children and their families travelling long distances. It should also include evaluation of the effectiveness of education and information provided to consumers and health professionals alike. Continued expansion of telepaediatric services combined with rigorous research and evaluation will determine the definitive place of telemedicine in the armamentarium of paediatric practice.

References

1   Black RE, Morris SS, Bryce J. Where and why are 10 million children dying every year? *Lancet* 2003; **361**: 2226–2234.
2   Tremblay RE, Nagin DS, Seguin JR, *et al.* Physical aggression during early childhood: trajectories and predictors. *Pediatrics* 2004; **114**: e43–e50.
3   Roberts R, O'Connor T, Dunn J, Golding J . The effects of child sexual abuse in later family life; mental health, parenting and adjustment of offspring. *Child Abuse and Neglect* 2004; **28**: 525–545.
4   Telemedicine for the Medicare population: pediatric, obstetric, and clinician-indirect home interventions. *Evidence Report/Technology Assessment (Summary)* 2001; **Aug** (24 suppl.): 1–32.
5   Spooner SA, Gotlieb EM for the Committee on Clinical Information Technology; Committee on Medical Liability. Telemedicine: paediatric applications. *Pediatrics* 2004; **113**: e639–e643.
6   Mair F, Whitten P. Systematic review of studies of patient satisfaction with telemedicine. *British Medical Journal* 2000; **320**: 1517–1520.
7   Marcin JP, Ellis J, Mawis R, *et al.* Using telemedicine to provide pediatric subspecialty care to children with special health care needs in an underserved rural community. *Pediatrics.* 2004; **113**: 1–6.
8   Kopel H, Nunn K, Dossetor D. Evaluating satisfaction with a child and adolescent psychological telemedicine outreach service. *Journal of Telemedicine and Telecare* 2001; **7** (suppl. 2): 35–40.
9   Elford DR, White H, St John K, *et al.* A prospective satisfaction study and cost analysis of a pilot child telepsychiatry service in Newfoundland. *Journal of Telemedicine and Telecare* 2001; **7**: 73–81.
10 Dick PT, Filler R, Pavan A. Participant satisfaction and comfort with multidisciplinary pediatric telemedicine consultations. *Journal of Pediatric Surgery* 1999; **34**: 137–41; discussion 141–2.
11 Blackmon LA, Kaak HO, Ranseen J. Consumer satisfaction with telemedicine child psychiatry consultation in rural Kentucky. *Psychiatric Services* 1997; **48**: 1464–1466.

Index